REVIEW OF

Nutrition and diet therapy

MOSBY

TIMES MIRROR

THE C. V. MOSBY COMPANY
11830 WESTLINE INDUSTRIAL DRIVE
ST. LOUIS, MISSOURI 63141

For prompt service, call (314) 872-8370

Instructor's Copy

This text is sent to you with the compliments of The C. V. Mosby Company. Examine it at your leisure and see how effectively it can fulfill your course requirements. We would greatly appreciate any comments you may have.

REVIEW OF NUTRITION AND DIET THERAPY by Sue R. Williams

COMMENTS:

Name

Course _____ Enrollment

School

City _____ State

FF-371

REVIEW OF
Nutrition and diet therapy

SUE RODWELL WILLIAMS, M.R.Ed., M.P.H.

Instructor in Nutrition and Clinical Dietetics, Kaiser Foundation
School of Nursing; Nutrition Consultant and Program Coordinator,
Health Education Research Center, Kaiser-Permanente Medical Center,
Oakland, California; Lecturer, Nutritional Science and Community
Nutrition, College of Alameda, Alameda, California; Lecturer,
Nutrition Education, School of Human Development and Education,
California State Polytechnic University, San Luis Obispo, California;
Field Faculty, M.P.H.-Dietetic Internship Program,
University of California, Berkeley, California

With 40 illustrations

THE C. V. MOSBY COMPANY
SAINT LOUIS   1973

To
LAURA CARR KERANEN
health educator, colleague, friend
who has taught me much about
human need and nurture

Preface

We are living in a rapidly changing world. Life styles and values as well as concepts of health and disease are changing. Among health professionals and consumers alike there is an increasing concern for *positive* health, a preventive approach, which provides opportunity for personal development, productivity, and self-fulfillment. For such a state of positive health, nutritional care is fundamental.

The health team is charged with the responsibility of providing such a level of quality care, not only as the baseline in health through energy, growth, and regulation of body processes, but also through its relation to disease. Nutritional therapy plays a vital role in the course, cause, cure, control, or prevention of disease.

In this emerging role of nutrition in health care, the nutritionist bears a primary responsibility, in collaboration with other members of the health team—physician, dentist, nurse, social worker, nutrition assistant, health educator, and other therapists. It is for all these practicing health professionals—and for the patient for whom they care in a variety of clinical and community settings—that this review manual is written. Its basic goal is to provide a ready reference for busy clinicians and practitioners to meet needs and to deal with problems and questions encountered in daily practice.

To meet these needs, this *Review* offers general background information in a broad overview of nutrition and its applications. A different format is used. Questions are posed that emphasize or clarify basic nutri-tional principles and relate them to various clinical and community problems and situations. Throughout an effort is made to look behind the label or signpost to discover and understand the human processes with which we are involved. To the degree that we relate nutritional principles to processes and practices will our daily nutritional care of persons with needs be valid and effective.

The material presented is organized, therefore, into three main sections. The first section, Nutritional Science, reviews some basic scientific principles of nutrition, with emphasis on their significance in human health. The two remaining sections, Community Nutrition and Clinical Nutrition, apply these principles to the life cycle and to a variety of community and clinical problems.

I am indebted to many colleagues too numerous to name who have contributed to the ideas and applications expressed here. To my students and to my patients I am especially grateful for the many insights they have given me through my years of teaching and clinical practice. From them I have learned much that is reflected here.

I am also grateful to George Straus whose diagrammatic illustrations have brought both clarification and beauty to the scientific concepts presented, to my typists, Elizabeth Carlson and Annette Brehmer, who through numerous drafts produced the final typescript, and to my family, without whose patience and constant support none of this would have been possible.

S. R. W.

Contents

I

Nutritional science

1 Nutrition and health

Caring for persons and their individual health needs is at the heart of the health professions. The role of nutrition in meeting these needs is becoming increasingly apparent. As health professionals in the midst of a rapidly changing world, we are charged with two responsibilities—to know our subject and to know our patient. Sound knowledge must be our tool; genuine concern for human need must be our motive; and amid the realities of life we must practice our art.

If the quality of life thus has a nutritional foundation, relevant integration of nutrition throughout the fabric of health care becomes a necessity. The nutrition specialist—nutritionist or dietitian—bears the major responsibility for nutritional care of persons in communities or in clinical settings. However, each member of the health team shares in this overall responsibility in a variety of ways. We are beginning to hear an increased number of concerned cries for more comprehensive, less fragmented care, for greater awareness of personal need, of concern for the "whole man." To this end team effort in the application of scientific nutrition in human terms, in terms of persons in real life situations of daily living as well as in times of stress, takes on new dimensions. It is within these dimensions that nutrition must be applied to help solve problems of health and disease.

CHANGING CONCEPTS OF HEALTH AND HEALTH CARE

■ How are concepts of health and disease changing?

Over the course of man's developing civilization, scientific knowledge has gradually replaced primitive superstition in the treatment of disease. As a result, public and personal hygiene has improved, therapy for specific diseases has become more scientific and skilled, and many of the most lethal childhood diseases have been eliminated. Faced now with the so-called gift of longer life, man has begun to view health increasingly in qualitative terms. Health concepts are moving from the wholly negative view of absence of disease (the curative approach) to a more positive view of optimum productivity (the preventive approach). This positive view was written into the preamble of the World Health Organization Constitution in 1946: "Health is a state of complete physical, mental, and social well-being, and not merely the absence of disease or infirmity."

Health, however, is a relative concept in any culture, and it must be viewed in relation to man's total wants and needs. Health competes with other values and is relative to a culture's way of life. The kind and degree of physical health required for success in one culture differs from that needed to succeed in another. This recognition of difference in needs extends the concepts of health to include moral, religious, and philosophical dimensions. Perhaps, then, a more realistic goal for world health effort would be a level of physical and mental health that would make for social well-being within the social system in which the individual must live, and that would provide opportunity for personal productivity and self-fulfillment.

3

■ **What are the causes of these changes in concepts of health and disease?**

A number of factors in the rapidly evolving society have contributed to changes in health values and practices:

1. *Scientific knowledge explosion.* Knowledge is increasing at an exponential rate. Consider the potential for growth of information in the following statistics:

Twenty-five percent of all the people who ever lived are alive today.

Ninety percent of all the scientists who ever lived are alive today.

The amount of technical information available doubles every 10 years.

Fifty percent of what we now know about chemistry has been learned since 1950.

Approximately one hundred thousand journals are currently being published around the world in more than sixty languages, and the number of them doubles every 15 years.

This burgeoning knowledge is reflected in all areas of health care. However, the necessary specialization that has followed has too often meant increased fragmentation of services. The patient often feels that no one member of the health team sees him as a whole person.

2. *Population explosion.* A recent book by Paul Erlich is aptly named *The Population Bomb.* The repercussions of this bomb are being felt in all of society. The approximately 3.5 billion people of the world are multiplying so fast that, if the present rate continues, the population will double about every 30 years. Within 200 years the world population would be approximately 230 billion—nearly 70 times the present total.

Not only is this population increase reflected in total numbers but also in percentage shifts in age and location. There is an increasing proportion of older people and there is greater overall mobility. Urban-suburban trends have created changes in individual psychologic patterns, in family patterns, and in community and national social patterns. All of these changes affect health needs and social values.

3. *Social revolution.* Radical changes in family and community relations have resulted within this development of an urban-suburban complex in a highly industrialized society. Crowded city housing contrasts with sprawling suburbs and rural blight. While the food-eating population grows, the food-bearing potential of the land diminishes. Economic affluence, higher costs of living, more emphasis on higher education—all in the face of poverty pockets in city ghettos and rural "Appalachias" —have changed human goals, human values, and medical care programs.

EFFECT OF CHANGE ON HEALTH CARE PRACTICES

■ **What basic changes are developing in health care?**

Whatever the ultimate forms and systems, health care in America in the 1970s is changing in four basic ways:

1. Change in *focus* to the social issues involved, without which a viable system cannot exist.

2. Changes in *systems of delivery* of health care based on two ideas:

a. A health team for primary care, composed of a family physician, nurse-practitioner, nutritionist, and family health worker, bringing in other specialists as needed.

b. Stations for service, such as satellite clinics or health centers surrounding a central core medical center or hospital.

3. Changes in *relations with consumers,* involving them in community control, planning, and decision making.

4. Changes in *payment for services* to some form of National Health Insurance Program.

■ **What are the roles of the various health team members in relation to nutritional care?**

According to need in a variety of situations, different members of the health team may assume differing degrees of responsibility for nutritional care at different times. By and large, however, the major responsibility falls to the nutrition specialist. This responsibility includes assessment of nutritional needs and planning of nutritional care and education, in consultation with the physician and integrated with his plan for medical management. Assisting the nutritionist in planning and carrying out nutritional care is the nurse, who integrates this aspect of care in total patient care. Other team members, such as the social worker, physical therapist, and health educator, also function as consultants in planning care.

In each case the goal of the health team, under the guidance of the nutrition specialist, is to gain sound relevant knowledge of the science of human nutrition, to translate the scientific principles of nutrition into clear concepts that can be applied to *person-centered* care.

2 Carbohydrates

Throughout its life-span the human body faces a major problem—energy procurement. Energy is necessary to sustain life processes; hence, it is the basic life force. It is constantly being transformed and recycled. Two major types of nutrients, carbohydrates and fats, provide the major fuel source of this vital power. It is no surprise, therefore, that the metabolic processes involving these two nutrients are closely interrelated. Questions concerning what these nutrient substances are and how they interact form a basic beginning point to an understanding of human nutrition.

CARBOHYDRATES: NATURE AND FUNCTION

■ **From what sources are the basic dietary carbohydrates, starches and sugars, formed?**

Plants are the main sources of starches and sugars in the human diet. In the plant, through the process of *photosynthesis,* carbon dioxide and water combine in the presence of sunlight and the plant's chlorophyll to produce carbohydrates. Animals produce some lesser sources of carbohydrate, such as lactose (milk sugar) and fructose (the sugar in honey).

■ **What is the chemical nature of carbohydrates?**

The basic chemical elements of carbohydrates are carbon, hydrogen, and oxygen. In starch these elements are combined in a complex structure with many branching chains. However, in simple sugars three to seven carbon atoms form a chain, with the hydrogen and oxygen atoms attached singly and in alcohol ($-OH$) or aldehyde ($=O$) groups. The most common carbon chain length is the hexose, or six carbons. Of the hexoses, glucose ($C_6H_{12}O_6$) is the most common example.

■ **According to chemical structure, how are carbohydrates classified?**

Monosaccharides the simplest form, a "single sugar."

Disaccharides more complex sugars made up of two monosaccharides.

Polysaccharides far more complex, branching structures composed of many monosaccharide units.

■ **What monosaccharides are most important nutritionally? How do they compare in sweetness, sources, and use in the body?**

The three nutritionally important monosaccharides are glucose, fructose, and galactose. *Glucose* (also called dextrose because it is the *dextro*rotatory form of the molecule) is moderately sweet. It is found preformed in foods (such as corn syrup) or is formed in the body from starch digestion. In human metabolism all other sugars are converted to glucose. Glucose (blood sugar) is finally oxidized by the cells to give energy.

Fructose (also called levulose because it is the *levo*rotatory form of the molecule) is the sweetest of the simple sugars. Dietary sources include fruits and honey. In the body fructose is converted to glucose to be oxidized for energy.

Galactose is not found free in foods but is produced in the body from lactose (milk sugar). It, too, is then converted to glucose to be oxidized for energy. During lactation glucose may be reconverted to galactose for breast milk production.

■ **What disaccharides are significant in human nutrition?**

The three main disaccharides, with their two component monosaccharides, are:

> Sucrose = glucose + fructose
> Lactose = glucose + galactose
> Maltose = glucose + glucose

Sucrose (common table sugar) is the most prevalent dietary disaccharide, contributing about 25% of the total carbohydrate calories. Its many forms include granulated sugar (made from sugar cane and sugar beets), brown and powdered sugar, sorghum cane and molasses, and maple syrup. The large consumption of sucrose in countries such as America and Great Britain—annually about 100 pounds per person—has become a growing concern to health practitioners. For example, the United States produces and consumes more candy than any other country in the world —an annual average of 17 to 20 pounds per person. Excess dietary sucrose bears a direct relationship to dental caries. Moreover, it has been implicated by several investigators in the incidence of atherosclerosis (see p. 224).

Lactose is the sugar in milk. Since it is the least sweet of the dietary disaccharides, about one sixth as sweet as sucrose, it is often used in high carbohydrate, high calorie liquid feedings, when the needed quantity of sucrose could not be tolerated.

Maltose occurs in malt products and in germinating cereals. As such it is a negligible dietary carbohydrate. However, it is important as an intermediate product of starch digestion.

■ **How do polysaccharides contribute to human nutrition?**

Starch is the most significant polysaccharide in human nutrition. It is a compound made up of glucose chains, hence it yields only glucose upon hydrolysis or digestion. This breakdown of starch is accomplished physiologically as a normal part of the body's digestion (starch → dextrins → maltose → glucose), or commercially by a process of acid hydrolysis. Starch is by far the most important source of carbohydrate in the diet, accounting for approximately 50% of the total carbohydrate intake in the American diet. In other countries, in which carbohydrate is the staple food substance, it may comprise an even higher proportion of the total diet. Major food sources include cereal grains, potatoes, and other root vegetables and legumes.

Cellulose is a form of polysaccharide that is resistant to the digestive enzymes in man. It remains in the digestive tract and contributes important bulk to the diet. This bulk helps to move the digestive food mass along and stimulates peristalsis. Since cellulose forms the supporting framework of plants, its main sources are the stems and leaves of vegetables, seed and grain coverings, skins, and hulls.

Pectins are nondigestible, colloidal polysaccharides. They are found mostly in fruits and possess a thickening quality.

Glycogen, often called "animal starch," is synthesized in the body from glucose and is stored in the liver and muscle tissue. Chief food sources of stored glycogen, therefore, are animal foods—meat and seafood. Since stored glycogen is formed from glucose, it yields only glucose upon metabolism.

Inulin, a polysaccharide composed of fructose units, has little dietary significance. It is found only in a few common foods, such as onions, garlic, and artichokes. However, although inulin is of small dietary significance, it is of importance because it provides a test of renal function. Since inulin is filtered at the glomerulus, but is neither secreted nor reabsorbed by the tubule, it can be used to measure glomerular filtration rate. This test is called the *inulin clearance test*.

■ **Why do the body tissues require a constant dietary supply of carbohydrate to meet their energy demands?**

There are three main reasons. First, the amount of carbohydrate in the body (circulating as blood sugar and stored as glycogen) is relatively small. For example; a man weighing 70 kg. would have these approximate amounts:

Liver glycogen	110 gm.
Muscle glycogen	245 gm.
Extracellular blood sugar	10 gm.
Total	365 gm.
	(1,460 calories)

This amount of 365 gm. of available glucose would provide energy sufficient for only about 13 hours of moderate activity. Thus, carbohydrate must be ingested regularly and at moderately frequent intervals to maintain this constant source of supply to meet the body's energy needs.

Second, without sufficient carbohydrate for energy demands the body turns to its other stores, first to fat and then to protein (muscle mass). However, products from carbohydrate metabolism such as pyruvate and oxaloacetate are necessary for the proper oxidation of fat for energy through the Krebs cycle. Therefore, if sufficient carbohydrate is not present to maintain the running of the body's main final metabolic pathway for energy production (the Krebs cycle), the metabolic products of fat breakdown, *active acetate*, will go instead into another pathway to form ketones. Ketosis, or keto-acidosis, results (see p. 22). Thus, adequate dietary carbohydrate exerts an *antiketogenic effect* and prevents a damaging excess of ketone formation and accumulation.

Third, sufficient dietary carbohydrate prevents the channeling of too much protein for energy demands. This *protein-sparing action* of carbohydrate allows a major portion of protein to be used for its basic structural purpose of tissue building.

■ **In addition to serving as the body's main energy source or as a part of this basic function, what special functions does carbohydrate perform in vital organs?**

As part of its role as chief energy source, carbohydrate serves several specific metabolic functions in vital organs. *In the liver*

carbohydrate is not only oxidized as fuel but also protects the tissue by being present as glycogen and by participating in specific detoxifying metabolic pathways. For example, a glucose derivative, glucuronic acid, conjugates with certain toxic drugs to produce harmless forms for excretion. Also, as indicated above, carbohydrate has a regulating influence on fat and protein metabolism through its antiketogenic and protein-sparing actions.

In the heart glycogen in cardiac muscle provides a constant important emergency source of contractile energy. In a damaged heart poor glycogen stores or a low carbohydrate intake may cause cardiac symptoms or angina.

In the central nervous system a constant amount of available glucose is necessary for functional integrity, since its regulatory center, the brain, contains no stored supply of glycogen. Therefore, it is dependent on a minute-to-minute supply of glucose from the blood. Sustained and profound hypoglycemic shock may cause irreversible brain damage.

DIGESTION-ABSORPTION-METABOLISM OF CARBOHYDRATES

In order to secure vital energy from its major fuel sources, carbohydrate foods, the body faces a large task. It must change this food in its variety of forms to entirely different forms of potential energy as chemical compounds. The changes along the way and the processes through which they are accomplished present a fantastic array of chemical achievements.

■ **What initial digestive processes change carbohydrate foods into a basic form that can be absorbed into circulation?**

The digestion of carbohydrate proceeds through the successive parts of the gastrointestinal tract aided by both mechanical and chemical processes. The mechanical processes include mastication and peristalsis. The chemical processes involved are enzymatic in nature. These basic processes of carbohydrate digestion are summarized in Table 2-1.

Table 2-1. Summary of carbohydrate digestion

Organ	Enzyme	Action
Mouth	Ptyalin	Starch → Dextrins → Maltose
Stomach	None	(Above action continued to minor degree)
Small intestine	Pancreatic	
	Amylopsin	Starch → Dextrins → Maltose
	Intestinal	
	Sucrase	Sucrose → Glucose + Fructose
	Lactase	Lactose → Glucose + Galactose
	Maltase	Maltose → Glucose + Glucose

■ **After digestive processes change complex carbohydrate foods into simple sugars, how do these sugars get into the bloodstream?**

These simple sugars—glucose, galactose, and fructose—are absorbed by the mucous membrane of the small intestine into the villi capillaries and enter the portal circulation for transportation to the liver. After a carbohydrate meal or snack, when the sugar concentration is greater within the intestinal lumen than in the mucosal cells and in turn in the blood plasma, glucose can easily be absorbed by *simple diffusion.* However, if a constant supply of blood glucose to cells is necessary for energy production, as we have seen, regardless of how small the intake may be at times, there must be some additional mechanism to ensure this absorption, even when the osmotic pressure gradient is not sufficient for diffusion to occur. This is indeed the case. A second mechanism of *active transport* is present. This finely balanced homeostatic mechanism operates on energy supplied by metabolic processes within the mucosal cells and absorbs glucose independently of the intestinal concentration. This active transport of glucose is accomplished through a metabolic "pump," which involves sodium and potassium.

■ **What factors influence absorption of digestive carbohydrates?**

Several interrelated physiologic factors influence carbohydrate absorption. These include the rate of entry into the intestine,

the type of food mixture present, the condition of intestinal membranes, the length of time the carbohydrate is held in contact with the absorbing membrane surface, and normal endocrine activity.

■ **How may clinical conditions affect these absorption factors?**

Several types of conditions may influence absorption of digested carbohydrate:

1. *Rate of entry.* Hypermotility of the stomach and malfunction of the duodenal sphincter muscle (pyloric valve) may cause loss of control of normal passage of food material and too rapid an entry of food mass into the intestine.

2. *Type of food mixture present.* With a concentrated carbohydrate meal, the competition for absorbing sites and available carrier transport systems may cause some passage of unabsorbed carbohydrate. Rates of absorption vary among the monosaccharides. Glucose and galactose are absorbed fairly rapidly, but fructose has a relatively slower rate because it lacks a "pump" to carry it "uphill."

3. *Condition of intestinal mucosa.* Any abnormality of the mucosal tissue, such as enteritis, celiac disease, or sprue, prevents normal absorption.

4. *Time carbohydrate is held in contact with mucosa.* Any condition, such as diarrhea, which causes abnormally rapid movement of the carbohydrate along the intestine, will hinder absorption.

5. *Endocrine activity.* Normal activity of the anterior pituitary and the related

functioning of the thyroid through the TSH hormone is necessary for normal absorption. In addition, the adrenal cortex hormones regulate the body's sodium exchange, which indirectly influences the operation of the sodium pump.

Metabolism of carbohydrates

Metabolism is the sum of the physical and chemical processes in a living organism by which energy is made available for the functioning of the organism and by which protoplasm, the basic substance of cells and tissues, is produced, maintained, or destroyed. A *metabolite* is a product of a specific metabolic process. The human organism is a whole made up of many parts and processes that possess unequalled specificity and flexibility. Intimate metabolic relationships exist among all the basic nutrients and metabolites, and it is impossible to understand any one of man's metabolic processes without viewing it in relationship to the others that comprise the whole. Thus, a basic concept emerges. It is the vital concept of *wholeness,* or integrity, of the human organism. Without an understanding of this basic concept no real appreciation of human nutrition is possible.

After the products of the digestion of dietary carbohydrate, the monosaccharides are absorbed and transported to the liver, the fructose and galactose are converted to glucose, and the glucose is in turn converted to glycogen for storage. The glycogen is reconverted to glucose as needed by the body.

The liver is the major site of this fascinating metabolic machinery that handles glucose, and much of the chemical activity takes place there. However, other tissues, such as adipose fat tissue, muscle tissue, and renal tissue, play important roles; and energy metabolism in general goes on in all cells.

Glycemia refers to blood sugar. Hence hyperglycemia means blood sugar levels that are above the normal range, and hypoglycemia indicates blood sugar levels below the normal range. It becomes apparent that

another major concept concerning carbohydrate metabolism is that of *balance.* Questions concerning carbohydrate metabolism, therefore, will revolve around mechanisms involved in supplying sources of blood glucose, taking glucose from the blood, hormones that control these mechanisms, and and processes by which energy is produced from the glucose.

■ **What are the sources from which glucose enters the blood?**

Sources of blood glucose may be divided into carbohydrate and noncarbohydrate substances. The carbohydrate sources include:

Dietary carbohydrates, which are starches and sugars that have been ingested, digested, and absorbed into the bloodstream.

Glycogen, which has been stored mainly in the liver, and as needed may be reconverted to form blood glucose. This conversion of glycogen to form glucose is called *glycogenolysis.*

Products of intermediary carbohydrate metabolism, such as lactate and pyruvate.

The noncarbohydrate sources are protein and fat. Certain amino acids are *glucogenic*, that is, they form glucose upon metabolic breakdown. After deamination (removal of the amino group) the remaining carbon chain forms the skeleton for glucose. This conversion process is catalyzed by adrenocortical steroids, such as cortisone. These steroids have, therefore, been called the S-hormones, or sugar-forming hormones. About 58% of the protein in a mixed diet is composed of these glycogenic amino acids. Thus, more than half of the dietary protein, although consumed primarily for its tissue building function, is available for use as energy.

Fat is also converted into glucose. After the breakdown of neutral fat into fatty acids and glycerol, the glycerol portion, upon hydrolysis, may be converted into glycogen in the liver and made available for glucose formation. Since glycerol comprises only about 10% of the fat, it normally

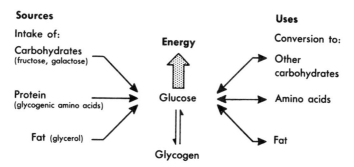

Fig. 2-1. Sources and uses of glucose.

contributes very little available glucose. The production of glucose from protein, fat, and various intermediate carbohydrate metabolites is called *gluconeogenesis*.

■ **After glucose has entered the blood-stream, what means does the body have for using it to keep the blood sugar balanced within a normal range?**

The constant, major use of blood sugar is for energy needs. In the cells various metabolic pathways are used to convert glucose, through a series of chemical changes, into energy. These pathways are the *Embden-Meyerhof glycolytic pathway* (EMP), the *hexose monophosphate shunt* (HMS), and the *Krebs cycle*.

Additional glucose may be drawn off and stored for reserve use. Two major processes convert glucose to storage forms: *glycogenesis*, which is conversion to liver and muscle glycogen; and *lipogenesis*, which is conversion to adipose fat tissue.

Some glucose is used in interconversion products of metabolism to form other carbohydrate compounds. These compounds include the sugars, ribose and deoxyribose for use in RNA and DNA, and lactose formed during lactation. Also, certain amino acids that are synthesized in the body derive their carbon skeletons from glucose or its metabolites.

Hence, these sources and uses of glucose act as checks and balances to maintain the blood sugar within its normal range of 70 to 120 mg./100 ml., by adding sugar to the blood or by removing it so that the body maintains a fairly constant internal environ-

ment. This sort of dynamic balance enables it to meet changing demands and stresses. This is but one more example of the remarkable *homeostatic* mechanisms of the body, built in to sustain life and promote health (Fig. 2-1).

■ **What hormone controls the blood sugar level by lowering it?**

Insulin is the only hormone that lowers the blood sugar. Insulin is produced by the beta cells in the islets of Langerhans in the pancreas. It is believed to stimulate use of blood sugar in several ways:

1. Insulin fosters *glycogenesis* by conversion of glucose to glycogen in the liver, where the glycogen has been stored.

2. Insulin fosters *lipogenesis*, the formation of fat.

3. Insulin increases cell *permeability to glucose* and allows glucose to pass from the extracellular fluids into the cells for oxidation to supply needed energy. When glucose enters the cell, potassium enters with it. Hence, treatment for patients with diabetic acidosis requires replacement potassium therapy. Apparently the cells' dependence on insulin for glucose entry differs in various tissues. For example, glucose uptake is unaffected by the absence of insulin in the brain, red blood cells, intestinal mucosa, kidney tubules, and probably the liver. Tissues dependent on the presence of insulin for glucose uptake are skeletal muscle, adipose tissue, cardiac muscle, eye lens, the aqueous humor, and pituitary tissue.

4. Insulin is also believed to influence

phosphorylation. Phosphorylation is the initial and necessary phosphorus-coupling step that allows glucose to enter the cell's metabolic pathway to produce energy. Insulin acts on antagonists to the reaction to prevent them from inhibiting the action of glucokinase, the specific hexokinase needed to catalyze glucose phosphorylation.

5. Insulin also promotes *protein synthesis.* This may be an indirect result of the increase in energy available for tissue building, which has been facilitated by glucose oxidation.

■ **What hormones control the blood sugar level by raising it?**

According to the body's need, certain hormones act to raise the blood sugar by stimulating release of stored carbohydrate sources. These hormones and their actions include:

Glucagon, produced by the alpha cells in the islets of Langerhans in the pancreas, stimulates *hepatic glycogenolysis,* the breakdown of liver glycogen to glucose.

Steroid hormones of the adrenal cortex stimulate *gluconeogenesis,* releasing glucose-forming carbon units from protein.

Epinephrine, produced by the adrenal medulla, also stimulates *glycogenolysis,* releasing a quick source of glucose from liver glycogen.

Growth hormone (GH) and *adrenocorticotrophic hormone* (ACTH), secreted by the anterior pituitary gland, raise the blood sugar level by acting as insulin antagonists.

Thyroxin, produced by the thyroid gland, has an elevating effect on blood sugar, probably because it influences the rate of insulin destruction, increases glucose absorption from the intestine, and liberates epinephrine.

■ **Once glucose gets into the cell, how does it produce energy?**

In the cell glucose undergoes a series of chemical reactions by which it is broken down through successive processes into the end products of carbon dioxide and water. In this process of breaking down glucose, large amounts of energy are generated. Three main chemical pathways are used for glucose oxidation by the cell: two major ones, the Embden Meyerhof pathway and the Krebs cycle, and one alternative shunt to the Embden-Meyerhof pathway.

■ **What systems of chemical change does the cell provide to accomplish this task?**

For energy to be produced from glucose (a six-carbon chain) and other interrelated metabolites such as fatty acids (multiple-carbon chains), the cell must solve several problems. It does this through three basic stages. First, the cell must produce a "common molecule," smaller two-carbon fragments activated with high-energy bonds for strong chemical combining power, a common point where the various energy sources (especially carbohydrate and fat) may converge. This vital "common molecule" is *active acetate,* or *acetyl CoA.* Thus the cell provides an initial chemical pathway through which glucose (a six-carbon chain) may be processed to an important three-carbon product, *pyruvate,* which in turn forms a substrate for the production of the "common molecule." This series of initial chemical processes, the Embden-Meyerhof pathway, takes place out in the cell cytoplasm. An alternative shunt to this pathway is also provided—the hexose monophosphate shunt (HMS).

Second, the cell must provide a final common energy-producing metabolic pathway through which the "common molecule" and other energy metabolites may be completely oxidized to carbon dioxide and ultimately to water. This the cell does in its "powerhouses," the *mitochondria.* Here a system of enzymes accomplishes this task in the Krebs cycle.

Finally, the cell must also provide a system of catalysts for "capturing" the energy derived from this tissue oxidation. This system binds the liberated energy in the form of high-energy intermediate compounds, adenosine triphosphate (ATP). These systems of collaborating catalysts, enzymes

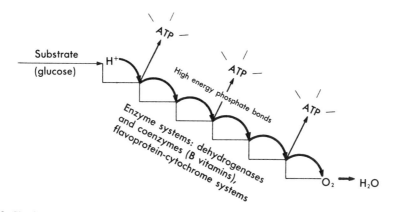

Fig. 2-2. The bouncing hydrogen ion—biologic oxidation in the cell to produce energy. Energy in the form of ATP (high-energy phosphate bonds) is produced through transfer of H+ and electrons by means of enzyme systems (dehydrogenases and coenzymes, the B vitamins, and the flavo protein-cytochrome systems). These enzyme chains are coupled with the glycolytic pathway and the Krebs cycle.

and co-enzymes, are called *respiratory chains*. At several points along the Krebs cycle, for example, respiratory chains using coenzyme factors involving the B vitamins, niacin and riboflavin, and iron transfer hydrogen ions along a series of steps to the final reaction with oxygen to form water (Fig. 2-2).

Thus, in this stepwise, efficient, and controlled transfer the free energy resulting from the oxidation of foodstuffs is made available and "captured" in the high energy chemical bonds of ATP. The remaining free energy is liberated as heat to help maintain the body temperature. Therefore, in this stepwise system the cell provides a highly efficient (40% to 50%) and controlled system for energy production and conservation.

■ **What basic coenzyme systems play a part in this hydrogen ion transfer in the respiratory chains to yield energy?**

The three systems involved are:

1. The *dehydrogenases*, with niacin as part of the coenzyme (nicotinamide-adenine dinucleotide → reduced nicotinamide-adenine dinucleotide [NAD → NADH]; nicotinamide-adenine dinucleotide phosphate [NADP → NADPH]).

2. The *flavoprotein system*, containing riboflavin coenzymes.

3. The *cytochrome system* (a "cousin" of hemoglobin), containing iron.

In summary the cell provides, through its Embden-Meyerhof pathway, Krebs cycle, and respiratory chains, several important metabolic functions:

1. The body's major source of energy
2. Glycogen formation and release
3. Intermediates for fat formation (lipogenesis)
4. Intermediates for synthesis of some amino acids (protein synthesis)

These systems provide for tremendous efficiency in the production of energy, an overall efficiency rate of 42%. It has been calculated that the oxidation of one mole of glucose through this overall system produces 38 high-energy phosphorus bonds (ATP), eight in the initial Embden-Meyerhof glycolytic pathway and 30 in the final common Krebs cycle and respiratory chains. This is equivalent to an energy output of 288,800 calories!

3 Fats

For constant, readily available, quick energy, man's prime food source is carbohydrates. However, to further solve his problem of energy procurement, man also needs a more concentrated storage form of available fuel. For this he turns to fats and in some cultures uses a relatively large amount of it. For example, about 40% to 45% of the total caloric intake of Americans is from fat and a large part of it—over half—is saturated fat. In comparison a number of other population groups consume far less fat. For example, in the general Japanese diet fat contributes 6% to 10% of the total calories.

Some nutrition authorities believe that the rich amount of dietary fat in the American diet is excessive, in view of its possible relationship with arteriosclerotic heart disease. The Food and Nutrition Board of the National Research Council recommends an intake of fat at about 25% of the total calories, with an increased ratio of unsaturated fat. However, the human body appears to be able to function on a wide range of fat intake. The answers to questions concerning man's use of fats, primarily as a fuel for energy, seem to revolve around quality as well as quantity and individual life needs.

■ **If carbohydrates and fats both supply energy to the human body, how do they differ?**

It is true that carbohydrates and fat are both composed of the same basic structural elements—carbon, hydrogen, and oxygen. In fat, however, the relatively larger ratio of hydrogen makes fat a more concentrated potential or "storage" form of energy. Fat has better than twice the energy value of carbohydrate. Also, the storage capacity for fat in the human body is far greater than that of carbohydrate as glycogen, as we have seen. Fats also differ from carbohydrate in that they are insoluble in water.

■ **Since fats are relatively insoluble in water, how can they be transported in the blood, a water solution?**

Because of this solubility problem, fats never travel free in the body. They must be attached to some sort of "carrier" substance. Usually this substance is protein. Thus, the basic vehicular compounds of fat are the lipoproteins, a group of lipids containing varying ratios of fat and protein. These compounds are cellular and blood constituents.

■ **What are lipids?**

The general name *lipids* is given to a large group of heterogeneous compounds related in some way, either actually or potentially, to fatty acids. Chemical compounds in this group may vary from such obvious members as oils, fats, and waxes, to less apparent ones, such as certain vitamins and hormones. Their one common property is a relative insolubility in water.

■ **If lipids are so varied in nature, how may they be classified?**

Since lipids, by definition, have in common some sort of relationship to fatty acids, they are most commonly grouped according to the degree of complexity of their structure and the nature of this relationship to fatty acids:

1. *Simple lipids.* Esters of fatty acids and glycerol. An ester is a combination of an alcohol and an acid. Common fats, whether a solid fat or a liquid oil, are compounds of three fatty acids, with glycerol as a base. Hence, they are called triglycerides

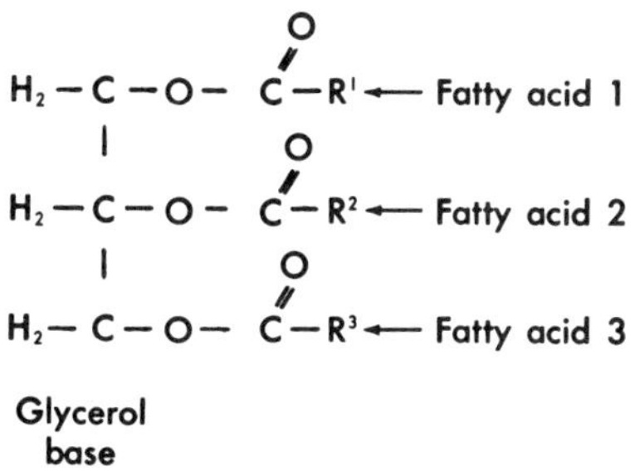

$$H_2 - C - O - \overset{\overset{\displaystyle O}{\nearrow}}{C} - R^1 \longleftarrow \text{Fatty acid 1}$$

$$H_2 - C - O - \overset{\overset{\displaystyle O}{\nearrow}}{C} - R^2 \longleftarrow \text{Fatty acid 2}$$

$$H_2 - C - O - \overset{\overset{\displaystyle O}{\nearrow}}{C} - R^3 \longleftarrow \text{Fatty acid 3}$$

Glycerol
base

Fig. 3-1. Triglyceride.

(Fig. 3-1). Examples of hard fats are the waxes, which are combinations of fatty acids with higher alcohols than glycerol.

2. *Compound lipids.* Combinations of fat with other components, for example, phospholipids, glycolipids, and lipoproteins.

3. *Derived lipids.* Fat substances derived from simple and compound lipids by hydrolysis or enzymatic breakdown; for example, fatty acids, glycerol, steroids.

■ **What is the nutritional significance of fats?**

Fats are important dietary constituents, not only for their high energy value but also because they supply fat-soluble vitamins and essential fatty acids. Stored in the body as adipose tissue, fat serves as an efficient source of direct and potential energy to meet day-to-day needs and provide a reserve for periods of stress. Certain vital tissue, such as nerve tissue has a particularly high amount of fat as reserve, and fatty acids are the preferred fuel for other vital tissue, such as cardiac muscle. Also, fat provides insulating material in subcutaneous tissues to help maintain body temperature and supplies supportive and protective tissue around vital organs, such as the kidneys.

■ **What is the chemical nature of fatty acids?**

Fatty acids are the basic structural units of fats. They are composed of single carbon chains varying from 4 to 24 carbon atoms. The chemical characteristics of a given fat

are determined by the nature of its constituent fatty acids. These fatty acids may be saturated or unsaturated fatty acids.

■ **What is the concept of saturation or unsaturation as applied to fatty acids?**

The terms "saturation" or "unsaturation" are used with fatty acids to refer to the ratio of hydrogen atoms to carbon atoms in the basic carbon chain that forms the individual fatty acid. In terms of chemical combining power, carbon has a *valence* of 4, meaning that *four* other atoms may attach themselves to positions on the carbon atom when various carbon compounds are formed. In a given fatty acid, if all the available valence bonds of a basic carbon chain are filled with hydrogen, the fatty acid is said to be completely *saturated with hydrogen.* However, if at one point along the carbon chain there are two fewer hydrogen atoms, the two involved carbon atoms take up their two available valence bonds to make one mutual bond. When this newly created mutual bond is added to the already existing bond between them, a double bond between the two carbon atoms is created. If only one such double bond occurs along the carbon chain, the fatty acid is called a *monounsaturated* fatty acid. If two or more double bonds occur along the carbon chain of the fatty acid, it is called a *polyunsaturated* fatty acid.

Compare the basic structures of representative examples of each form of fatty acid as shown in Fig. 3-2.

■ **How is this saturation factor reflected in different kinds of food fats?**

According to degree of saturation of its

constituent fatty acids, the physical nature of a food fat varies along a spectrum of hard-to-soft-to-liquid form. The more saturated the fat the more dense and hard it tends to be. Such harder fats come usually from animal sources—the meat fats. The more unsaturated the fat the less dense and more soft or liquid it tends to be. Such liquid fats come from plant sources—the vegetable oils.

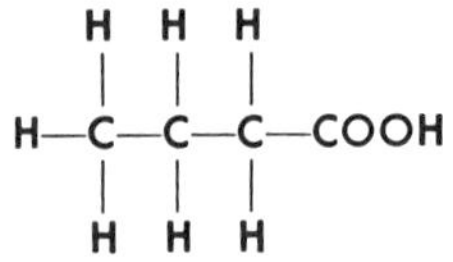

$$\underset{\displaystyle \text{H}}{\overset{\displaystyle \text{H}}{\text{C}}}$$

Saturated—butyric acid, as found in butter (4 carbons, no double bond)

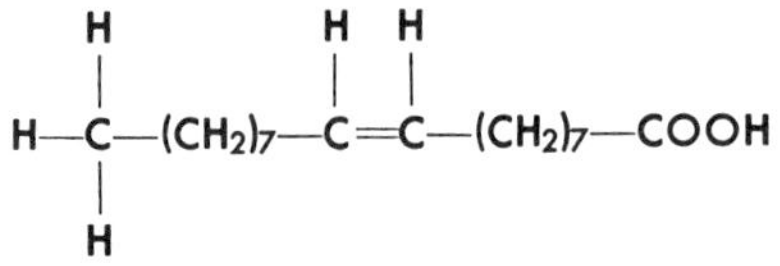

Monounsaturated—oleic acid, component fatty acid in olive oil (18 carbons, 1 double bond)

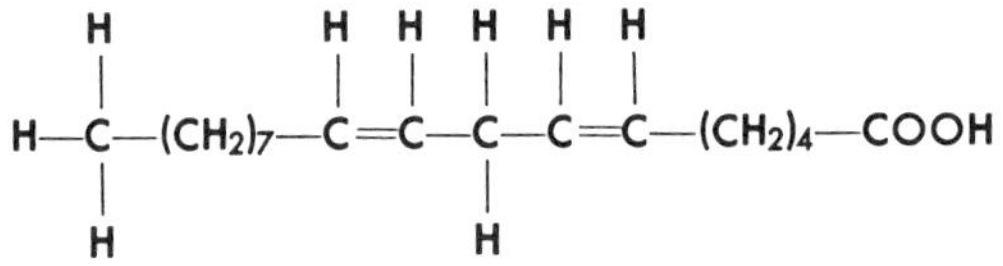

Polyunsaturated—found in various vegetable oils
Linoleic acid (18 carbons, 2 double bonds)

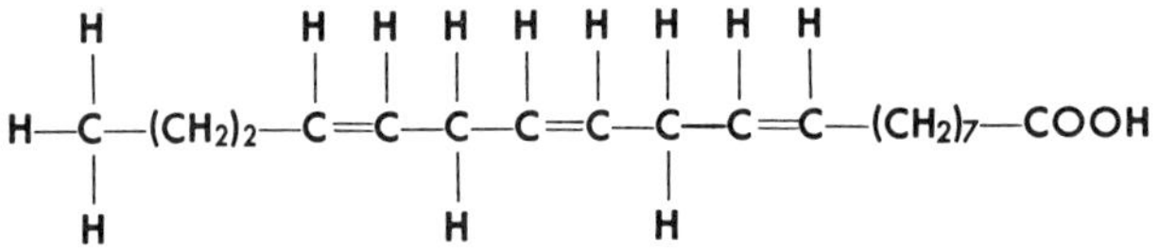

Polyunsaturated linolenic acid (18 carbons, 3 double bonds)

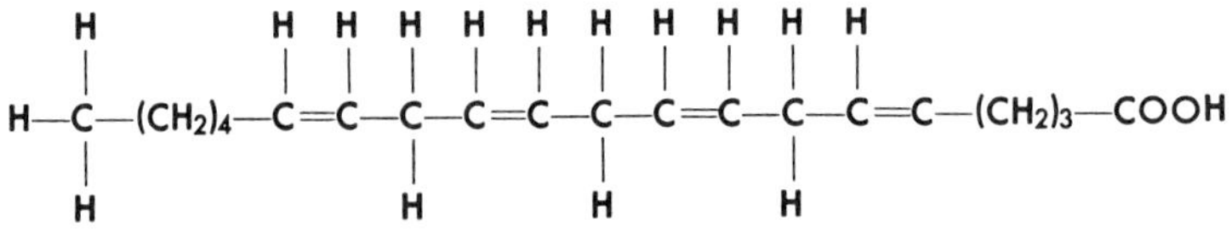

Polyunsaturated arachidonic acid (20 carbons, 4 double bonds)

Fig. 3-2. Chemical structures of fatty acids.

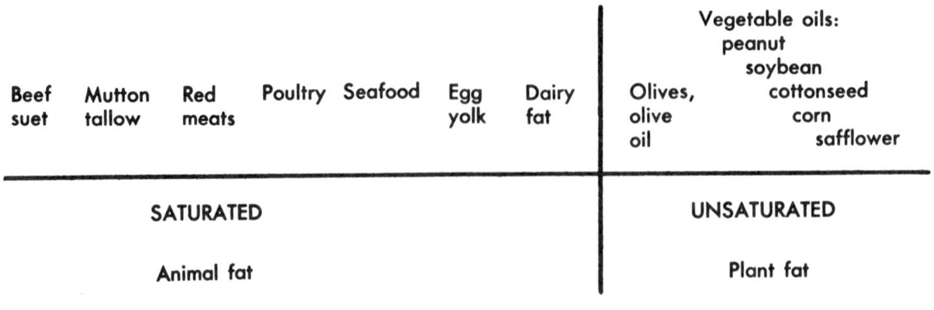

Beef suet	Mutton tallow	Red meats	Poultry	Seafood	Egg yolk	Dairy fat	Olives, olive oil	Vegetable oils: peanut soybean cottonseed corn safflower
SATURATED							UNSATURATED	
Animal fat							Plant fat	

Fig. 3-3. Spectrum of food fats according to degree of saturation of component fatty acids.

Compare these food fats on a general saturated-unsaturated spectrum as shown in Fig. 3-3.

■ **What are essential and nonessential fatty acids?**

The terms "essential" or "nonessential," when applied to fatty acids, refer to a twofold physiologic fact: (1) a fatty acid is essential if the body cannot manufacture it and must obtain it from the diet; (2) a fatty acid is essential if its absence will create a specific deficiency disease. For example, a type of eczema in infants is caused by lack of linoleic acid in the diet.

Three polyunsaturated fatty acids—linoleic acid, linolenic acid, and arachidonic acid—are usually termed essential fatty acids. However, *linoleic acid* may be considered the one essential fatty acid for two reasons: linolenic acid has relatively little effect in relieving the skin lesions originally associated with a deficiency of essential acids, and arachidonic acid can be synthesized by the body from linoleic acid and therefore does not have to be supplied as such in the diet.

■ **What important functions does the essential fatty acid, linoleic acid, serve?**

Linoleic acid serves several important functions in the body:

1. Strengthens capillary and cell membrane structure, which helps prevent increase in skin permeability.
2. Combines with cholesterol to form cholesterol esters. It is also part of the phospholipid and glycoprotein complexes.
3. Lowers serum cholesterol. Some investigators suggest that linoleic acid may play a key role in the transport and metabolism of cholesterol, although just what this role may be is not known at this time.
4. Prolongs blood clotting time and increases fibrinolytic activity.

■ **What is the relationship between linoleic acid, or the degree of saturation of fat, and the critical tissue changes in the artery disease atherosclerosis?**

The precise relationship between these unsaturated fatty acids and food fats and the disease process involved in atherosclerosis has not been determined. Recent research seems to indicate that increased dietary sources of linoleic acid have a cholesterol-lowering effect. Also, the amount of saturated fat (triglycerides) and cholesterol in the diet seems to have some relationship to the production of various forms of lipoproteins that may accumulate in abnormal levels in the blood. Five types of these lipid disorders (hyperlipoproteinemia) have been identified (see p. 226).

■ **What is hydrogenation?**

The process of hydrogenation introduces hydrogen gas into the available double bond linkages of unsaturated fats. Industrially, nickel is used as a catalyst. The process is also known as "hardening." It has commercial value, since it converts liquid fats, such as vegetable oils, into a solid form for use as vegetable shortening and margarines.

DIGESTION-ABSORPTION-METABOLISM OF FATS

Because of their relative insolubility in water and more varied complex structure, fats pose a larger digestion-absorption-metabolism task for the body than do carbohydrates. After initial enzymatic breakdown in digestion, a number of highly specific resynthesis processes occur during absorption. Finally, fats are conveyed by way of the lymphatic system to the liver and adipose tissue for the many interconversions involving lipids with other nutrients.

■ **What initial digestive processes change fat foods into forms ready for absorption into circulation?**

The digestion of fats proceeds through the successive parts of the gastrointestinal tract aided by both mechanical and chemical processes. Except for the small action of a gastric lipase (tributyrinase) or butterfat (tributyrin), chemical aspects of fat digestion, however, do not occur until the food mass reaches the small intestine. Here, with agents from the liver, the gallbladder, and the pancreas, fats are broken down successively into smaller fragments in preparation for their absorption.

Table 3-1. Summary of fat digestion

Organ	Enzyme	Activity
Mouth	None	Mechanical; mastication
Stomach	Gastric lipase (tributyrinase)	Mechanical separation of fats as protein and starch digested out
Small intestine	Gallbladder	Butterfat (tributyrin) to di- and mono-glycerides
	Bile salts (emulsifier)	Emulsifies fats
	Pancreatic	
	Lipase (steapsin)	Triglycerides to di- and monoglycerides in turn, then fatty acids and glycerol
	Cholesterol esterase	Free cholesterol + fatty acids to cholesterol esters
	Intestinal	
	Lecithinase	Lecithin to glycerol, fatty acids, phosphoric acid, choline

■ **What is the function of bile in the digestion of fats?**

Bile is produced in the liver and then is concentrated and stored in the gallbladder, ready for use in the handling of fats. Its function is that of an emulsifier. Emulsification is an important first step in the preparation of fats for digestion by the enzymes. This emulsifying process has a two-fold nature: (1) it breaks the fat into small particles or globules, which greatly enlarges the surface area available for action of the enzymes; and (2) it also lowers the surface tension of the finely dispersed and suspended fat globules, thus allowing greater ease of penetration of the enzymes. This is similar to the "wetting action" of detergents. The bile also provides an alkaline medium necessary for the action of lipase.

■ **How is the secretion of bile from the gallbladder regulated when it is needed?**

The presence of fat in the duodenum stimulates the secretion of *cholecystokinin* from glands in the walls of the intestines. Cholecystokinin is the triggering hormone for the secretion of bile. It provides the stimulus for the contraction of the gallbladder, relaxation of the sphincter, and subsequent secretion of bile salts into the intestine by way of the common bile duct.

■ **What enzymatic breakdown of fats occurs in the small intestine?**

The major fat splitting enzyme is pancreatic lipase (steapsin). In a stepwise fashion, pancreatic lipase breaks off one fatty acid at a time from the glycerol base of neutral fats. After this initial breaking off of the first fatty acid, each succeeding step of this breakdown is effected with increasing difficulty. In fact, separation of the final fatty acid from the remaining monoglyceride is such a slow process that less than one third of the total fat present actually reaches complete breakdown. Thus, the final products of fat digestion presented for absorption are fatty acids, diglycerides, monoglycerides, and glycerol. There are also two additional enzymes that act in the small intestine. An enzyme from the pancreas, *cholesterol esterase*, catalyzes the combining of free cholesterol with fatty acids to form cholesterol esters. Another enzyme, from the intestinal glands, *lecithinase*, catalyzes the breakdown of lecithin (a phospholipid) to glycerol, fatty acids, phosphoric acid, and choline. These various digestive changes are summarized in Table 3-1.

■ **How are these various products of fat digestion absorbed?**

The intestinal wall, with its vast mucosal absorbing surface and its serosal surface contiguous with blood and lymph vessels, is a highly active metabolic organ. This fact is particularly evident in its handling of fats through three distinct stages:

Stage 1. The absorbing surface of the small intestine, with its millions of small villi, handles the products of fat digestion in the various ways:

a. *Glycerol.* Because it is water soluble, glycerol is easily absorbed into the portal blood system and carried to the liver.

b. *Short- and medium-chain fatty acids.* These shorter fatty acids are relatively soluble in water and thus may also be absorbed directly into the portal vein and carried to the liver.

c. *Diglycerides, monoglycerides, unhydrolyzed triglycerides, and long-chain fatty acids.* These products of fat digestion are insoluble in water and hence pose the greatest problem for absorption. They require a wetting agent to facilitate this process. Bile salts perform this vital function and act as a ferry system to transport these products of fat digestion into the intestinal wall. With the monoglycerides and fatty acids, bile acids form a micellar complex so fine that it is almost a clear solution, and the fat particles rendered are about 1/100 the size of those that first entered the intestine. With the remaining unhydrolyzed triglycerides and diglycerides, bile forms an emulsion for absorption. This process is shown in Fig. 3-4.

Electron microscopic observations indicate that this neutral fat complex may be absorbed by a process called *pinocytosis,* a direct engulfing of the globule by the cell membrane.

d. *Cholesterol.* Cholesterol may be taken in as such in the diet (exogenous

cholesterol) or it may be synthesized by the body (endogenous cholesterol). One of the major sites of cholesterol synthesis is intestinal tissue. Here in initial absorption, dietary cholesterol is absorbed with the aid of bile salts as free or unesterified cholesterol. Most of it, however, has been esterified with fatty acids by the enzymatic action of cholesterol esterase in the intestine and is absorbed as cholesterol esters.

e. *Phospholipids.* Phospholipids, mainly lecithin, may also be taken in as such in the diet, or may be synthesized in intestinal tissue. Preformed dietary phospholipid, because of its *hydrophilic* nature (strong affinity for water), may be absorbed directly into portal blood. Endogenous phospholipid synthesized in intestinal tissue becomes part of the lipoprotein complex (chylomicron) that is absorbed into the lymphatic system. It then passes to the liver by way of the thoracic duct.

Stage 2. Intestinal wall action.

a. *Bile.* Bile in the micellar complex is separated out and absorbed through the portal blood for return to the liver and recirculation. This cycle, the *enterohepatic circulation of bile salts,* forms an efficient system for conserving bile and maintaining a constant supply of this necessary substance as needed.

b. *Glycerides.* Monoglycerides, diglycerides, and triglycerides are further hydrolyzed by an *enteric lipase* that is present within the cells of the intestinal wall. This enzyme continues the enzymatic hydrolysis of these remaining glycerides to their constituent fatty acids and glycerol.

c. *Triglyceride resynthesis.* Fatty acids are activated and combined with an active form of glycerol produced from glucose via the Embden-Meyerhof pathway (see p. see p.

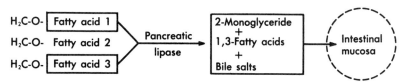

Fig. 3-4. Micellar complex of fats with bile salts for transport of fats into intestinal mucosa.

11). Thus new triglycerides are formed ready for use by the tissues.

d. *Cholesterol and phospholipids.* Cholesterol and phospholipids, mainly lecithin, are further synthesized in the cells of the intestinal wall.

Stage 3. Final absorption and transport of fat.

a. *Chylomicron formation.* The problem now is to convey this load of triglyceride, which is insoluble in water, through the blood, which is a water medium. Provision for this final absorption of fat is made by combining it with a small amount of protein to form a *lipoprotein complex* called *chylomicrons.* The chylomicron particles are fat droplets containing mostly triglycerides (about 81%) and fat-related products (cholesterol 9%, phospholipid 7%, fatty acids 1%) and some "carrier" protein (2%). These chylomicrons penetrate the intercellular spaces of the intestinal mucosa and enter the abdominal lacteals. They apparently can cross the cell wall intact and are carried by the lymphatic system to the portal blood.

b. *Lipoprotein lipase activity.* Following a meal, chylomicrons accumulate in the lymphatic vessels and plasma. However, these lipoproteins disappear rather quickly from the plasma into various tissues for oxidation or storage. The efficient clearing factor is an enzyme, another lipase called *lipoprotein lipase,* which begins its action in the plasma but continues it mainly in the tissue taking up the fat. It releases fatty acids after their hydrolysis from depot fats. As one would expect, a large amount of the enzyme is present in adipose tissue, but none has been found in liver, where fat is not stored.

Metabolism of fats

Following the unique work of the intestinal wall in absorbing and resynthesizing lipids and then transporting them via the lymph into portal circulation, the remaining metabolic work in handling fats is achieved through a constant balance between fat breakdown (lipolysis) and fat synthesis (lipogenesis). Two major metabolic organs—the liver and adipose fat tissue—maintain this metabolic balance. This dynamic interplay has been called the "liver-adipose tissue axis."

■ **What factors work together to control the level of plasma lipids?**

The interacting factors constantly at work to control the level of plasma lipids include:

1. Diet
2. Synthesis of fat in the tissues
3. Mobilization of fat from the depots
4. Rate of oxidation in the various body tissues
5. Deposition of fat in adipose tissue and the liver

■ **What is the function of the liver in fat metabolism?**

The liver's main function in handling fat is one of producing needed lipoproteins to transport fat in the body. Its other synthesis functions involve cholesterol, fatty acids, and triglycerides. It also does some oxidation of fatty acids to produce energy. Its functions may be summarized as follows:

1. *Synthesis of lipoproteins.* Three additional forms of lipoproteins are synthesized in the liver, the pre-beta, beta, and alpha lipoproteins. These are compounds containing a little less fat than the chylomicrons and a little more protein. They are the forms of lipoproteins that may accumulate excessively in specific lipid disorders. The purpose of this synthesis of lipoproteins is to provide additional transport forms for the fat coming into the liver in order that it may not remain in the liver and produce a pathologic condition—a fatty liver. Thus to prevent abnormal accumulation of fat in the liver, certain *lipotropic* factors are active in this organ. By a process of *transmethylation* these lipotropic agents promote the production of lipoproteins, which transfer the fatty acids and fats out of the liver. A major example of such a lipotropic agent is choline, a component of the phospholipid, lecithin. Choline, sometimes classified as a B-complex vitamin, is synthesized from methionine, an essential amino acid. The therapeutic effect of protein in early liver disease may derive in some mea-

sure from its lipotropic constituent amino acid, methionine.

2. *Cholesterol synthesis.* The liver is the other body tissue besides intestinal wall tissue where cholesterol may be synthesized from active acetate.

3. *Fatty acid and triglyceride synthesis.* The liver also snythesizes fat from fatty acids and glycerol produced from carbohydrates, although it does less of this than does adipose tissue. This is the process of lipogenesis.

4. *Phospholipid synthesis.* Some phospholipid is synthesized by the liver from the fatty acids and glycerol present.

5. *Fatty acid oxidation.* Lipolysis of fatty acids is achieved in the liver through a process of beta oxidation. In this process fragments of fatty acids are broken off and active acetate is formed, which then enters the Krebs cycle to produce energy for the body's work.

6. *Bile synthesis and circulation.* The liver recirculates bile and synthesizes additional amounts as needed.

■ **What is the function of adipose tissue in the metabolism of fats?**

Adipose tissue is by no means the static storage reserve of fat it was once thought to be. It is now known to be one of the most metabolically active body tissues. It maintains a constant turnover, synthesizing and depositing fat and breaking down and mobilizing fat.

1. *Lipogenesis.* The most active site of lipogenesis in the human body is adipose tissue. Here triglycerides are formed from fatty acids and glycerol. The needed fatty acids may come either from the diet or from synthesized fatty acids made in the tissues from precursors, such as carbohydrate and its metabolites (glucose, pyruvate, and active acetate). The synthesized fat is then deposited in three major body sites: (1) subcutaneous connective tissue, (2) abdominal cavity, and (3) intermuscular connective tissue. These three general types of fat deposits in the body are collectively called adipose fat tissue.

2. *Lipolysis.* Lipolysis also takes place in adipose tissue, since depot fat is constantly being mobilized by the body. The fat is again broken down into glycerol and fatty acids. The glycerol is released, is converted in the liver to glycogen, and is eventually oxidized as glucose. The free (unesterified) fatty acids released are transported to various cells as needed to be oxidized for energy. The turnover rate of these free fatty acids is high. They are the metabolically active forms of lipids. All tissues can oxidize them completely to carbon dioxide and water. They are even the preferred form of fuel for some tissues, such as the myocardium. Hence, the major function of fat is to supply energy for the body.

■ **What is the relationship between fat metabolism and carbohydrate metabolism?**

Fat metabolism is closely interdependent with carbohydrate metabolism and indicates that adipose tissue is in fact one of the major sites of insulin activity. Carbohydrate metabolism provides three major substances related closely to fat metabolism:

1. *Activated glycerol.* In the Embden-Meyerhof glycolytic pathway for glucose metabolism, an activated form of glycerol is produced, which is necessary for lipogenesis. Since adipose tissue lacks the activating enzyme to produce this material (glycerokinase), this active form of glycerol (α-glycerophosphate) must come from the glycolytic pathway of glucose metabolism.

2. *NADPH.* NADPH is the niacin-containing coenzyme required for the synthesis of fatty acids from pyruvate and active acetate. It is produced through the pentose shunt of the Embden-Meyerhof glycolytic pathway. Tissues active in lipogenesis, such as adipose tissue and the lactating mammary glands, have a very active pentose shunt pathway. This helps to explain why glucose and insulin are necessary for lipogenesis. The required coenzyme, NADPH, is produced by glucose oxidation through this shunt.

3. *Oxaloacetate.* Oxaloacetate is produced through the Embden-Meyerhof path-

way from glucose oxidation to constantly refuel and maintain the Krebs cycle for oxidizing active acetate, formed from fat breakdown, to produce energy. Thus oxalo-acetate is the necessary carbohydrate fuel to keep the process going, for with each complete cycle of reaction in the Krebs cycle by which active acetate is broken down to produce carbon dioxide, water, and energy, another unit of oxaloacetate is produced, which begins the process again. If there is not adequate oxaloacetate from carbohydrate to maintain the cycle efficiently, active acetate from fat cannot be handled properly and is diverted to form ketone bodies.

■ **What are ketones?**

Under usual circumstances ketones may be considered normal intermediates of fat metabolism. However, when the amount of glucose available is insufficient to perpetuate the Krebs cycle, fat is broken down so rapidly that it cannot be used for fuel. Without the necessary carbohydrate to handle the fat properly through the Krebs cycle, the ketones accumulate, causing ketosis. These ketones are acids (acetoacetic acid, acetone, and beta-hydroxybutyric acid), and the accumulation of these strong acids upsets the normal acid-base balance in the body and acidosis results. Diabetic acidosis, for example, clearly demonstrates the interrelationship of the nutrients and their metabolites. When glucose cannot be properly oxidized because insulin is lacking or unavailable, the oxaloacetate that is necessary to the maintenance of the Krebs cycle is not provided and the active acetate from fat cannot be handled. Instead, it is converted into ketones.

■ **What hormones influence fat metabolism?**

Since fat and carbohydrate metabolism are so closely interrelated, the same hormones that affect carbohydrate metabolism also affect fat metabolism.

1. Growth hormone (GH), adrenocorticotrophic hormone (ACTH), and thyroid-stimulating hormone (TSH), which are all secreted by the pituitary gland, increase the release of free fatty acids from adipose tissue by imposing energy demands on the body.

2. Cortisone and hydrocortisone, which are secreted by the adrenal gland, cause the release of free fatty acids. Epinephrine and norepinephrine stimulate lipolysis, the breakdown of triglycerides.

3. The important lipogenic activity of insulin, which is secreted by the pancreas, has been described. Glucagon, also secreted by the pancreas, has an opposite effect by increasing the release of free fatty acids from adipose tissue.

4. Thyroxin, which is secreted by the thyroid gland, affects fat metabolism by stimulating adipose tissue release of free fatty acids. It also lowers blood cholesterol.

■ **What is the effect of body temperature on fat metabolism?**

Lowering of body temperature stimulates the release of fatty acids. These fatty acids then supply the necessary fuel to return the body temperature toward normal.

■ **What is cholesterol and how does it enter into fat metabolism?**

Cholesterol is a fat-related compound, a sterol ($C_{27}H_{45}OH$). It has a complex cyclic ring structure with an attached fatty acid. It is a normal constituent of bile and a principal constituent of gallstones. In body metabolism cholesterol is important as a precursor of various steroid hormones, such as sex hormones, and adrenal corticoids. It has been associated with atherosclerosis, a disease of blood vessels characterized by the formation of localized plaques within or beneath the intimal surface of the vessel wall. Cholesterol is one of the major components of these fatty plaques. Cholesterol can be synthesized by the liver and the intestinal wall tissue. It is widely distributed in nature, especially in animal tissue, such as glandular meats and egg yolks.

The blood level of cholesterol is nor-

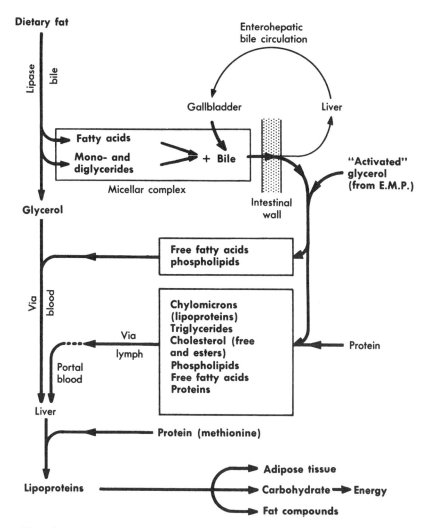

Fig. 3-5. Summary of fat metabolism. (E.M.P. = Embden-Meyerhof glycolytic pathway.)

mally maintained at 150 to 300 mg./100 ml. Cholesterol is excreted by the liver in bile. The liver, therefore, has a major cholesterol-regulating role, since it adds and removes cholesterol from the blood as needed.

A summary of fat metabolism is given in Fig. 3-5 for review and reference.

4 Proteins

Proteins are well named. The word comes from the Greek *proteios*, meaning "primary, holding first place." Proteins are indeed primary to life as we know it, for they make up the basic structure of all living cells. Hence they provide the essential life-forming and life-sustaining ingredient of the diet of all animal organisms.

In countries with adequate nutrition protein contributes from 10% to 15% of the total calories. In more restricted diets it may contribute less, leading to varying degrees of protein malnutrition. In the average American diet, protein contributes approximately 14% of the total calories.

TISSUE BUILDING AND REBUILDING: A CONTINUOUS PROCESS

Since protein is the basic structure of all living cells, its primary importance is to help man solve his continuous problem of tissue building and rebuilding—growth and maintenance. It is with this basic task that the processes of protein metabolism are involved.

■ **How does protein differ from carbohydrate and fat, enabling it to provide the growth element of life?**

Like carbohydrate and fat, protein contains carbon, hydrogen, and oxygen; but protein is unique in that it also contains *nitrogen*. Sixteen percent of its total composition is made up of nitrogen. It often contains other elements, such as sulfur. Also, the structure of protein is different from that of either carbohydrate or fat. The proteins are much more complex compounds, with high molecular weights that range from a few thousand to a million or more.

■ **What is the basic structural unit of protein?**

Proteins are organic substances, which, upon hydrolysis or digestion, yield their constituent unit building blocks—*amino acids.* Early in the 1800's scientists recognized that proteins could be broken down into a number of smaller structural units. Because these substances seemed to behave chemically with a dual nature—both acid and base—they were given the seemingly contradictory name *amino* (base) *acids.* Proteins should be viewed, then, in terms of their building blocks, amino acids, for it is these structural units that will constantly be encountered in clinical practice.

■ **What is the significance of an amino acid's dual nature?**

As indicated by its name, an amino acid has a chemical structure that combines both acid and base (amino) factors. This important chemical structure gives to amino acids a unique *amphoteric* nature (Gr. *amphoteros*, both). This dual nature can be seen in the fundamental pattern of an amino acid as shown in Fig. 4-1.

The acid factor is the carboxyl group (COOH) and the base factor is the amino group (NH_2). A radical that is specific for the individual amino acid is grouped with the acid and base radicals around a central carbon atom.

As a result of its dual nature, therefore, an amino acid in solution can *ionize* (dissociate or separate into its constituent ions). Thus it may behave either as an acid or as

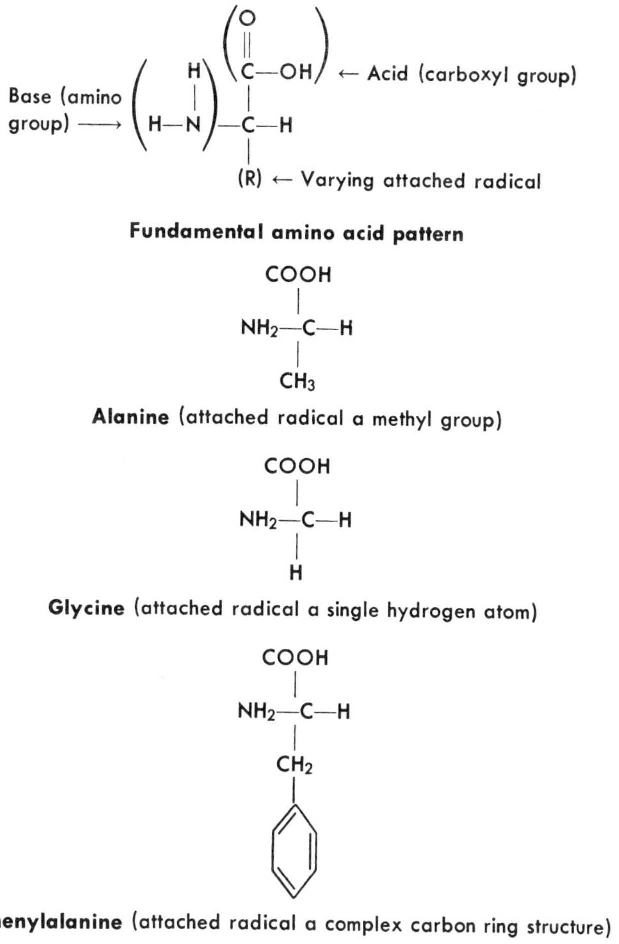

$$\text{Base (amino group)} \longrightarrow \left(\begin{array}{c} \text{H} \\ | \\ \text{H---N} \end{array} \right) \overset{\displaystyle \left(\begin{array}{c} \text{O} \\ \| \\ \text{C---OH} \end{array} \right)}{\underset{\displaystyle (R)}{\begin{array}{c} | \\ \text{C---H} \\ | \end{array}}} \leftarrow \text{Acid (carboxyl group)}$$

← Acid (carboxyl group)

(R) ← Varying attached radical

Fundamental amino acid pattern

$$\begin{array}{c} \text{COOH} \\ | \\ \text{NH}_2\text{---C---H} \\ | \\ \text{CH}_3 \end{array}$$

Alanine (attached radical a methyl group)

$$\begin{array}{c} \text{COOH} \\ | \\ \text{NH}_2\text{---C---H} \\ | \\ \text{H} \end{array}$$

Glycine (attached radical a single hydrogen atom)

$$\begin{array}{c} \text{COOH} \\ | \\ \text{NH}_2\text{---C---H} \\ | \\ \text{CH}_2 \end{array}$$

Phenylalanine (attached radical a complex carbon ring structure)

Fig. 4-1. Comparative structure of amino acids: the basic amino acid pattern and three examples of amino acids—alanine, glycine, phenylalanine.

a base, depending on the pH of the solution. This means that amino acids have a great *buffer* capacity, which is an important clinical characteristic. The interesting term commonly used for this unique phenomenon is *zwitterion*. The term is taken from the German word *Zwitter*, meaning "hybrid" and the Greek word *ion*, meaning "wanderer." Amino acids behave like "hybrid wanderers," either acid or base, depending on the buffering need presented by a particular solution.

■ **How are amino acids joined together to form proteins?**

This acid-base chemical nature of amino acids also enables them to join in the char-

acteristic chain structure of proteins. The amino group of one amino acid joins the carboxyl group of another. This characteristic chain structure of amino acids is called a *peptide linkage*. Long chains of amino acids that are linked in this manner are called *polypeptides*.

■ **How are these polypeptide chains arranged to structure particular types of proteins?**

These long polypeptide chains may be coiled or folded back upon themselves in a spiral shape called a *helix*. These coiled chains are held together in some instances by additional cross-links of bonds involving sulfur and hydrogen. The helical shapes of these coils may be of two types: (1) *fibrous*—a protein that coils and unfolds on contraction and relaxation (for example, myosin in muscle fiber); (2) *globular*—a protein forming a dense compact coil (for example, serum albumin or serum globulin and the hormone insulin).

The various component structures within the total structure of the protein molecule may be grouped according to increased complexity of arrangement. The *primary structure* is the basic polypeptide chain. The *secondary structure* is the helix with its coils linked to one another by crossbonds, usually of hydrogen or sulfur. The *tertiary structure* is the characteristic arrangements of helices, which form specific layers on fibers of specific proteins.

■ **How do the different tissues of the body maintain their unique structure and nature?**

A given protein contains a *specific* number of *specific* amino acids linked in a sequence that is *specific* for that protein. It is this very *specificity* of protein structure in a definite amino acid sequence that gives various tissues their unique form, function, and character. If any single amino acid required for a specific protein structure is missing in the body, that particular protein will not be synthesized at that time. This is known as the law of "all or none" in protein synthesis.

■ **What is the difference between "essential" and "nonessential" amino acids?**

Amino acids are termed "essential" or "nonessential" according to two factors: (1) whether the body can manufacture the particular amino acid, and (2) whether the amino acid is essential for normal growth and development. It is apparent, therefore, that in man the protein requirement must be considered on the basis of the quality and not merely the quantity of the protein. It is obviously not just a matter of total amount of protein needed, but of the specific amino acids needed.

On the basis of these distinctions in body dependence, eight amino acids have been demonstrated to be essential for adults. The approximately twelve remaining amino acids are nonessential or dispensable. The body can manufacture them. The following is a listing of the essential and nonessential amino acids.

Essential	Nonessential
Threonine	Glycine
Leucine	Alanine
Isoleucine	Aspartic acid
Valine	Glutamic acid
Lysine	Proline
Methionine	Hydroxyproline
Phenylalanine	Cystine
Tryptophan	Tyrosine
	Serine
	Arginine
	Histidine

The last named nonessential amino acids, arginine and histidine, are necessary during growth but not during adulthood. Therefore they may be called "semiessential." Three other amino acids, cysteine, citrulline, and hydroxylysine, may be added to the nonessential list. Although not naturally occurring, they are nonetheless metabolically active in the body. Therefore in total there are some 22 amino acids in the body, eight of which are essential and must be obtained in the diet.

■ **What are "complete" and "incomplete" proteins?**

It naturally follows, therefore, that food proteins are classified as having high biologic value or not according to their constituent amino acids. Proteins are called "complete" proteins if they contain all of the eight essential amino acids in sufficient quantity and specific ratio to supply the body's needs. These proteins are of animal origin: meat, milk, cheese, and egg.

However, incomplete proteins are those deficient in one or more of the essential amino acids. They are of plant origin: grains, legumes and nuts, and certain seeds. In a mixed diet animal and plant proteins supplement one another.

■ **How may a vegetarian secure "complete" proteins if such proteins are found only in foods of animal origin?**

Some vegetarians allow milk and egg in

their diet. They would have no problem, therefore, in securing complete protein. Other more strict vegetarians, however, the so-called "Vegands," who eat only plant foods, would need to eat enough different plant food sources to supplement one another and thus assure a correctly proportioned supply of all eight essential amino acids. In a mixed diet animal and plant proteins supplement one another, but even a mixture of plant proteins may provide an adequate balanced ratio of amino acids if it is planned wisely. The value of variety in the diet is therefore evident.

■ **What kinds of protein make up the body?**

Proteins may be classified into seven broad categories according to their function in the body. These seven types with some examples are given below:

Structural proteins—collagen
Contractile proteins—muscle
Antibodies—gamma globulin
Blood proteins—albumin, fibrinogen, globulin, and hemoglobin
Hormones—insulin
Enzymes—lipase
Nutrient proteins—food sources of essential amino acids

■ **Other than its primary use for building and rebuilding tissue, does protein have any other function?**

Yes. Protein also contributes to the body's overall energy metabolism. After removal of the nitrogenous portion of the constituent amino acids, the amino acid residue may be either glycogenic (capable of being converted to carbohydrate) or ketogenic (capable of being converted to fatty acids). Only leucine, phenylalanine, and tyrosine are fully ketogenic; and isoleucine is weakly so. The remaining amino acids are glycogenic. It has been estimated that, on an average, 58% of the total dietary protein becomes available as glucose and is oxidized as such to yield energy.

■ **Are there individual amino acids that have special physiologic functions in addition to general tissue building and energy functions?**

Yes. Two may serve as examples: (1) *tryptophan* is the precursor of the vitamin nicotinamide (niacin) and the precursor of the vasoconstrictor serotonin; (2) *phenylalanine* is the precursor of the nonessential amino acid tyrosine. Together with tyrosine, phenylalanine leads to formation of the hormones thyroxine and epinephrine.

DIGESTION-ABSORPTION-METABOLISM OF PROTEINS

In order to build tissue the first task of the body is to procure the raw building material and convert it into the necessary structural units that the cells can use. These structural units are the amino acids. The raw building material is the dietary protein. The dietary protein supplies the appropriate numbers and types of amino acids for efficient synthesis of specific cellular tissue proteins. In addition, protein supplies amino acids for other essential nitrogen-containing substances, such as enzymes and hormones.

■ **What initial digestive processes change protein foods into the basic forms that can be absorbed into circulation?**

Chemical digestion of protein begins in the stomach. In fact, the stomach's chief digestive function in relation to all foods is the partial enzymatic breakdown of protein. Three agents contained in the gastric secretions participate in different ways in this beginning hydrolysis. These agents are pepsin, hydrochloric acid, and rennin.

Protein digestion continues in the alkaline medium of the small intestine. A number of enzymes from both pancreatic and intestinal secretions take part. Through this overall system of protein splitting enzymes, the pancreatic and intestinal secretions break down the large, complex proteins into progressively smaller peptide chains; and amino acids are split off from the ends of these chains. The end products of protein digestion, the amino acids, are then ready for absorption by the intestinal mucosa. These changes in food protein to render the necessary amino acids for absorption are summarized in Table 4-1.

Table 4-1. Summary of protein digestion

Organ	Enzyme			Digestive action
	Inactive precursor	Activator	Active enzyme	
Mouth			None	Mechanical only
Stomach (acid)	Pepsinogen	Hydrochloric acid	Pepsin	Protein → proteoses and peptones
			Rennin (infants) (Ca necessary for activity)	Casein → coagulated curd
Intestine (alkaline)				
Pancreatic juice	Trypsinogen	Enterokinase	Trypsin	Protein, proteoses, peptones → polypeptides, dipeptides
	Chymotrypsinogen	Active trypsin	Chymotrypsin	Proteoses, peptones → polypeptides, dipeptides Also coagulates milk
			Carboxypeptidase	Polypeptides → simpler peptides, dipeptides, amino acids
Intestinal juice			Aminopeptidase	Polypeptides → peptides, depeptides, amino acids
			Dipeptidase	Dipeptides → amino acids

■ **How are the amino acids absorbed and transported to their distribution center and building sites?**

Since amino acids are water soluble, they are absorbed rapidly from the small intestine directly into the portal blood system through the fine network of villous capillaries. Most of this amino acid absorption probably takes place in the proximal portion of the small intestine. An active and selective transport system is present, which is energy dependent. The amino acids in their natural forms are transported by this active system; their isomers may be absorbed by free diffusion.

Vitamin B_6 (pyridoxine) in the form of pyridoxal phosphate (B_6-PO_4) appears to be intimately involved in the active transport of amino acids from the intestinal mucosa to the serosa. This vitamin also seems to play a role in the transport of amino acids into the cells for eventual metabolism.

A few larger fragments of short-chain peptides may remain after digestion and be absorbed as such. Even whole proteins are sometimes absorbed intact. These larger molecules apparently cannot be used in protein synthesis as can free amino acids, but they may play a part in the development of immunity and sensitivity. For example, antibodies in the mother's colostrum (the premilk breast secretion) are passed on to her nursing infant.

Metabolism of proteins

In human nutrition the amino acids derived from the digestion of proteins are the metabolic currency of the body. It is with the fate of these vital compounds that the metabolism of protein is ultimately concerned. These metabolic activities in large measure can be summarized under the basic concept of *balance*.

Throughout the body many interdependent checks and balances exist. There is a constant ebb and flow of materials, a building up and breaking down of parts, and a depositing and mobilizing of constituents. Many body mechanisms maintain internal physiologic stability (equilibrium). The body has built-in controls that operate as coordinated responses of its parts to any situation that tends to disturb its normal condition or function. The resultant state of equilibrium is called *homeostasis,* and the various mechanisms designed to preserve it are called *homeostatic mechanisms.* This balance between body parts and functions is life sustaining. Older ideas of a rigid body structure are giving way to this concept of dynamic equilibrium. All body constituents are in a constant state of flux, although some tissues are more actively engaged than others. This concept of dynamic equilibrium can be seen in carbohydrate and fat metabolism; however, it is especially striking in protein metabolism.

The adult body's state of stability, then, is the result of a balance between the rates of protein breakdown and protein resynthesis. In periods of growth the synthesis rate is higher, so that new tissue can be formed. In conditions of starvation and wasting diseases and more gradually as the aging process advances in the elderly, the rate of breakdown exceeds that of synthesis and the body deteriorates.

■ **How does the body ensure a ready source of amino acids needed at a particular time for a particular protein synthesis?**

The liver may be thought of as a distribution center for amino acids. After absorption the amino acids are carried through the portal circulation to the liver for distribution to various tissues as needed. Thus amino acids derived from endogenous tissue breakdown and the amino acids from dietary protein both enter a common metabolic pool of amino acids. This metabolic pool serves as a reserve backup to ensure needed proteins being available. Thus a balance of amino acids is maintained to supply the body's total needs.

Shifts and balances between tissue breakdown and dietary protein ensure the constant availability of a balanced mixture of amino acids. From this amino acid pool specific amino acids are supplied as needed for specific tissue protein synthesis and to make up body losses.

■ **What is nitrogen balance?**

The words "nitrogen balance" refer to the balance between intake and output of nitrogen in the body. Nitrogen is found in other compounds than amino acids. Nonprotein nitrogen is present, for example, in urea, uric acid, ammonia, creatine, creatinine, and other body tissues and fluids. Total nitrogen balance involves all these sources. Thus the term *negative nitrogen balance* is used to indicate that the output of nitrogen exceeds its intake. *Positive nitrogen balance* is that state in which the intake of nitrogen exceeds its output. Thus *total nitrogen balance* is the net result of all nitrogen gains and losses in all protein compartments. However, it gives no picture of the shifts in distribution of nitrogen. For example, a tissue involved in a malignant neoplastic process may be robbing other tissues of nitrogen; yet this loss would not be reflected in total nitrogen balance. Nonetheless, the total nitrogen balance is a useful general measure of body equilibrium. Nonprotein nitrogen (nitrogen from sources other than amino acids) plays a role in protein synthesis through its sparing effect on some amino acid requirements. By providing the amino group for transamination, it relieves the need for amino acid food sources to supply the nitrogen radical.

■ **How is tissue built in the body?**

The building or synthesis of tissue protein is governed by a unique *specificity* with respect to the amino acid constituents that are required to produce a specific protein. This has been called the law of "all or none." All the necessary amino acids for a given protein must be present at the same time or the protein will not be formed. Specific selection and supply of amino acids are mandatory. This specific selection is governed by gene control. Specific genes have specific control over the building of specific proteins. The material in the gene that exercises this control has been identified as DNA.

■ What is DNA?

DNA is deoxyribonucleic acid. It is the controlling mechanism by which genetic design is passed from generation to generation. It is the key material in the chromosomes of the cell nucleus. Each gene is probably composed of a complex nucleic acid molecule. DNA is a large double chain *polymer* (a compound of high molecular weight made up of many parts). It is composed of nitrogenous bases called nucleotides (purines, pyrimidines), a sugar (deoxyribose), and a phosphate group. DNA forms the basic pattern of the message code in each cell. This code or pattern for sequence of amino acids to structure a specific protein thus determines what specific protein will be synthesized.

■ What is messenger RNA?

RNA is ribonucleic acid. It is formed by DNA in the cell nucleus and receives its specific pattern imprint from DNA, in a similar manner that plastic poured into a mold receives the imprint of the mold. RNA differs from DNA, however, in that it is only a single strand structure; whereas DNA is a double strand, ladderlike helix. RNA also has a different sugar and one of its nitrogen bases is a different compound. Once RNA is formed in the cell nucleus by the DNA, it carries the message pattern out into the cell cytoplasm. This type of RNA has been called "messenger RNA." Out in the cell, messenger RNA uses one of the membranous tubules of the endoplasmic reticulum as its working site. Here it attaches itself to the row of reticular granules that are called ribosomes as an anchor point for its operations.

The ribosomes form the specific building site in the cell for the synthesis of protein. The messenger RNA strand from the nucleus attaches itself to the ribosome and thus forms a template or mold to direct the lining up of amino acids in the exact se-

quence necessary to fit the master pattern for the desired protein. This is part of the marvelous specificity of protein synthesis at work. This preparation, therefore, in the cell nucleus by which DNA transfers a specific protein pattern to messenger RNA is the first stage in the process of protein synthesis.

■ After the message pattern is set on "messenger RNA," what are the remaining stages of protein synthesis?

The remaining stages of protein synthesis involve activated amino acids and "transfer RNA."

Stage 2. Activated amino acids must be produced before they can enter into protein synthesis. This means that they must be energized in order to be capable of combining chemically with other substances. This is done in the cell's cytoplasm by an activating enzyme that is specific for each amino acid plus an energizing phosphate compound, ATP (adenosine triphosphate) or AMP (adenosine monophosphate). The complex thus formed (enzyme + ATP + amino acid) produces an activated amino acid that is ready to go into its position in the protein molecule.

Stage 3. Transfer RNA occurs free in the cell's cytoplasmic fluid. These are many short-chain fragments of RNA. There appears to be a specific transfer RNA molecule for each amino acid that is to be used. Each transfer RNA molecule attaches itself to its specific amino acid partner and carries it into position of the strand of messenger RNA. The amino acids slip perfectly into their correct slots, one beside another along the grid of the ribosomal template, guided into place by the transfer RNA fragments.

Stage 4. Finally the amino acids are lined up side by side in precise sequence and are joined to each other by peptide linkages to form long polypeptide chains. This is the specific polypeptide chain of the protein originally designated by the pattern coded on the DNA in the cell nucleus. The newly formed polypeptide chain breaks free from the ribosome and the transfer RNA molecules are freed from the messenger RNA template. The transfer RNA molecules are now available to perform the same process all over again. These successive stages in protein synthesis may be visualized in the diagram in Fig. 4-2.

■ **What processes are involved in the breaking down of tissue protein?**

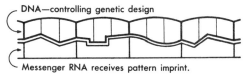

Stage 1: Preparation in cell nucleus: DNA transfers specific protein pattern to messenger RNA

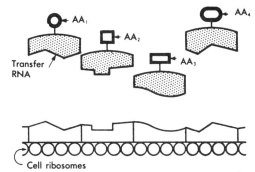

Stage 2: Activated amino acids in cell cytoplasm attach to transfer RNA partner

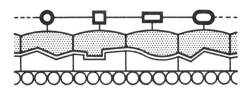

Stage 3: Transfer RNA carries the active amino acids into position, and peptide linkage forms

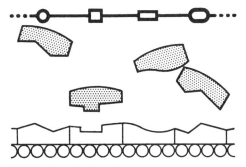

Stage 4: Newly formed polypeptide chain breaks free; transfer RNA is released to repeat process

Fig. 4-2. Stages in protein synthesis.

In a constantly balanced interplay with tissue synthesis, tissue protein is being degraded and its constituent amino acids are being released. If any amino acid is not then reused in tissue protein synthesis, it may be degraded in turn or oxidized to use energy. The two parts rendered from this breaking down of amino acid are the nitrogenous group (NH_2) and a non-nitrogen residue, a "carbon skeleton."

Nitrogenous group (NH₂). The first step in the metabolic breakdown of amino acids is the splitting off of the nitrogenous portion (the amino group, NH_2) by hydrolysis. This process, which takes place chiefly in the liver, is called *deamination*. The ammonia (NH_3) that is formed may be handled in several ways. It may be converted into urea in the liver and excreted by the kidney in the urine. This conversion in the liver is completed by a special urea cycle. Also, the ammonia may be used in the production of purines and other nitrogen-containing compounds. Or the ammonia may be combined with various carbohydrate derivatives of amino acid residues to form still other amino acids. Such amino acids would be termed "nonessential" because the body can manufacture them. This process of transferring the amino group from an amino acid to a carbohydrate derivative or an amino acid residue is called *transamination*. The process is catalyzed by specific enzymes called *transaminases*. A vitamin B_6 derivative (pyridoxal phosphate) acts as a coenzyme. When tissue is damaged, transaminases are released and their level in plasma rises. Finally, ammonia may also be taken up by an amino acid to produce still another form of that acid, the *amine* form. This process is called *amination*. For example, a glutamic acid molecule may take up an NH_3 radical to form glutamine. The NH_3 radical may then be liberated in the distal tubules of the kidney and excreted. This process of amination and deamination provides an efficient way of removing a toxic substance (NH_3, ammonia) from the body.

Non-nitrogen residue. The non-nitrogen residue, "carbon skeleton," is called a *keto-acid*. The residue of a given amino acid is either glycogenic (leading to the formation of carbohydrate), or ketogenic (leading to the formation of fat). The ketogenic amino acids are phenylalanine, tyrosine, and leucine; isoleucine residue is also weakly ketogenic. The remaining ones, the majority of the amino acids, are glycogenic.

Thus, the intermediate metabolites from

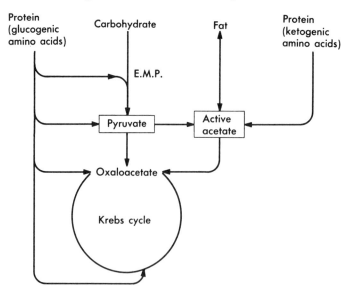

Fig. 4-3. Converging of glucogenic and ketogenic amino acids with carbohydrate and fat in the Embden-Meyerhof glycolytic pathway and the final common Krebs cycle for energy production.

protein, carbohydrate, and fat enter a common metabolic pool. There is constant interplay between this pool and the amino acid pool. Finally, metabolites from all three basic nutrients enter the Krebs cycle and produce energy, with the end products of carbon dioxide and water. These interrelationships between the basic nutrients are shown in Figs. 4-3 and 4-4.

■ **What is the meaning of the terms "anabolism" and "catabolism"?**

The term "anabolism" is used to designate the process of building up tissue, protein synthesis. This condition prevails during periods of positive nitrogen balance or physiologic growth periods or the constant balance of tissue synthesis for maintenance purposes. The term "catabolism" is applied to the tissue breakdown process. It prevails in periods of negative nitrogen balance during wasting diseases or starvation or more gradually in the aging process. Catabolism is constantly going on in a balancing relationship with anabolism to maintain tissue in a dynamic state.

■ **Why does carbohydrate have a protein-sparing effect?**

During a fasting period glycogen stores from carbohydrate metabolism are rapidly depleted. Fat stores in adipose tissue are then reduced more slowly. Only as the fat stores are depleted does the body, in its attempt to maintain itself, begin to break down tissue protein. For this reason a diet that contains a sufficient amount of carbohydrate calories to supply day-to-day energy demands has a protein-sparing effect in that it supplies energy needs so that protein will not be diverted for this purpose. A healthy diet, therefore, should have a balanced quantity of both protein and energy materials from carbohydrate and fat.

■ **What hormones influence protein metabolism?**

The anabolism and catabolism of protein is regulated by certain hormones. Those hormones having an anabolic, or tissue-building, effect are pituitary growth hormone (GH), androgens (gonadotrophins), insulin, and normal amounts of thyroid hormone. Hormones that have a catabolic, or tissue breaking-down, effect are adrenal steroids, such as glucocorticoids (cortisone and hydrocortisone), and large amounts of thyroid hormone.

A summary of the metabolic interrelationships among protein, carbohydrate, and fat is given in Fig. 4-5 for review and reference.

■ **How are individual protein requirements determined?**

A number of individual factors must be considered in determining a person's individual protein requirements. These include age, physical health status, specific requirements for essential amino acids, nature of

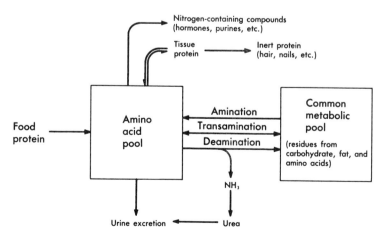

Fig. 4-4. Interrelationships between the amino acid pool and the common metabolic pool of residues from carbohydrates, fats, and amino acids.

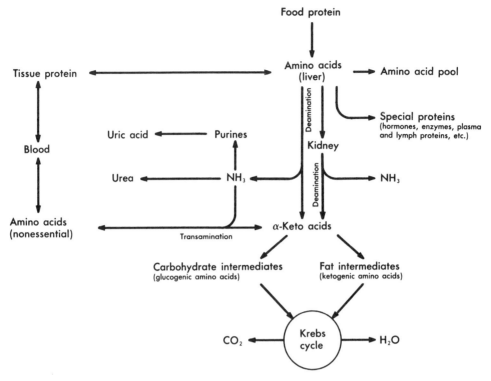

Fig. 4-5. Metabolic interrelationships between protein, carbohydrate, and fat.

the total diet (amount of carbohydrate and fat present), timing of meals, presence of tissue injury, disease, fever, surgery.

■ **What are the "recommended allowances" for protein?**

Two basic measures of protein requirement must be considered: quantity and quality. Protein quantity establishes the total protein requirement. The United States standard is generally set for adults at 0.9 gm. per kg. of body weight. This amounts to about 65 gm. (slightly more than 2 ounces) daily for a person weighing 70 kg. (143 pounds). A total of 65 to 75 gm. daily or more are needed during pregnancy and lactation. The requirements for infants and children vary according to growth patterns. This amount of protein recommendation in U. S. standards is based on the philosophy of allowing an excess margin for safety to cover a wide number of individuals and situations. It is usually set at approximately twice the minimum requirements.

It is evident, however, that total quan-

tity of protein alone is not a sufficient standard of reference. Since the value of protein is dependent on its content of essential amino acids, in the final analysis the measure of protein requirement must be based on *quality*, that is, on the essential amino acid content. Guides for this purpose are based on the ideal amino acid proportionality pattern of individual need.

■ **What is the "amino acid proportionality pattern"?**

This provisional amino acid pattern is a widely used guideline outlined by the Food and Agriculture organization, a division of the World Health Organization of the United Nations. This pattern is constructed according to the formula shown in Table 4-2.

The amino acid that is required by the body in the smallest quantity is tryptophan. Tryptophan is therefore assigned the value of 1.0. Values for the other essential amino acids express the ratio between the body's tryptophan requirement and its need for the other amino acids. On the basis of the

Table 4-2. Food and Agriculture Organization* amino acid proportionality pattern for the adult based on essential amino acid requirements

Amino acid	Requirement (mg.)	Proportionality pattern	Pattern simplified in common use†
Tryptophan	250	1.0	1.0
Threonine	500	2.0	2.0
Isoleucine	700	2.8	3.0
Lysine	800	3.2	3.0
Valine	900	3.6	3.0
Total sulfur amino acid	950	3.8	3.0
(Methionine minimum)	(325)	(1.3)	
Leucine	1050	4.2	3.4
Total aromatic amino acid	1550	6.2	
(Phenylalanine minimum)	(325)	(1.3)	2.0

*Food and Agriculture Organization, Protein requirements, FAO Nutritional Studies, No. 16, Rome, 1957 (adapted).
†Leverton, R. M.: Amino acids. In Stefferud, A., editor: Food, the yearbook of agriculture, 1959, Washington, D. C., 1959, U. S. Department of Agriculture.

provisional amino acid pattern thus determined, an ideal *proportionality pattern* of amino acid is constructed, against which the amino acid ratios in different foods may be measured. According to this method of study, egg and milk rank highest as reference proteins against which to measure other foods.

Protein quality in terms of essential amino acid content is of great practical significance in world health problems. In countries in which the diet is limited to a few foods and protein is available in only one main plant source, the protein intake could be made adequate by introducing other complementary plant proteins to make up the lacking amino acids.

■ **What is the National Research Council and how does it set recommended dietary allowances?**

The National Research Council is a section of the National Academy of Sciences. This is a private organization in the United States established for the study of nutrition and nutrient needs of the United States population. It is supported in part by grants from the National Institute of Health of the United States Public Health Service and from private donations. It is located in Washington, D. C.

Since 1940 the Food and Nutrition Board has developed formulations of daily nutrient intakes that were judged to be adequate for the maintenance of good nutrition in the population of the United States. These formulations are designated as "Recommended Dietary Allowances" (RDA). It must be remembered, however, that although these recommendations are based on existing knowledge of nutritional science and are constantly subject to revision as new knowledge becomes available, they are nonetheless value judgments. They are intended to serve only as recommendations designed to cover a wide range of need, and in order to provide a margin of safety to cover stress situations they are approximately double the minimum allowances. They are not absolute and rigid requirements but *flexible recommendations.* As such they should be used to serve only as rough guides and should be adapted as needed to the individual's need. Individuals whose diets do not meet the RDA are not necessarily suffering from malnutrition, and diets should not be judged as "poor" on an arbitrary figure based on comparison with the RDA. These standards are revised about every 5 years in order to include new research findings.

5 Energy metabolism

The human energy system is part of a far larger universal energy system that sustains life on this planet. The ultimate source of power in this larger system is the sun, with its vast reservoir of nuclear reactions. The study of nutrition is concerned with the basic question of how the human body transforms the elements of its food into energy. Energy is the basis of ongoing life. It is the power of an organism to do its work. Hence fundamental laws of physical existence ultimately must revolve around the production of energy.

The word energy comes from two Greek roots that together mean "work." The Greeks put these two roots together to form their word *energon,* meaning "active." Hence energy is that force or power that enables the body to carry on life-sustaining activities. The word *metabolism* also comes from two roots, *meta* meaning "beyond" and *ballein* meaning "to throw." The Greeks put these two roots together to form the noun *metabolé,* meaning "change." Thus metabolism is the total of all those chemical processes in the body by which substances initially in food are "thrown beyond themselves" to be changed over and over again into other substances. This very phrase gives the feel of the power involved in the processes that nurture and sustain life. *Energy metabolism* deals with the very real and dynamic concept underlying all of life —change. It is these constant, multiple changes in the forms of physiologic constituents that produce energy.

■ **How is energy measured?**

Energy is measured commonly by the unit of heat measure known as the *calorie.* In nutritional and physiologic studies the unit of measure is the large calorie, or kilocalorie, which is equal to 1,000 small calories. A kilocalorie is the amount of heat required to raise 1 kg. of water 1° C.

■ **How are the calorie values of various foods determined?**

The calorie value of various foods has been determined by the use of a metal instrument that is called a bomb calorimeter because its shape resembles that of a bomb. A weighed amount of food is placed into the core of the calorimeter, and the instrument is immersed in a large container of water. The food is then ignited by an electric spark in the presence of oxygen and burned. The resulting increase in temperature of the surrounding water indicates the number of calories given off by the oxidation of the food.

■ **What are the calorie values of the three major nutrients—carbohydrate, fat, and protein?**

The average calorie value of each of the three major nutrients is known as its respective *fuel factor.* One gram of carbohydrate yields four calories, 1 gm. of fat yields 9 calories, and 1 gm. of protein yields 4 calories.

■ **What is a joule?**

The joule is the unit of heat measure in the metric system. It was named for an English physicist, James Prescott Joule (1818 to 1889). He is credited with discovering the first law of thermodynamics, which states that energy is neither created nor destroyed. The majority of the world nations use the metric system in scientific and community life. Since the United States is beginning a transition period of converting to the metric system, it is important that students in the sciences begin to make these conversions in their own calculations and practices.

The conversion factor necessary to convert calories to joules in the metric system is the following: 1 calorie equals 4.184 joules. Thus in the metric system the fuel factors for the three major nutrients would be: 1 gm. of carbohydrate yields 17 joules, 1 gm. of fat yields 38 joules, and 1 gm. of protein yields 17 joules. This comparison is in reference to the large calorie and large joule, or kilocalorie and kilojoule.

■ **If energy, like matter, in our universal system can neither be created nor destroyed, how is energy in the human energy system cycled and transformed?**

It is clear that energy is not created. It exists in many forms and is constantly being transformed. In the human body energy is available in four basic forms for life

processes: chemical, electrical, mechanical, and thermal. It is constantly being cycled through these forms.

In this perpetual cycle of energy the ultimate source of power is the sun. Through the process of photosynthesis, with water and carbon dioxide as raw materials, plants transform the sun's energy into food storage forms. In the body these food sources are converted into the basic energy unit of glucose, which is burned to release energy. Water and carbon dioxide are the end products of this process of oxidation.

■ **What are the "transformers" in the body that change energy from one form to another?**

Metabolism is the sum total of all of the chemical processes that convert chemical energy to other forms of energy for the body's work. Hence the "transformers" in the human energy system are the metabolic

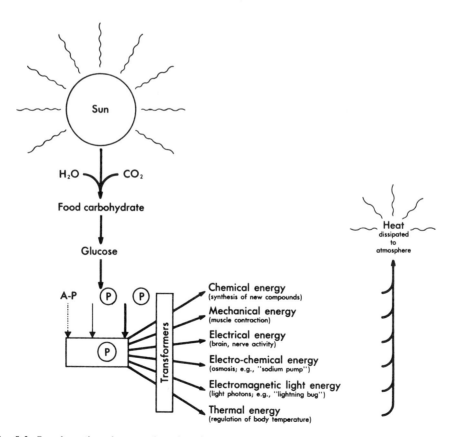

Fig. 5-1. Transformation of energy from its primary source (the sun) to various forms for biologic work by means of metabolic processes ("transformers").

processes involved in making change. The chemical energy is changed to electrical energy, as in brain and nerve activity; to mechanical energy, as in muscle contraction; to thermal energy, as in regulation of of body temperature; and to other types of chemical energy, as in the synthesis of new compounds. In all these work activities of the body, heat is given off. This cycling and transformation of energy is shown in the diagram in Fig. 5-1.

■ **What are "free" and "potential" energy?**

In human metabolism, as in any energy system, energy is always present as either free or potential energy. Free energy is the energy involved in any given moment in the performance of a task. It is doing work. It is unbound and in motion. Potential energy is the energy that is stored, or bound, in various chemical compounds and is available for conversion to free energy as needed. For example, energy stored in the sugar molecule is potential energy. When it is burned, free energy is released and work results. As the work is done, energy in the form of heat is given off.

Whether the energy system is electrical, mechanical, thermal, or chemical, in the course of the many reactions that comprise its operation free energy is decreased and the reservoir of potential energy is secondarily diminished. Therefore the system must constantly be refueled from some outside source. In the human energy system this source is food.

■ **How is the human energy system controlled?**

Without control, energy in any system would be destructive or unproductive. The mechanism by which energy is controlled in the human system is *chemical bonding.* The chemical bonds that hold the elements of the compounds together consist of energy. As long as that compound remains constant, energy is being exerted to maintain the atomic constellation that is characteristic for that molecule. It is in this sense that potential energy is stored in the compound. When the compound is broken into its parts, energy is released and becomes free energy. It is characteristic of free energy that it immediately involves itself in the bonding of other atoms, which then results either in a rearrangement of the atoms within the same compound or in the formation of new compounds. Three types of chemical bonds transfer energy in the body:

1. *Covalent bonds.* Covalence refers to the chemical combining power of an element. A common example of covalent bonds are those shared between neighbor carbon atoms in the core of an organic compound. Since carbon has a valence of 4, it may attach other radicals at four positions on its atom.

2. *Hydrogen bonds.* Hydrogen bonds are weaker bonds, which attach hydrogen to various compounds. They are less rich in energy than covalent bonds, but the very fact that they can be broken easily gives them physiologic importance. They can be moved around easily and thus alter molecular shapes, as in protein molecules; and they can be transferred or passed readily from one substance to another, thus forming new substances.

3. *High-energy phosphate bonds.* Phosphate (PO_4) bonds are the bonds that attach the phosphate radical to a compound. They play an important role in energy metabolism. Since the phosphate radical is highly labile, more energy is required to bind it than to bind carbon or most other radicals and hence more free energy is released when the phosphate bond is broken. Many phosphate bonds are referred to as high-energy bonds. The sign $\sim$ is used to indicate these bonds. An example of such a high-energy compound is ATP: $A - PO_4 \sim PO_4 \sim PO_4$.

■ **What is ATP?**

ATP is the chemical compound *adenosine triphosphate.* It has been called "the currency of the cell," which may be "cashed in" by the body for energy as needed to perform its work. Like storage batteries, these PO_4 bonds become the controlling force of any further energy needs. In a sense, then, the compound ATP is the means that the body has devised for trapping, storing, and releasing energy as it is needed in our basic biochemical energy system.

■ **How do enzymes control chemical reaction?**

In order to speed up reactions that would take years to produce energy, or to regulate and slow down reactions that would produce energy in a single explosion, control agents are necessary. These control agents are enzymes and their partners, the coenzyme factors. They control biologic oxidation of the cells. Hormones also play a regulatory role in this overall process.

All enzymes that have been isolated thus far are protein substances. They are produced in the cells, apparently under the control of specific genes. One specific gene controls the making of one specific enzyme, and there are thousands of enzymes in each cell.

The substance on which a particular enzyme works in a catalytic manner is called its *substrate*. Enzymes possess a remarkable and highly significant degree of specificity for their special substrates; that is, a particular enzyme will act only on its own particular substrate. Like the interlocking pieces of a jigsaw puzzle, the specific shapes, or molecular shapes, of enzyme and substrate must fit together perfectly or the reaction will not take place. In this vital lock and key mode of action the enzyme,

coenzyme, and substrate first combine in a complex, exert pressure on one another, then break apart and produce new reaction products and the original unchanged enzymes. While the substrate is locked in place with the enzyme, the enzyme places specific stress on it to break certain bonds and rearrange certain molecules. When the unlocking occurs, different reaction products are released and the enzyme breaks away unchanged, ready to perform its remarkable feat over and over again. This action is graphically shown in Fig. 5-2.

■ **What are coenzymes?**

The completion of reactions such as those involved in cellular oxidation to yield energy requires coenzymes. These are partners in the reaction necessary for it to take place. In many instances these coenzyme factors involve other nutrients, such as vitamins and minerals. For example, three such enzyme systems in cellular oxidation use vitamins or minerals as cofactor coenzymes: the dehydrogenases, with niacin as part of the coenzyme (NAD, NADP); the flavoprotein system, containing riboflavin coenzymes; the cytochrome system (a "cousin" of hemoglobin), containing iron.

An example of a dehydrogenase of clinical significance is *lactic dehydrogenase* (LDH). This enzyme catalyzes the change of lactic acid to pyruvic acid in muscle. When heart muscle is damaged, as in a myocardial infarction, the enzyme is released from the cells and accumulates in

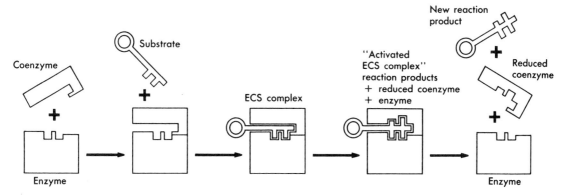

Fig. 5-2. Lock-and-key concept of the action of enzyme, coenzyme, and substrate to produce new reaction products.

the blood. Hence, a rise in the blood level of this enzyme is used as a diagnostic measure.

■ **How does cellular oxidation take place to produce the potential energy compound ATP?**

In respiratory chains for oxidation in the cells oxygen was originally thought to enter into the process and take part in the reactions. Hence the term oxidation has been used. It is now known, however, that energy is generated by a system of hydrogen ion transfer from product to product, with formation of high energy phosphate compounds of ATP along the way. The coenzymes act in this system as a series of accepters of the "bouncing hydrogen ion" until hydrogen finally combines with oxygen to form water (see Fig. 2-2, p. 13). The enzyme system that operates the respiratory chains is located in the mitochondria adjacent to those enzymes operating in the Krebs cycle. Hence the two systems operate together and complement one another.

■ **What role do hormones play in controlling energy metabolism?**

Hormones are secretions of the endocrine glands, and they perform many regulatory functions in the body. The word "hormone" comes from the Greek word *hormaein* meaning "to set in motion" or "to spur on." In energy metabolism hormones act as chemical messengers to trigger or control enzyme action. For example, the rate of oxidative reactions in the tissues (the body's metabolic rate) is controlled by thyroxine from the thyroid gland, which in turn is controlled by thyrotropic hormone from the anterior pituitary gland. Another familiar example is the controlling action of insulin from the pancreas on the rate of glucose utilization in the tissues. Steroid hormones also have the capacity to regulate the cell's ability to synthesize enzymes.

■ **What is energy balance?**

The concept of balance may also be applied to the body's energy system. The input of energy into the system is represented by the food or fuel one consumes. The output from the system is represented by the energy demands placed on the body. These energy demands are of two kinds: (1) basal energy demands, and (2) physical activity demands.

■ **What is the basal metabolic rate (BMR) of an individual?**

Basal metabolism is a measure of the energy produced in the maintenance of the body at rest after a 12 hour fast. The basal metabolic rate (BMR) is the rate of internal chemical activity of resting tissue.

Certain small but vitally active tissues—brain, liver, gastrointestinal tract, heart, kidney—together make up less than 5% of the total body weight, yet they contribute about 60% of the total basal metabolic processes. On the other hand, although resting muscle and adipose fat tissue are far larger in mass, they contribute much less to the body's BMR.

■ **How is the BMR measured?**

For clinical purposes, indirect calorimetry is used. This method measures the exchange of gases in respiration while the subject is at rest. Usually the calories are computed according to an average of the amount of oxygen consumed during two 6-minute periods. The metabolic rates are based, then, on the *respiratory quotient*. This is the ratio between the volume of carbon dioxide given off and the volume of oxygen consumed:

$$\frac{\text{Volume of CO}_2 \text{ produced}}{\text{Volume of O}_2 \text{ consumed}} = \text{RQ}$$

Energy calculated in this manner is equivalent to the heat given off by the body. The BMR is calculated for a given person in terms of the number of calories given off per hour per square meter of body surface area, with corrections for age, sex, height, and weight. The results are then expressed in percent of variation above or below the normal number of calories per square meter of body surface area for a person of like height, weight, age, and sex. The ranges usually given as normal are −10% to +10%, which includes about 75% of normal people, and −15% to +15%, which includes about 95% of normal people.

■ **What general factors influence one's BMR?**

Factors that increase the BMR include those that stimulate metabolic activity. For example, growth, pregnancy, lactation, sex (men tend to have higher rates because they have a larger body mass), climate (colder climates stimulate BMR to help regulate body temperature), and thyroxin from the thyroid gland.

Factors that tend to depress or decrease the BMR are situations in which overall metabolism is decreased. These situations include malnutrition and starvation. Obesity seems to have little effect on the BMR, although it may lower the rate somewhat.

■ **How does fever affect the BMR?**

Fever increases the BMR about 7% for each 1° F. rise in temperature. It is evident, therefore, that sufficient calories and especially protein must be included in the diet during such periods to counteract the catabolic effect of the fever.

■ **What additional factors affect one's total energy requirement?**

Other influences on total calorie requirements include physical activity, such as muscular work in general activities or exercise; emotional state (increased muscle tension, restlessness, and agitation of movement); diet (food intake increases the expenditure of calories for digestion and absorption). Protein especially has a high *specific dynamic action*, because it requires more metabolic work for handling. Mental effort, as in studying, demands few if any calories. Feelings of fatigue following periods of study, for example, are not caused by vast cerebral activity but by various amounts of muscle tension involved.

An individual's total daily energy requirement, therefore, is the number of calories necessary to replace daily basal metabolic loss, plus loss from exercise and other physical activities. These general calorie needs for various ages are indicated in the 1968 revisions of recommendations by the National Research Council. These recommendations are listed in the table in Appendix E.

6 Vitamins

Over the past six decades the discoveries of the vitamins have formed a fascinating chapter in nutrition history. The name vitamin was first applied in 1911 by Casimir Funk, a Polish chemist working at the Lister Institute in London. He discovered a nitrogen-containing material that he thought was an amine. Because it was apparently vital to life he called it *vitamine* ("vital-amine"). The final "e" was dropped later when other similarly vital substances turned out to be a variety of organic compounds. The name "vitamin" has been retained to designate compounds of this class.

Probably no other group of nutritional elements has so captured interest and stimulated concern among biochemists, members of the health professions, and the general public as has the vitamin group. New questions are currently being raised. One by one the list of vitamins has grown over the years. Two characteristics mark a compound for assignment to the vitamin group: (1) it must be a vital organic dietary substance that is neither a carbohydrate, fat, mineral, nor protein but is necessary in very small quantities for the performance of particular metabolic functions or for the prevention of an associated deficiency disease; and (2) it cannot be manufactured by the body and therefore must be supplied in food. Usually this amount required of a vitamin is a very small amount.

Vitamins are usually grouped according to solubility. Although this distinction is sometimes an arbitrary one, it is still used for want of a better basis. The fat-soluble group includes vitamins A, D, E, and K. The water-soluble group includes vitamins C and the B-complex vitamins.

FAT-SOLUBLE VITAMINS
Vitamin A (retinol)

■ **What is the nature of vitamin A?**

Chemically, vitamin A is a primary alcohol of high molecular weight ($CO_{20}H_{29}OH$). Because it has a specific function in the retina of the eye and because it is an alcohol, it has been given the name *retinol*. However, it is still commonly referred to by its letter name.

In its natural form vitamin A is found only in animal sources and is usually associated with lipids because it is fat soluble. As an ester with fatty acids, it is deposited in such tissues as kidney, lung, fat depots, and especially the liver.

■ **What is provitamin A?**

The ultimate source of all vitamin A is plants. The preformed sources in our diet have been produced in animals, which we then consume as food. The precursor of vitamin A—*provitamin A*—is a substance called carotene ($C_{40}H_{56}$), a pigment found in certain plants. Its name comes from the color of the pigment in which it was first discovered, a yellow pigment of carrots. Carotene occurs as crystals in plant cells. It is found in deep yellow and green plants.

■ **How is vitamin A absorbed?**

Vitamin A enters the body in two forms: as the preformed vitamin from animal sources and as the provitamin carotene. Three substances aid in the absorption of vitamin A and carotene by the body:

1. Bile salts. Vitamin A oxidizes readily and hence is easily destroyed upon contact with oxygen. Therefore the natural antioxidant effect of bile salts helps to stabilize the vitamin. Bile also aids in the absorption of vitamin A, as it does with other fat-related substances, since it serves as a vehicle of transport through the intestinal wall. Clinical conditions affecting the biliary system, such as obstruction of the bile ducts, infectious hepatits, and cirrhosis of the liver, hinder vitamin A absorption. This is caused more by the rapid oxidation of the unprotected vitamin than by any primary defect in the absorptive process itself.

2. *Pancreatic lipase.* The fat-splitting enzyme lipase is necessary for initial hydrolysis of vitamin A in the upper intestinal tract. This applies to oil solutions of the vitamin. However, if the vitamin is administered in an aqueous dispersion form, this enzyme is not required for its absorption. Therefore, in conditions in which secretions of pancreatic lipase are curtailed, such as in cystic fibrosis, the aqueous dispersion form is preferred.

3. *Fat.* The presence of some fat in the intestine, simultaneously absorbed, is apparently required for effective absorption of vitamin A. This seems to be more true of carotene than of preformed vitamin A.

After absorption, vitamin A and carotene are carried through the same route as fat. They enter the lymphatic system and are carried through the thoracic duct into the portal vein and then to the liver for storage and distribution. The liver is by far the most effective storage organ. It contains about 90% of the total vitamin A in the body. This amount is sufficient to supply the body's needs for 3 to 12 months. Liver stores, as well as plasma levels, are reduced, however, during periods of infectious disease, such as pneumonia and rheumatic fever. At such times supplements of vitamin A may be indicated. Vitamin E may be given with the supplement to help prevent rapid oxidation of vitamin A.

■ **What factors affect absorption and storage of vitamin A?**

Vitamin A absorption and utilization is diminished in intestinal diseases, such as celiac disease, sprue, and colitis, which cause changes in the absorptive surface tissue of the mucosa. Age is also a factor in vitamin A absorption. In the newborn infant, especially the premature infant, absorption is poor. With advancing age the elderly person may experience increasing difficulties with absorption also.

■ **What is the effect of mineral oil on vitamin A?**

A warning must be given about the nonfood fat, mineral oil. This oil is not digested by the body but goes through the gastrointestinal tract intact. If it is present in the intestine along with fat-soluble vitamins, such as A or carotene, it absorbs them and carries them out also. Therefore mineral oil should never be used with meals, nor should it be taken immediately before or after eating. The practice of making mineral oil salad dressings, therefore, should be avoided.

■ **What physiologic function does vitamin A serve in promoting vision?**

The ability of the eye to adapt to changes in light is dependent on the presence of a light-sensitive pigment, *rhodopsin* (commonly known as visual purple), in the rods of the retina. Rhodopsin is a conjugated protein made up of *opsin,* the protein part, and *retinene,* the nonprotein part. It is this latter nonprotein part of the pigment that is a vitamin A compound. When light hits the retina, rhodopsin is split into its two parts, opsin and retinene. In the dark the two components recombine to form visual purple again. Normally there is more than enough vitamin A in the pigment layer behind the rods and cones to ensure constant adjustments to variances in light. When the body is deficient in vitamin A, however, less retinene is available for formation of visual purple. The rods and cones become increasingly sensitive to light changes, which finally causes night blindness. This condition can usually be cured in a half hour or so by an injection of vitamin A, which is readily converted into retinene and then into visual purple.

■ **How does vitamin A relate to the health of epithelial tissue?**

Vitamin A has a vital role in the formation and maintenance of healthy, functioning epithelial tissue, which forms the body's primary barrier to infection. The epithelium includes not only the outer skin of the body but also the mucous membranes lining the ocular and oral cavities and the gastrointestinal, respiratory, and genitourinary tracts.

Without vitamin A the epithelial cells become dry and flat and gradually harden to form scales that slough off. This process is called *keratinization*. Keratin is a protein that forms dry, scalelike tissue, such as nails and hair. When the body is deficient in vitamin A many epithelial tissues may undergo keratinization:

1. *Eye.* The cornea dries and hardens. This condition, called *xerophthalmia*, may progress to blindness in extreme deficiency of vitamin A. The tear ducts dry, which robs the eye of its cleansing and lubricating means, and infection follows easily.

2. *Respiratory tract.* Ciliated epithelium in the nasal passages dries, and the cilia are lost. A barrier to entry of infection is therefore removed. The salivary glands dry and the mouth becomes dry and cracked, open to invading organisms.

3. *Gastrointestinal tract.* The secretory function of mucous membranes is diminished, so that tissue sloughs off, which affects digestion and absorption.

4. *Genitourinary tract.* Epithelial tissue breaks down, creating problems, such as urinary tract infections, renal calculi, and vaginal infections.

5. *Skin.* The skin becomes dry and scaly, and small pustules or a hardened, pigmented papular eruption may appear around the hair follicles. This condition resulting from vitamin A deficiency is called *follicular hyperkeratosis.*

■ **What relation does vitamin A have to tooth formation?**

Certain epithelial cells surounding tooth buds and fetal gum tissue become specialized cup-shaped organs (*ameloblasts*) for forming the enamel structure of the developing tooth. Each cell carries out the fascinating task of producing and depositing minute prisms of enamel substances that eventually form the erupted tooth. Inadequate vitamin A produces faulty enamel-forming epithelial cells, which impairs the soundness of the tooth structure. It is evident, therefore, that a woman's diet during pregnancy should have increased amounts of vitamin A to ensure this formation of tooth buds in the developing fetus.

■ **How is vitamin A related to growth?**

A number of observations have been made relating vitamin A deficiency to retarded growth, but the mechanism is unknown. It is almost unbelievable that we still do not fully understand the metabolic role of vitamin A outside of the clearly defined role in the visual cycle. Perhaps this is because in man nutritional deficiency usually involves multiple factors that make it difficult to isolate specific nutrient influences. Apparently, however, vitamin A contributes in some essential way to the growth of skeletal and soft tissue, perhaps through an effect upon protein synthesis, mitosis, or stability of cell membranes. Currently the search for the metabolic function of vitamin A outside the visual cycle has centered on its possible role in ensuring the normal structure and function of biologic membranes.

Frequently vitamin A deficiency is associated with protein malnutrition, kwashiorkor, or marasmus. For example, in India, Indonesia, and the Middle East a large percentage (30% to 50%) of patients with kwashiorkor or marasmus also suffer from vitamin A deficiency. The intake of protein, a high protein supplement, in therapy for treating kwashiorkor or marasmus apparently mobilizes the last reserves of vitamin A from the liver and thus precipitates the vitamin A deficiency. Therefore when feeding a high-grade protein to children to prevent or treat kwashiorkor, a supplement of vitamin A should also be given. It is very important to supplement skim milk with vitamin A because increased protein intake causes increased vitamin A requirements.

■ **How much vitamin A do we need?**

A number of variables influence one's requirements for vitamin A: the amount stored in the liver, the form in which it is taken (as carotene or as vitamin A), the medium in which taken (oil or aqueous dispersion), illness, and gastrointestinal defect. Thus, to cover such variables, the National Research Council's recommendations allow a margin of safety above minimal needs. The recommendation is set for adults at 5,000 International Units (I.U.) daily, with a daily addition of 1,000 I.U. for women during pregnancy and an additional 3,000 units during lactation. The need of infants during the first year is approximately 1,500 I.U., increasing gradually through the growth years, to reach the 5,000 unit requirement by age 18.

■ **Is it possible to get too much vitamin A?**

Yes. There are several reports in the literature of acute *hypervitaminosis A* in infants caused by single massive doses of vitamin A, usually given mistakenly by mothers who give a vitamin A concentrate (dosage prescribed in drops) in amounts required for liver oil forms (dosage prescribed in teaspoons). Acute vitamin A toxicity was first recognized in Arctic explorers who ingested large quantities of polar bear liver in which great amounts of vitamin A were stored.

The main manifestations of vitamin A toxicity are transient hydrocephalus and vomiting. There may also be joint pain, thickening of long bones, loss of hair, and jaundice. Thus, it is well to remember that vitamins are substances that are required in *small* amounts. These small amounts are vital, but too much of some vitamins can be dangerous.

■ **What are some good food sources of vitamin A?**

Food sources of preformed vitamin A are animal sources. These include liver, kidney, cream, butter, and egg yolk. The major dietary source, however, is carotene or provitamin A, which is found in yellow and green vegetables and fruits, such as carrots, sweet potatoes, squash, apricots, spinach, collards, broccoli, cabbage, and other dark leafy greens. A number of commercial products may be fortified with vitamin A. Margarine, for example, is forti-

fied with 15,000 I.U. of vitamin A per pound.

Vitamin D (calciferol, viosterol)

■ **What is the nature of vitamin D?**

Vitamin D is a group of sterols varying in potency. The two D vitamins most important in nutrition are D_2 and D_3. D_2 is formed by irradiating the provitamin D_2 (ergosterol), found in ergot and in yeast. The irradiated product is known as calciferol or viosterol. Vitamin D_3 occurs in fish liver oils (and also in human skin). Provitamin D_3 (7-dehydrocholesterol) is converted to the active form by sunlight.

Vitamin D is unique among the vitamins in two respects. It occurs naturally in only a few common foods, mainly in fish oils; and it can be formed in the body by exposure of the skin to ultraviolet rays either from the sun or from a lamp.

■ **How is vitamin D absorbed?**

Vitamin D is absorbed, along with calcium and phosphorus, in the small intestine. Since it is fat soluble, this absorption requires the presence of bile salts, as for other fats and fat-related products. As with vitamin A, diseases such as celiac syndrome, sprue, and colitis hinder its absorption.

After being ingested or produced on or in the skin in the presence of sunlight, vitamin D is absorbed and carried to the liver and other organs for use. A relatively small amount is stored in the liver, compared with the liver's much larger capacity for vitamin A storage. Vitamin D is excreted from the circulative blood by way of the bile.

■ **How does vitamin D work with calcium and phosphorus to build bone tissue?**

Vitamin D in the body is predominantly associated with calcium and phosphorus in the building of bone. It does this vital task in two ways:

1. *Absorption of calcium and phosphorus.* The primary action of vitamin D is to facilitate the absorption of calcium from the small intestine. This absorption apparently takes place by active transport

in the proximal segment of the small intestine and throughout the remainder of the intestine by passive diffusion. Phosphorus absorption follows that of calcium. Vitamin D probably is responsible for the more rapid absorption of calcium by making the cell membrane more permeable to calcium.

2. *Calcification.* After the absorption of calcium and phosphorus through the intestinal wall, vitamin D continues to work in partnership with calcium and phosphorus in the calcification aspect of bone formation. Vitamin D directly increases the rate of mineral accretion and resorption in bone by which the tissue is built and maintained.

■ **Does vitamin D have any effect on renal phosphate clearance?**

Yes. When the body is deficient in vitamin D, as in rickets, the renal threshold for phosphate excretion is lowered and the kidney excretes more phosphate than usual. Therapeutic doses of vitamin D raise the renal threshold by causing more tubular reabsorption, which conserves the plasma phosphate level.

This renal mechanism gives another interesting example of the bodys' tenacious effort to adapt to the presence of disease and to maintain the integrity of the blood even at the expense of the tissue. The initial problem in rickets is lack of calcium caused by an absence of vitamin D to facilitate its absorption. In order to preserve the vital balance between calcium and phosphorus in the blood, the kidney then lowers its threshold point for phosphate and excretes more of it. If this adjustment were not made, the vital ratio of calcium to phosphorus would not be corrected and tetany would resutlt.

■ **How much vitamin D do we need?**

Individual needs for vitamin D vary widely, depending on the food sources available and the degree to which the body is able to produce vitamin D in response to irradiation. Thus, one's way of living determines the degree of exposure to sunlight and would therefore influence one's individual need for additional vitamin D. For example, a city dweller living in a high-rise apartment or in a tenement and working indoors would need more vitamin D than a farmer who worked out of doors all day. Elderly people or invalids who do not go out of doors have a need for supplementary vitamin D. Also, growth demands in childhood and in pregnancy and lactation necessitate increased intake.

The National Research Council recommends 400 I.U. daily for children and for women during pregnancy and lactation. They make no statement concerning adult need, which indicates that in most instances general exposure to sunlight in adulthood is sufficient.

■ **Is it possible to get too much vitamin D?**

Yes. As with vitamin A, *hypervitaminosis D* is possible. This is a special danger in infants' eating practices where fortified milk, fortified cereal, plus variable vitamin supplements are used. The infant needs only 400 I.U. daily, whereas the amount in all of the above items could easily total 4,000 I.U. or more. Since vitamin D is now commonly added to many infant foods, it seems wise to reconsider the need for supplementation with vitamin D preparations.

Symptoms of vitamin D toxicity include calcification of soft tissue, such as lungs and kidney, and bone fragility. Renal tissue is particularly prone to calcify, thus affecting glomerular filtration and overall function.

■ **What are some good food sources of vitamin D?**

Unlike the other vitamins, there are few natural food sources of vitamin D. The two basic vitamins, D_2 and D_3, occur only in yeast and fish liver oils. Thus the main food sources are those to which crystalline vitamin D has been added or in which vitamin D has been produced by irradiation. Milk, because it is so commonly used, has proved to be the most practical carrier, and it is now a widespread commercial practice to standardize the added vitamin content at 400 I.U. per quart. Milk is also a good companion for the vitamin because it provides natural sources of calcium and phosphorus. Butter substitutes, such as margarines, are also fortified with vitamin D.

Vitamin E (tocopherol)

■ **What is the nature of vitamin E?**

Vitamin E is an alcohol and was discovered in animal research concerning reproductive processes. Hence it was named *tocopherol* from the Greek *tokos* meaning "childbirth" and *phero* meaning "to bring," with the suffix *ol* denoting its chemical nature as an alcohol. Since this discovery, tocopherol has come to be known as the antisterility vitamin. However, this function has been demonstrated only in the rat and not in man. A number of related compounds have since been discovered, and it is known that vitamin E is in reality a group of vitamins. Of these α-tocopherol is the most significant. Vitamin E is a stable material that is insoluble in water and that oxidizes very slowly. This antioxidant characteristic gives it one of its most important chemical functions?

■ **How is vitamin E absorbed?**

Since vitamin E is a fat-soluble vitamin, it requires bile salts and the presence of fats for optimum absorption to take place. Storage occurs in different body tissues, but particularly in adipose tissue.

■ **During pregnancy is there any maternal transfer of vitamin E to the infant?**

Apparently the amount of vitamin E that crosses the placenta is limited to immediate fetal needs. However, the amount transferred to the infant through mother's milk is apparently greater than that transferred through regular feeding of a formula of cow's milk. Vitamin E levels in breast-fed infants rise more rapidly than in bottle-fed infants. Vitamin E values in human colostrum and in human milk range about twice the value found in cow's milk formula in its regular dilution for infant feeding.

■ **What are the physiologic functions of vitamin E?**

Knowledge concerning the functions of vitamin E thus far has largely been learned through experiments and research with laboratory animals and animals important to commerce and industry. Some of these functions include:

1. *Reproduction.* Classic studies have established the role of vitamin E in the reproductive function of the rat. In the female rat a deficiency of vitamin E causes poor placental implantation with consequent fetal resorption. In the male rat a deficiency of vitamin E causes testicular degeneration, with atrophy of spermatogenic tissue and consequent permanent sterility.

2. *Muscle integrity.* Vitamin E also serves as a structural element in the building and functioning of smooth muscles, skeletal muscle, cardiac muscle, and vascular tissue. Muscles that are affected display various stages and forms of degeneration, such as pallor, fragmentation of fibers, edema, nuclear breakdown, necrosis, calcification, fibrosis, and pigmentation. In some animals cardiac muscle fibrosis leads to failure and death.

3. *Liver integrity.* Massive liver necrosis in rats was made worse by vitamin E deficiency and was improved by vitamin E treatment. The condition was induced by a low-protein diet that was especially low in cystine, an amino acid that contains sulfur. In these studies, if the diet was supplemented with cystine, vitamin E, and a newly discovered "factor 3" (a selenium compound), liver necrosis was prevented; if it had already occurred it was reversed. Just what the mechanism of this function is, is not understood.

4. *Red blood cell integrity.* The strong antioxidant nature of vitamin E gives it a value in protecting red blood cells against hemolysis. Vitamin E may preserve the integrity of the erythrocyte by inhibiting the action of the oxidase in hemoglobin on the unsaturated fatty acids of the cell membrane. In this manner it may protect cellular unsaturated lipids from oxidative breakdown. Polyunsaturated lipids, together with proteins and carbohydrates, constitute the principal structural components of living

cells. Hence these polyunsaturated lipids supply the food from which most of the membraneous structures of the cells are built. These lipids are also particularly useful in forming the endoplasmic reticulum in the cell, those rod-shaped structures that float about in the cell, and the mitochondria, which are the principal energy sources in the cell. Therefore these fatty acids are needed in relatively large amounts for cell structure. They make up about 17% of the total lipids in the American diet.

The aging of our bodies appears to be influenced by radiation bombardment that occurs during our lifetime. This radiation causes gradual deterioration in the cell by penetrating throughout the body and entering every cell, striking the polyunsaturated lipids present as a structural component. If enough vitamin E is not present the destructive process will proceed more rapidly by these energetic rays as they strike the lipid molecules and cause complete oxidation. This lipid peroxidation (complete oxidation) is believed to be the mainspring in the aging process.

Already this antioxidant property of vitamin E is being made use of in commercial products to retard spoilage. For example, butylated hydroxytoluene (a synthetic antioxidant that has vitamin E activity) is widely used in preventing polyunsaturated lipid peroxidation in foods. Also, vitamin E is added to therapeutic forms of vitamin A to protect the vitamin A from oxidizing before it is absorbed. In any event it is evident that increased intakes of polyunsaturated fatty acids in the diet increase the requirement for vitamin E.

■ **How may these findings be applied to human beings?**

Although vitamin E may not be a panacea for all ills, it certainly has been demonstrated that it is an essential element in human nutrition. Several areas of its possible physiologic function are:

1. *Aging process.* The antioxidant nature of vitamin E may well prove to be the clue to the puzzle of the aging process in man. Its presence may protect the poly-

unsaturated lipid structure of the cells from deterioration and destruction.

2. *Anemias.* Low plasma vitamin E levels have been found in some newborn infants, and erythrocytes tested in dilute hydrogen peroxide have shown increased hemolysis. These malnourished infants with macrocytic anemia have responded to vitamin E therapy with a favorable hematologic response.

3. *Malabsorption and muscle defects.* Patients with cystic fibrosis of the pancreas accompanied by steatorrhea demonstrate low plasma vitamin E levels and increased red blood cell hemolysis. Low plasma vitamin E levels and skeletal muscle lesions have also been reported in patients with kwashiorkor.

4. *Relation to unsaturated fatty acid metabolism.* This definite correlation indicating vitamin E's protective role of unsaturated fatty acids, especially linoleic acid, in the body has been demonstrated.

■ **How much vitamin E do we need?**

Although the exact mechanism by which vitamin E functions in the body is as yet unknown, it is an essential nutrient and as such a recommended dietary allowance has been indicated by the National Research Council's revised statement in 1968. About 5 I.U. of vitamin E is recommended for infants during the first year, with a gradual increase through the growth years to reach approximately 30 I.U. in adulthood.

■ **What are the main food sources of vitamin E?**

The richest sources of vitamin E are the vegetable oils. These also are the richest sources of polyunsaturated fatty acids. Other food sources include milk, eggs, muscle meats, fish, cereals, and leafy vegetables.

Vitamin K

■ **What is the nature of vitamin K?**

Vitamin K was named by its discoverer, Professor Henrik Dam, biochemist at the University of Copenhagen, as he was studying hemorrhagic disease in chicks fed a fat-free diet. Because he determined that the absent factor responsible was a blood-clotting vitamin, he called the substance "Ko-agulationsvitamin," or vitamin K. Later he succeeded in isolating and identifying the vitamin from alfalfa. In 1943 he was awarded the Nobel Prize for physiology and medicine in recognition of his work.

As with most of the vitamins, vitamin K is actually a group of substances with similar biologic activity. There are three main K vitamins. Two occur in nature and are fat soluble: K_1 (phylloquinone or phytonadione), and K_2 (farnoquinone), which was isolated from putrefied sardine meal by other investigators. Vitamin K_3 (menadione) has been made synthetically and has wide clinical use in patients in whom a fat-soluble form would be less readily metabolized.

■ **What is the main source of vitamin K?**

The main source of vitamin K is endogenous. It is synthesized by the normal intestinal bacteria so that an adequate supply is generally present. Examples, therefore, of inadequate vitamin K include the newborn infant, since the intestine at birth is sterile. The supply of vitamin K is inadequate until normal bacterial flora of the intestine develop about the third or fourth day of life.

■ **How are dietary sources of vitamin K absorbed?**

As with other fat-soluble materials, vitamins K_1 and K_2 require bile salts for absorption. Afterward they enter the metabolic system by way of the abdominal lacteals into the lymphatic system and then into portal blood in the liver. Vitamin K is apparently stored in very small amounts, since considerable quantities are excreted after administration of therapeutic doses.

■ **What is the physiologic function of vitamin K?**

As was indicated by its discovery during the study of hemorrhagic disease, the major function of vitamin K is its participation in the blood-clotting mechanism. Vitamin K catalyzes the synthesis of prothrombin by the liver. Without vitamin K the whole vital process of blood clotting cannot be initiated. It accomplishes this initiation of blood clotting by acting either as an enzyme or a coenzyme for the production of prothrombin. This mechanism for the production of prothrombin in the liver is not known, but in the absence of functioning liver tissue, vitamin K cannot act. When liver damage has caused hypoprothrombinemia, and this in turn has led to hemorrhage, vitamin K is an ineffective therapeutic agent. This relation of vitamin K to the overall blood-clotting mechanism is shown in the diagram in Fig. 6-1.

■ **How does this major blood-clotting function of vitamin K relate to clinical problems, and what vitamin K therapy may be indicated?**

A number of clinical situations have important relationships with vitamin K.

1. *Obstetrics.* Since the intestinal tract of the newborn is sterile, the infant has no vitamin K during the first few days of life until his normal bacterial flora develops. During this immediate postnatal period hemorrhage may therefore occur. This condition is called *hemorrhagic disease of the newborn.* Vitamin K therapy may be given to the mother before delivery, but the effectiveness of placental transfer is debatable. Therefore a prophylactic dose of vitamin K is usually given to the infant soon after birth.

2. *Biliary disease and surgery.* Any condition of the biliary tract affecting the flow of bile will prevent the proper absorption of vitamin K. Since vitamin K is a fat-soluble material, bile is necessary for its absorption. Thus bleeding tendencies would be enhanced in obstruction of the bile ducts, jaundice, gallbladder disease, hepatic injury, or liver disease. In such cases water-soluble forms of vitamin K, such as menadione, are available for therapeutic use. Parenteral use of menadione or oral administration of bile salts together with vitamin K, may be indicated to counteract the delayed clotting.

Surgical procedures involving the biliary tract, such as operations on the common bile duct or removal of the gallbladder (cholecystectomy), usually necessitate

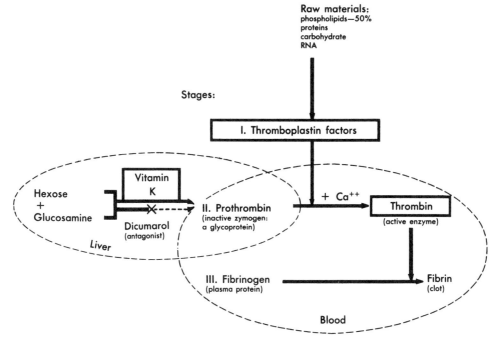

Fig. 6-1. The three stages of blood clotting. Note the role played by vitamin K in the production of prothrombin. Dicumarol, an anticlotting drug, acts as an antagonist (antimetabolite) to vitamin K and therefore inhibits the clotting mechanism at the start.

vitamin K therapy to prevent excessive hemorrhage.

3. *Intestinal disease.* Vitamin K deficiency is common in diseases such as celiac disease, sprue, and colitis, which affect the absorbing mucosa of the small intestine, or other diarrheal diseases, such as ulcerative colitis, that cause rapid loss of intestinal contents. In such cases intravenous administration of vitamin K may be indicated.

4. *Antibiotic therapy.* Prolonged use of antibiotics may adversely affect the normal bacterial flora of the intestine, so that vitamin K deficiency occurs.

5. *Anticoagulant therapy.* The use of heparin or *bishydroxycoumarin* (Dicumarol) in anticoagulant therapy for coronary thrombosis or thrombophlebitis may counteract the action of vitamin K. Dicumarol has a molecular structure so similar to that of vitamin K that it can act as an antimetabolite or antagonist to vitamin K because of the lock-and-key concept of enzyme action (see Fig. 5-2, p. 39). Dicumarol al-

most fits into vitamin K's spot in the enzyme substrate complex. Therefore it gets in the way and prevents the normal reaction of vitamin K and prothrombin. This accounts for Dicumarol's anticoagulant action. In case of an overdose of the anticoagulant, vitamin K may be used as an antidote.

■ **How much vitamin K do we need?**

No requirement for vitamin K has been stated, since a deficiency of vitamin K is unlikely except in the clinical situations indicated. An adequate amount is usually ensured because (1) the intestinal bacteria constantly synthesize a supply, and (2) the amount the body needs is apparently very small. The liver, however, must produce prothrombin if vitamin K is to be effective. Without a functioning liver, vitamin K cannot act.

■ **What are some food sources of vitamin K?**

Although vitamin K is mainly supplied by intestinal bacteria, there are a few food

Table 6-1. Summary of fat-soluble vitamins

Vitamin	Physiological functions	Results of deficiency	Requirement	Food sources
A (retinol)	Production of rhodopsin (visual purple)	Xerophthalmia	Adult: 5,000 I.U.	Liver
Provitamin A (carotene)	Formation and maintenance of epithelial tissue Toxic in large amounts	Night blindness Keratinization of epithelium Follicular hyperkeratosis Skin and mucous membrane infections Faulty tooth formation	Pregnancy: 6,000 I.U. Lactation: 8,000 I.U. Children: 1,500 to 5,000 I.U. depending on age	Cream, butter, whole milk Egg yolk Green and yellow vegetables Yellow fruits Fortified margerine
D (calciferol)	Absorption of calcium and phosphorus Calcification of bones Renal phosphate clearance Toxic in large amounts	Rickets Faulty bone growth Osteomalacia in adults	400 I.U. (children; pregnant or lactating women)	Fish oils Fortified or irradiated milk
E (tocopherol)	Related to action of selenium Antioxidant with vitamin A and unsaturated fatty acids Hemopoiesis Reproduction (in animals)	Hemolysis of red blood cells; anemia Possible protection of unsaturated fatty acids Sterility (in rats)	Adult: 25 to 30 mg.	Vegetable oils
K (menadione)	Blood clotting, necessary for synthesis of prothrombin Possible coenzyme in oxidation phosphorylation Toxic in large amounts	Hemorrhagic disease of the newborn Bleeding tendencies in biliary disease or surgical procedures Deficiency in intestinal malabsorption (sprue, celiac disease, colitis) Prolonged antibiotic therapy Anticoagulant therapy (Dicumarol counteracts)	Unknown	Green leafy vegetables Cheese Egg yolk Liver

sources. These include green leafy vegetables, such as cabbage, spinach, kale, and
cauliflower. Lesser amounts are found in
tomatoes, cheese, egg yolk, and liver.

A summary of the fat-soluble vitamins is
given in Table 6-1 for review and reference.

WATER-SOLUBLE VITAMINS
B-complex vitamins

It was the continuing search for a cure
to the age-old disease of the orient, beriberi, that led finally to the successive discoveries of the B vitamins in the early
1900s. Clues from a number of observations by workers in Japan and the Dutch
East Indies pointed to a food factor as the
related agent. An American chemist working in the Philippines first used this factor
in the form of extracts of rice polishings to
cure infantile beriberi. Then in 1916 E. V.
McCollum at the University of Wisconsin
named the food factor "water-soluble B"
because he thought at first it was a single
vitamin. Continuing study proved, however, that vitamin B was not a single substance but about a dozen vitamin and vi-
tamin-related factors. The B complex family of vitamins is now recognized.

The B vitamins, originally believed to be
important in preventing the deficiency diseases that led to their discovery, have now
been identified with many important metabolic functions. For example, they serve as
vital partners in many reactions as coenzyme factors in energy metabolism. Group-
ing them according to their function is
therefore a useful step in understanding
the significance of each vitamin in relation
to human nutrition.

Group I: Classic disease factors
 1. Thiamine (vitamin B_1)—antiberiberi
    factor or antineuritic vitamin, called
    "aneurin" in Europe and some other
    areas; essential in carbohydrate me-
    tabolism
 2. Riboflavin (vitamin B_2, formerly
    known as G)—essential in tissue res-
    piration, hence in growth; and essen-
    tial to the prevention of various skin

disorders such as cheilosis (cracking
at the corners of the mouth)
 3. Niacin—nicotinic acid, originally
    called P-P factor (pellagra-prevent-
    ing factor); a coenzyme essential to
    tissue oxidation and cell metabolism

Group II: More recently discovered coenzyme factors
 1. Pyridoxine (vitamin B_6)—essential
    coenzyme in amino acid metabolism;
    need for pyridoxine is increased in
    high protein diets.
 2. Pantothenic acid—essential part of
    coenzyme A or active acetate; a pivo-
    tal key compound in the metabolism
    of carbohydrate, fat, and protein
 3. Lipoic acid—coenzyme associated
    with thiamine in carbohydrate me-
    tabolism; a fatty acid, not a true vita-
    min
 4. Biotin (formerly vitamin B_7 or H)—
    coenzyme in carbon dioxide fixation
    reactions in energy metabolism

Group III: Cell growth and blood-forming
factors
 1. Folic acid (formerly vitamin B_9 or
    B_{10})—a group of factors essential to
    the growth and reproduction of cells;
    associated with anemias because of
    their vital role in formation of red
    blood cells
 2. Para-aminobenzoic acid (PABA)—
    part of the folic acid molecule; sul-
    fonamide antagonist; not a true vita-
    min
 3. Cobalamin (vitamin B_{12})—red, co-
    balt-containing vitamin group; the
    antipernicious anemia factor; extrin-
    sic factor (Castle)

Group IV: Other related nutrition factors
(pseudovitamins)
 1. Inositol—lipotropic agent in animal
    nutrition
 2. Choline—essential metabolite, nerve
    mediator, lipotropic agent

Thiamine

■ **What is the nature of thiamine?**
Thiamine hydrochloride is a white crystalline material, sometimes described as

having a nutlike and yeasty odor. It is water soluble and stable when dry, but is destroyed by alkalis. Thus it is absorbed more readily in the acid medium of the proximal duodenum than in the lower duodenum, where the acidity of the chyme is counteracted by alkaline intestinal secretions.

■ **Is thiamine stored in the body?**

The capacity of the body for storing thiamine is limited. It is present mainly in the heart, liver, and kidneys and in lower concentration in skeletal muscle and brain. When thiamine is administered, there is an increase in the tissues but within certain limits. On the other hand, on a thiamine-free diet, the tissue content is depleted rapidly, indicating the need for providing an adequate daily supply. The tissue content is highly relevant to heightened metabolic demand, such as fever, increased muscular activity, pregnancy, and lactation, or to the composition of the diet. Increased intake of carbohydrate increases the need for thiamine, whereas fat and proteins spare thiamine. When normal amounts of thiamine are ingested (1 to 2 mg. daily), about 10% of it is excerted in the urine. The remainder is apparently phosphorylated and utilized for metabolic functions.

■ **What is the physiologic function of thiamine?**

The major role of thiamine in metabolism is that of coenzyme factor in carbohydrate metabolism. When actively combined with phosphorus as thiamine pyrophosphate (TPP), thiamine plays a key role as a coenzyme in two main reactions in carboydrate metabolism:

1. In the oxidation of glucose thiamine serves as a coenzyme factor during the decarboxylation reaction in which pyruvate is converted into active acetate and carbon dioxide is removed. The enzyme controlling this reaction is called a *decarboxylase.* Thiamine pyrophosphate (TPP) acts as a *cocarboxylase.* This reaction enables pyruvate to enter into the Krebs cycle to produce vital energy.

2. In the hexose monophosphate shunt pathway for glucose oxidation, thiamine pyrophosphate (TPP) also acts as a coenzyme factor in the important reaction that provides active glyceraldehyde. This is the key link providing activated glycerol for lipogenesis, the conversion of glucose to fat. The process here is called *transketolation* (keto-carrying), and the enzyme controlling the reaction is a *transketolase.* Thiamine pyrophosphate (TPP) is the key activator for this reaction, which provides the high energy phosphate bond. Ionized magnesium (Mg^{++}) is another cofactor present.

■ **What are the clinical effects of thiamine deficiency?**

If thiamine is not present in sufficient amounts to provide the key energizing coenzyme factor in the cells, clinical effects will be reflected in several body systems:

1. *Gastrointestinal system.* Thiamine deficiency is manifested by such symptoms as anorexia, indigestion, severe constipation, gastric atony, and deficiency hydrochloric acid secretion. The cells of the smooth muscles and secretory glands of the gastrointestinal tract are not able to receive sufficient energy from glucose. Therefore they cannot do their proper work in digestion to provide still more glucose for the body, and a vicious cycle ensues as deficiency continues.

2. *Nervous system.* The central nervous system is extremely dependent on glucose for energy to do its work. If sufficient thiamine is not present to provide this need for energy, neuronal activity is impaired, alertness and reflex responses are diminished, and general apathy and fatigue result. If the thiamine deficiency continues, increasing damage or degeneration of myelin sheaths of nerve fibers causes increasing nerve irritation. This degeneration produces pain and prickly or deadening sensations. Eventually paralysis may result if the process continues unchecked in a severe deficiency state.

3. *Cardiovascular system.* With persisting thiamine deficiency, the heart muscle weakens and cardiac failure may result.

Also, smooth muscle of the vascular system may be involved, causing peripheral vasodilation. As a result of the cardiac failure, edema may occur in the extremities.

■ **How much thiamine do we need?**

Since thiamine is directly related to the metabolism of carbohydrate in the production of energy, the requirements for thiamine in human nutrition are usually stated in terms of the direct relation of thiamine to carbohydrate or energy metabolism. This relation is usually expressed in caloric intake. The National Research Council allowances recommend 0.5 mg./1,000 calories, with a minimum of 1.0 mg. for any intake between 1,000 and 2,000 calories.

■ **Are there clinical situations in which one would need more than the recommended allowance of thiamine?**

Yes, several important situations influence thiamine requirements and should be recognized: (1) during growth periods of infancy, childhood, and especially adolescence, thiamine needs are increased; (2) thiamine needs are increased during gestation because of the increased metabolic rate characteristic of pregnancy and the production of milk; (3) the larger the body and its tissue volume, the greater its cellular energy requirements, hence its requirements for thiamine; and (4) fevers and infections increase cellular energy requirements, which also increase thiamine needs. Elderly patients and those with chronic illness or debilitating disease require particular attention to avoid deficiencies.

■ **What are the main food sources of thiamine?**

Thiamine is distributed throughout the plant kingdom, occurring in the highest concentration usually in the seed, but also being present in the leaf, root, stem, and fruit. In cereal grains it is concentrated in the outer germ and bran layers, which are often discarded during the milling process. However, there is replacement of the vitamin in the enrichment of the refined grain. Good sources of thiamine include lean pork, beef, liver, whole or enriched grains, and legumes. Eggs, fish, and a few vegetables are fair sources. Thiamine is somewhat less widely distributed in food than some of the other vitamins, such as A and C, and the quantities of thiamine in the foods that supply it are less than the naturally available quantities of vitamins A and C. Therefore thiamine deficiency is a real possibility in the average diet, especially when calories are markedly curtailed, as in some strict weight-reduction regimes or in some highly inadequate special therapeutic diets.

Riboflavin

■ **What is the nature of riboflavin?**

The name riboflavin was officially adopted for this B vitamin because of its color (L. *flavus*, yellow) and carbohydrate component, a pentose sugar d-ribose. Riboflavin is a yellow-green, fluorescent pigment that forms yellowish brown needlelike crystals. It is water soluble, relatively stable to heat, but easily destroyed by light and irradiation. In acid media, however, it is stable and not easily oxidized. In strong alkalis it is destroyed. Absorption seems to occur, therefore, in the upper section of the small intestine where the acid content of the chyme is greater. This absorption is facilitated by combining the riboflavin with phosphorus in the intestinal mucosa.

■ **Is riboflavin stored in the body?**

Storage of riboflavin is relatively limited, although some amounts are found in the liver and kidney. Day-to-day tissue turnover needs must be supplied by the diet. Urinary excretion varies according to intake and the state of tissue depletion. When larger amounts of riboflavin are administered, as much as 50% may be eliminated in the urine. The capacity of the body for utilizing and retaining riboflavin is reduced in the presence of a negative nitrogen balance, for example, low-protein intake, excessive protein catabolism. Apparently flavoproteins are more labile than most other body proteins.

■ **What is the main physiologic function of riboflavin?**

Just as thiamine is a partner in carbohydrate metabolism, riboflavin is a vital factor in protein metabolism. It, too, combines with phosphorus to form essential coenzymes in tissue respiration systems. The enzymes of which riboflavin is an important constituent are called *flavoproteins.* Two such riboflavin enzymes operate at vital reaction points in the respiratory chains of cellular metabolism:

1. *Flavin mononucleotide* (FMN) is riboflavin phosphate activated with a high-energy phosphate bond. It participates in the enzyme systems that remove the amino group (NH_2) from certain amino acids. This process is called deamination (see p. 32).

2. *Flavin adenine dinucleotide* (FAD) is a riboflavin enzyme that contains two high-energy phosphate bonds. It is a highly active form, operating in many reactions affecting amino acids, fatty acids, and carbohydrates. For example, it aids in the deamination of glycine, an assential amino acid, and in the oxidizing of some of the lower fatty acids, such as butyric acid. It also acts in one of the systems of H^+ transfer in cellular oxidation (see p. 39).

■ **What are the clinical effects of riboflavin deficiency?**

Since riboflavin is closely related to protein metabolism, manifestations of its deficiency center around tissue inflammation and breakdown:

1. *Wound aggravation.* Minor tissue injuries easily become aggravated and do not heal easily.

2. *Mouth.* Cheilosis develops and the lips become swollen, crack easily, and characteristic cracks develop at the corners of the mouth.

3. *Nose.* Cracks and irritation develop at nasal angles.

4. *Tongue.* The tongue becomes swollen and reddened (glossitis).

5. *Eyes.* Extra blood vessels develop in the cornea (corneal vascularization); and the eyes burn, itch, and tear.

6. *Skin.* A scaly, greasy eruption may develop, especially in skin folds (seborrheic dermatitis). Riboflavin deficiencies seldom occur alone, but rather, as part of multiple deficiencies. They are especially likely to occur in conjunction with deficiencies of other B vitamins and protein.

■ **How much riboflavin do we need?**

The requirement for riboflavin is related to body size, metabolic rate, and rate of growth, all of which are related to protein intake. The lower the protein intake the more riboflavin is excreted and lost. The general recommendations of the National Research Council for riboflavin have, therefore, been stated in terms of *metabolic body size:* 0.07 mg./kg.$^{0.75}$.

■ **In what circumstances is the need for riboflavin increased?**

Additional amounts of riboflavin are needed under circumstances involving tissue building: after severe injury or burn, during increased protein catabolism, and during acute illness and early convalescence. Apparently these increased needs are related to the active participation of riboflavin in anabolic or tissue-building processes of protein synthesis. It is apparent, therefore, that attention should be given to certain high-risk groups or clinical situations in which this increased need for riboflavin may be present or where deficiencies are more likely to occur. These situations include:

1. Cheap, high-starch diets that are limited in protein foods, such as milk, meat, and vegetables, may be deficient in riboflavin.

2. Gastrointestinal disorders or chronic illness may result in a riboflavin deficiency because food intake in such circumstances is affected by anorexia, poor tolerance, or by prolonged use of a too-limited special diet. Disorders that affect absorption of nutrients can also cause riboflavin deficiency.

3. Wound healing, as in surgical procedures, trauma, and burns, increases the need for riboflavin because of the increased need for protein.

4. Periods of normal body stress, such as growth periods, pregnancy, and

lactation, increase the need for ribo-flavin.

■ **What are the main food sources of ribo-flavin?**

As with thiamine, the riboflavin content of cereal grains is concentrated in the germ and the bran layers, which are often discarded in the milling process. Therefore cereals are poor sources of riboflavin unless they are enriched. The most important food source of riboflavin is milk. One of the pigments in milk, *lactoflavin,* is the milk form of riboflavin. Each quart of milk contains 2 mg. of riboflavin, which is more than the daily requirement. Other good sources include active organ meats, such as liver, kidney, and heart. Some vegetables contribute additional amounts. However, since riboflavin is water soluble and destroyed by light, considerable loss can occur in open, excess-water cooking. Therefore covered containers and limited water usage are indicated.

Niacin (nicotinic acid, nicotinamide)

■ **What disease is associated with niacin deficiency?**

The discovery of niacin was the result of a search for the cause of the age-old disease pellagra. Pellagra is characterized by a typical dermatitis and often has fatal effects on the nervous system. Observations of pellagra were first recorded in the eighteenth century in Spain and Italy where it was endemic in populations subsisting largely on corn. In the early 1900s Joseph Goldberger, a United States Public Health Service physician studying the problems of pellagra, observed incidences of the disease in the majority of children in an orphanage as compared with a few of the children who were healthy. He traced the absence of pellagra in the few that were healthy to their pilfering of milk and meat from the orphanage's limited supply. Later in 1911 Casimir Funk, in London, isolated nicotinic acid from rice polishings but did not recognize its disease-preventive significance. It was not until 1937 that Conrad Elvehjem, a scientist at the University of Wisconsin,

definitely associated the vitamin with pellagra by using it to cure the related disease, black tongue, in dogs.

■ **How is niacin related to tryptophan?**

In 1945 at the University of Wisconsin Willard Krehl discovered that tryptophan is a precursor of niacin. Here again is demonstrated a vital link of a B vitamin with protein through the essential amino acid, tryptophan. Milk prevents pellagra, not because it is high in niacin (it is actually low in niacin), but because it is high in tryptophan. Almost exclusive use of corn contributes to pellagra because corn is low in tryptophan. Populations subsisting on diets that are low in niacin may never have pellagra because they happen to be consuming adequate amounts of tryptophan.

This tryptophan-niacin relation led to the development of a unit of measure called *niacin equivalent.* It was calculated that in persons with average physiologic needs, approximately 60 mg. of tryptophan produces 1 mg. of niacin. Hence, this amount of tryptophan—60 mg.—was designated as a niacin equivalent. Dietary requirements are now usually given in terms of total milligrams of niacin and niacin equivalents.

■ **What is the nature of niacin?**

Niacin, or nicotinic acid, derives its name from the fact that it can be prepared by oxidation of nicotine, although it differs strikingly from nicotine in its pharmacologic effects. Two forms of niacin exist. Niacin or nicotinic acid is easily converted into its amide form, *nicotinamide,* which is water soluble, stable to acid and heat, and forms a white powder when crystallized.

■ **What is the physiologic function of niacin?**

Niacin is a partner with riboflavin in the cellular coenzyme systems (NAD, NADP) that convert proteins and fats to glucose, and that oxidize glucose to release controlled energy. These tissue-oxidation enzyme systems are called the dehydrogenases (see p. 39). Energy is formed and stored in the compound ATP through a series of reactions that transfer hydrogen ion. These ions are passed down the line between the successively simpler compounds that comprise these oxidative systems to the eventual receiver oxygen, and the end product is water.

■ **What are the clinical effects of niacin deficiency?**

General niacin deficiency is manifested as weakness, lassitude, anorexia, indigestion, and various skin eruptions. More specific manifestations involve the skin and nervous system. Skin areas exposed to sunlight are especially affected and they develop a dark, scaly dermatitis. If the deficiency of niacin continues, the central nervous system becomes involved and confusion, apathy, disorientation, and neuritis develop.

Since riboflavin and niacin have close interrelationships in cell metabolism, clinical manifestations of their deficiency closely parallel each other. Furthermore, if one of these two components is deficient, the other is usually deficient as well.

■ **What is the pharmacologic action of niacin?**

Niacin is unique among the vitamins in that it has a rather marked pharmacologic action when given in relatively large doses. Both niacin and nicotinamide have a stimulating effect on the central nervous system. In therapeutic doses nicotinic acid (but not nicotinamide) produces pronounced transient vasodilation, with flushing of the face, neck, and arms. This is accompanied by an increase in peripheral blood flow and skin temperature, with a frequently uncomfortable sense of warmth and at times burning and itching. Wide individual variations in this response occur. Nicotinic acid may also reduce the plasma lipid concentration in certain cases of hyperlipemia. The mechanism for this effect is unknown.

■ **How much niacin do we need?**

Human requirements for niacin indicate that the minimum for necessary tissue stores is about 9 mg./1,000 calories. The National Research Council recommendations are for 6.6 mg./1,000 calories and not less than 13 niacin equivalents at intakes of less

than 2,00 calories. This is about 50% higher than minimum requirements, and provides a margin of safety to cover variances in individual needs. These recommendations also allow for the contribution of tryptophan in terms of niacin equivalents from the dietary protein sources. Many factors affect these general requirements. Indications for increased amounts are age and growth periods, pregnancy and lactation, illness, tissue trauma, body size, and physical activity.

■ **What are the main food sources of niacin?**

Meat is a major source of niacin. Peanuts, beans, and peas are also good sources. Enrichment improves refined cereal grains as a source of niacin, since the natural vitamin is removed in the milling process. Corn and rice are poor sources of niacin because they are low in tryptophan. Oats are also low in niacin. Fruits and vegetables generally are rather poor sources.

Pyridoxine (B$_6$)

■ **What is the nature of pyridoxine?**

Pyridoxine was so named because its chemical structure is that of a pyridine ring. Like many of the other B vitamins, pyridoxine is not one substance but several. Three forms of vitamin B$_6$ occur in nature —pyridoxine, pyridoxal, and pyridoxamine. In the body all three of these forms are converted to pyridoxal phosphate. The term *pyridoxine* or vitamin B$_6$ is generally used to designate the entire group as well as any one of its components. The phosphate derivative of the vitamin, pyridoxal phosphate (B$_6$-PO$_4$), is by far the most potent and active form of the vitamin in vitamin tablets.

Pyridoxine is a water-soluble, heat-stable vitamin that is sensitive to light and to alkalis. Hence, as with other B vitamins, it is absorbed in the upper portion of the small intestine where the acid media facilitates passage. After absorption it is distributed throughout the body tissues, which is evidence of its many essential metabolic activities.

■ **What is the physiologic function of pyridoxine?**

The metabolic functions of pyridoxine are closely related primarily to the metabolism of protein. In the absorption of protein, B_6 is believed to facilitate this initial absorption through the intestinal wall. Pyridoxine is also believed to participate in an active transport system that carries amino acids across the cell walls. The other area of basic physiologic function of pyridoxine is that of a coenzyme factor in protein metabolism. Among these coenzyme functions, for example, are actions related to deamination, transamination, and heme formation.

■ **Does pyridoxine have a role in carbohydrate and fat metabolism as well?**

Yes, but to a much lesser extent than it does with protein metabolism. By way of the transfer systems involving pyridoxine in protein metabolism, such as decarboxylation and transamination, carbon metabolites are provided for energy-producing fuel in the Krebs cycle. In fat metabolism, B_6-PO_4 participates in the conversion of the essential fatty acid, linoleic acid, to another fatty acid, arachidonic acid.

■ **What are the clinical effects of pyridoxine deficiency?**

Since pyridoxine has such a wide use in metabolic activities, it is understandable that it holds a key to a number of clinical problems:

1. *Anemia.* A hypochromic, microcytic anemia has been observed in several patients even in the presence of a high serum iron level. In these cases a deficiency of B_6-PO_4 was demonstrated by a tryptophan load test, and the anemia was subsequently cured by supplying the deficient vitamin. The role of pyridoxine in heme formation relates it in general to any anemia.

2. *Central nervous system disturbances.* Since pyridoxine plays a vital role in the formation of two regulatory compounds in brain activity, serotonin and aminobutyric acid, B_6-PO_4 has a significant place in control of related neurologic conditions. For example, in infants deprived of the vitamin there is increased hyperirritability that progresses to convulsive seizures. A classic case occurred in the early 1950s when infants fed a commercial milk formula in which most of the pyridoxine content had been inadvertently destroyed by high-temperature autoclaving subsequently developed convulsions. The seizures ceased soon after a B_6-supplemented formula was used.

3. *Physiologic demands of pregnancy.* Pyridoxine deficiencies during pregnancy have also been demonstrated by tryptophan load tests. These deficiencies were subsequently alleviated by supplementation with the vitamin. Fetal growth, in addition to creating greater maternal metabolic demands, increases the pyridoxine requirement. In past years, vitamin B_6 has been used to treat the hyperemesis of pregnancy, but there is no real evidence to substantiate this practice.

■ **What relation does pyridoxine have to tuberculosis therapy?**

The chemotherapeutic agent for tuberculosis, isoniazid (isonicotinic acid hydrazide; INH), has been shown to be an antagonist for pyridoxine. By inhibiting the conversion of glutamic acid (the only amino acid the brain metabolizes), isoniazid has caused a side effect of neuritis in some patients. Treatment with large doses (50 to 100 mg. daily) of pyridoxine prevents this effect.

■ **How much pyridoxine do we need?**

The amount of pyridoxine required by the body is very small, so that a deficiency in usual circumstances is unlikely. Some of the vitamin is provided by bacterial synthesis in the intestine, but just how much is available from this source is unknown. The need for vitamin B_6 varies with the dietary protein intake because it is intimately involved in amino acid metabolism. For adults approximately 1 mg. daily is minimal. However, to assure a safety margin for various individual needs, the National Research Council has set its recommended allowance for pyridoxine at 2 mg./day for adults.

■ **What are the major food sources of pyridoxine?**

Pyridoxine is widespread in nature, but

many of the sources provide very small amounts. Most of its food sources are associated with protein, a would be expected. These sources include yeast, wheat and corn, liver and kidney, egg yolk, and meat. There are limited amounts in milk and vegetables.

Pantothenic acid

■ **What is the nature of pantothenic acid?**

Pantothenic acid gets its name from the fact that it is so widely distributed in nature. It is present in all forms of living things and is found throughout body tissues. Pantothenic comes from the Greek word *pantothen*, which means "in every corner" or "from all sides." Intestinal bacteria synthesize considerable amounts of the vitamin. This, together with its widespread natural occurrence, makes a deficiency unlikely. Most of the study done on deficiency states has, for the most part, been by inducing them in animals.

■ **What is the physiologic function of pantothenic acid?**

The coenzyme role of pantothenic acid is vital to overall body metabolism. This coenzyme role is closely associated with the active metabolite of carbohydrate and fat, acetyl CoA or active acetate. In the metabolism of carbohydrate, active acetate is the point at which important reactions in a number of directions can involve carbohydrates, fats, and proteins. Pantothenic acid is an essential constituent of this vital enzyme CoA, which forms active acetate and as such has extensive metabolic responsibility as an activating agent. The process of *acetylation* by the enzyme CoA is one of the prime chemical reactions of the body. Thus examples of the vital role of pantothenic acid is tied to activating reactions involving active acetate.

■ **How much pantothenic acid do we need?**

No requirement for pantothenic acid has been established since a deficiency is unlikely. Studies with adults have shown that daily excretion rates range from 2.5 to 9.5 mg. The daily intake of pantothenic acid in an average American diet of from 2,500

to 3,000 calories is about 10 to 20 mg. Therefore it is only perhaps under extreme metabolic stress that a deficiency may be encountered.

■ **What are the major food sources of pantothenic acid?**

As indicated by its name, sources of pantothenic acid are widespread. Yeast and metabolically active tissues such as liver and kidney are rich sources. Egg yolk and skimmed milk contribute more. Additional sources include lean beef, milk, cheese, legumes, broccoli, kale, sweet potatoes, and yellow corn.

Lipoic acid

■ **What is the nature of lipoic acid?**

In the continuing study of thiamine as a coenzyme in carbohydrate metabolism, it was discovered that this metabolic system required other coenzyme factors in addition to thiamine. One of these new factors proved to be a fat-soluble acid and was named lipoic acid from the Greek word *lipos*, meaning "fat." However, subsequent study of its structure in natural sources proved it to be a sulfur-containing fatty acid ($LipS_2$ or LSS). Thus, lipoic acid is not a true vitamin. Because of its coenzyme function, however, it is sometimes classified with the B-vitamin group.

■ **What is the physiologic function of lipoic acid?**

Lipoic acid is an essential coenzyme that functions with thiamine in the initial decarboxylation step of pyruvate. Pyruvate is a key product in carbohydrate metabolism formed in the beginning pathway of glucose oxidation through the Embden-Meyerhof glycolytic pathway. This key reaction enables pyruvate ultimately to enter the Krebs cycle to produce energy. Lipoic acid has two sulfur bonds of high-energy potential (LSS). It combines with the active thiamine coenzyme with two high-energy phosphate bonds (thiamine pyrophosphate, TPP) to reduce pyruvate to active acetate, thus preparing it for the final energy cycle.

■ **Are other nutrients related to this key reaction of oxidative decarboxylation along with lipoic acid?**

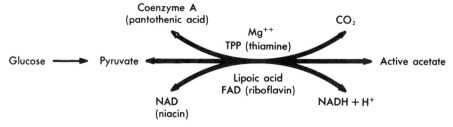

Fig. 6-2. Conversion of pyruvate to active acetate (acetyl CoA), illustrating the team action of five B vitamins and one mineral (magnesium).

Yes. In fact, if one looks closely at this reaction one can see that not one but *five* B vitamins are involved in this one reaction, together with ionized magnesium (Mg^{++}). This one key reaction helps to provide for needed energy production. It is an excellent example of team reaction among the nutrients. This team reaction is shown in Fig. 6-2.

■ **What is the requirement for lipoic acid?**

A requirement for lipoic acid in human nutrition has not been established. Only a minute amount appears to be needed for this significant reaction of oxidated decarboxylation, and lipoic acid is wide spread in active tissues. Continued study may prove that this coenzyme is of even greater siginficance than is now known.

■ **What are the food sources of lipoic acid?**

Lipoic acid is found in many biologic materials, including yeast and liver.

Biotin

■ **What is the nature of biotin?**

Biotin is a water-soluble vitamin factor, a member of the B-complex group of vitamins. It has been called a "micronutrient" because such minute traces of it perform its metabolic task. However, its potency is great and a natural deficiency is unknown. It is widespread in both plant and animal tissues and is also synthesized by intestinal bacteria. Thus man is not dependent on dietary sources to ensure a supply. Biotin has been called the "anti-egg white injury" factor because it was first discovered in relation to its effect in counteracting an injurious substance in egg

white, *avidin*, a carbohydrate-containing protein. Apparently avidin combines with biotin in the intestine and prevents its absorption. Biotin deficiency in human beings from this cause is certainly unlikely, unless one had an unusual taste for large amounts of raw eggs!

■ **What is the physiologic function of biotin?**

The coenzyme role of biotin in metabolism is its main function. Even in very small amounts it appears to be needed in two main types of reaction:

1. *Carboxylation.* This is the reaction that fixes or adds carbon dioxide to a compound. Biotin serves as a coenzyme with active acetate in reactions that transfer carbon dioxide from one compound and fix it to another. Examples of this combination of cofactors at work are: (1) initial steps in synthesis of some fatty acids, (2) conversion reactions involved in synthesis of some amino acids, and (3) carbon dioxide fixation in forming purines.

2. *Deamination.* Biotin serves as a coenzyme with deaminases in splitting off the amino group from certain amino acids (aspartic acid, serine, threonine).

■ **What is the requirement for biotin?**

The human requirement for biotin has not been established, since the amount needed for metabolism is so small. Moreover, a deficiency is highly unlikely because the vitamin occurs in many natural foods and is apparently synthesized by intestinal bacteria.

■ **What are some of the food sources of biotin?**

Examples of excellent food sources of

biotin include egg yolk, liver, kidney, tomatoes, and yeast.

Folic acid

■ **What is the nature of folic acid?**

Folic acid or folicin, was named from the Latin word *folium* meaning "leaf" because a major source of its extraction was dark, green, leafy vegetables, such as spinach. As with a number of the B vitamins, folic acid is not one but a group of related compounds with similar activities. It is a water-soluble material, a conjugated substance made up of three acids, one of which is the amino acid glutamic acid. Folic acid is absorbed throughout the small intestine and some amount apparently is synthesized by intestinal bacteria.

■ **What is the physiologic function of folic acid?**

Folic acid functions as one of the major coenzyme factors. Its major task is that of single carbon transfer. A number of key compounds are formed by these conversions:

1. *Hemoglobin.* Folic acid performs its basic carbon carrier role in the formation of heme, the iron-containing protein in hemoglobin. This important function relates folic acid with blood cell formation and anemias.

2. *Purines.* Purines are part of a group of materials called *nucleoproteins.* These are essential constituents of all living cells. Because the nucleoproteins are intimately related to the nuclear substance of the cell, they are involved in cell division and in the transmission of inherited traits. It is evident, then, that any factor involved in the formation of nuclear proteins, such as folic acid, would play a vital role in cell growth and reproduction. Purines are found in large quantity, therefore, in tissues with very active cellular growth and reproduction, such as glandular tissue.

3. *Thymine.* Thymine is an essential nuclear protein material that forms a key part of DNA (deoxyribonucleic acid), the important material in the cell nucleus that is responsible for transmitting genetic char-acteristics (see p. 30). Folic acid participates in the reactions that synthesize this important material.

■ **What is the relationship of folic acid to pernicious anemia?**

In the beginning study of pernicious anemia, folic acid was used in therapy and was found to help with needed blood cell regeneration in patients with pernicious anemia. However, its effect was not permanent, and it did not control the degenerative neurologic problems associated with the disease. Continued study of pernicious anemia revealed that vitamin B_{12}, discovered after folic acid, proved to be the fully effective agent both for blood regeneration and for the neurologic defect. Therefore, the American Medical Association and the Food and Drug Administration have recommended that no more than 0.4 mg. of folic acid be included in nonprescriptive multivitamin preparations, since this would suffice for common needs, while at the same time it would not mask the development of pernicious anemia to prevent its diagnosis.

■ **Is there an anemia directly related to simple folic acid deficiency?**

Yes. A nutritional megaloblastic anemia caused by simple folic acid deficiency has been clearly described. A report of seven cases indicated low serum folic acid in the face of normal serum B_{12} levels. A rapid hematologic response followed treatment with folic acid alone.

■ **Is folic acid needed during pregnancy?**

Yes, because of its vital role in heme formation for hemoglobin synthesis. In fact, the recent report of the National Research Council on the relation of nutrition to the course of pregnancy indicated a need for supplementation with folic acid. Some cases of macroctyic anemia of pregnancy have been attributed to dietary folic acid deficiency. A similar megaloblastic anemia of infancy has also been reported. In one instance a mother with macrocytic anemia and her 3-month-old nursing infant with megaloblastic anemia both responded to folic acid given to the mother alone. It is evident, then, that folic acid is secreted in breast milk.

■ **Is folic acid related to gastrointestinal disease?**

Yes. Folic acid has been shown to be effective in the treatment of sprue, a gastrointestinal disease characterized by intestinal lesions, malabsorption defects, diarrhea, macrocytic anemia, and general malnutrition from lack of absorbed nutrients. Response to folic acid has been excellent in these cases. Both the blood-forming and gastrointestinal defects have been corrected by the vitamin.

■ **Is the folic acid antagonist, _aminopterin_, effective in the treatment of leukemia?**

No, because its initial effect is not sustained. This potent folic acid antagonist, aminopterin, has been used in some cases of malignant neoplastic disease such as leukemia. Unfortunately, however, although temporary remissions have been achieved with aminopterin, the leukemic cells seem to develop a resistance to the antagonist with continued use, and its effectiveness is overcome.

■ **What is the requirement for folic acid?**

The National Research Council stated a requirement for folic acid for the first time in its 1968 recommendations. The average American diet contains about 0.6 mg. of total folic acid activity. Thus, to cover variances in need and in the amount of available folic acid in food, the recommendation for adults is set at 0.4 mg. daily. Because of the greater need during pregnancy, however, a recommendation is made for 0.8 mg. daily; for lactation, 0.5 mg. daily is recommended. Stress, such as disease and growth, also increases the requirement.

■ **What are the main food sources of folic acid?**

As indicated by its name, folic acid is widespread in green, leafy vegetables. Other sources include liver, kidney, and asparagus. Relatively poor sources, though adding some folic acid, are fruit, milk, poultry, and eggs.

■ **What is PABA?**

PABA is para-aminobenzoic acid, a structural unit of folic acid. Sometimes PABA is listed as a separate factor because it is essential to the growth of certain microorganisms. However, its main role in human nutrition is related to that of folic acid in its role as an essential component in folic acid formation.

PABA in therapeutic doses is used in the treatment of some rickettsial diseases. Its use in treating such diseases is based on the concept of metabolic antagonism. PABA acts as an antagonist to a recently discovered material essential to the small parasites of the genus _Rickettsia_. It is antagonistic to the material essential to these organisms, paraoxybenzoic acid. The rickettsial organisms are killed because PABA blocks their essential metabolite.

Cobalamin (vitamin B$_{12}$)

■ **What is the nature of vitamin B$_{12}$?**

The generic name, _cobalamin_, has been given to vitamin B$_{12}$ because of its unique chemical structure. B$_{12}$ is the only vitamin that contain cobalt. It is a complex, red crystalline compound of high molecular weight with a single cobalt atom at its core. It occurs as a protein complex in foods so that its food sources are mostly of animal origin. The ultimate source, however, might be designated as microorganisms in the gastrointestinal tract of herbivorous animals. Such microorganisms are found in large amounts in the rumen (first stomach, containing cud) of cows. Apparently some synthesis occurs in the intestinal bacteria of man, also, although the amount supplied from this source is unknown.

The discoverey of B$_{12}$ resulted from the continued search for a specific agent in the control of pernicious anemia. When folic acid was found to be lacking in full effectiveness for controlling the disease, a later factor proved to be able to control both the blood-forming defect and the neurologic involvement in pernicious anemia. This agent was vitamin B$_{12}$.

■ **How is B$_{12}$ absorbed?**

The absorption of B$_{12}$ has proved to be the key defect in pernicious anemia. An agent is required for this absorption, *intrinsic factor* (IF)—a mucoprotein enzyme that is secreted by glands in the fundus and cardia of the stomach but not in the pylorus. It is when this intrinsic factor is absent that pernicious anemia occurs because B_{12} cannot be absorbed without this specific carrier. Absorption of B_{12} takes place in the ileum. However, it is prepared for absorption by two gastric secretions. Hydrochloric acid in the stomach begins to split the B_{12} from its peptide bonds and this splitting is continued by a group of enzymes in the intestine. The free B_{12} then combines with the intrinsic factor and is absorbed in the ileum and carried by the blood to various organs, where it is utilized.

■ **Can vitamin B_{12} be stored?**

Yes. It is this storage capacity that is indicated by delay in the appearance of pernicious anemia after removal of the stomach in gastrectomy. When the stomach is removed, there is a loss of gastric secretions necessary for the absorption of vitamin B_{12} but this anemia does not become apparent until 3 to 5 years after the gastrectomy. Organs holding the greatest amount of B_{12} are the liver, kidney, heart, muscle, pancreas, testes, brain, blood, spleen, and bone marrow. These organs are related to red blood cell formation. Even though the amounts stored in these tissues are very minute, they are vital; the body apparently holds tenaciously to this supply, and stores are very slowly depleted.

■ **What is the physiologic function of vitamin B_{12}?**

Vitamin B_{12} appears to have many metabolic interrelationships with the basic nutrients. The requirement for B_{12} increases as protein intake increases. It is also related to the utilization of fat and carbohydrate. The manner in which B_{12} is related to these aspects of general metabolism is associated with the process of *methylation,* the forming or transferring of key methyl groups (CH_3). In this role B_{12} participates in the synthesis of nucleic acid and vital cell proteins. Hence B_{12} is closely related to normal growth and tissue development. The other well-established role of vitamin B_{12} is its participation in the formation of red blood cells and therefore in the control of pernicious anemia.

■ **What is the relationship between vitamin B_{12} and folic acid in the control of pernicious anemia?**

It has been postulated that B_{12} has an indirect effect on blood cell formation through activation of folic acid coenzymes. Within the developing red blood cell, activities that are dependent on folic acid are indirectly controlled by vitamin B_{12}. Perhaps this link with folic acid explains why the folic acid may alleviate pernicious anemia only temporarily and why the folic acid must be supplemented by vitamin B_{12} if the pernicious anemia is to be corrected over a long period of time.

■ **How is vitamin B_{12} administered to control pernicious anemia?**

Usually a patient with pernicious anemia is given from 15 to 30 μg. of B_{12} daily in intramuscular injections during a relapse. He can be maintained afterward by an injection of about 30 μg. every 30 days. This controls both the blood cell-forming disorder and the degenerative effects on the nervous system.

■ **Is vitamin B_{12} also effective in the treatment of sprue?**

Like folic acid, vitamin B_{12} has been effective in the treatment of the intestinal syndrome sprue. However, it seems most effective when used in conjunction with folic acid. Therefore, its role may be indirect in that it facilitates the action of the folic acid.

■ **What is the requirement for vitamin B_{12}?**

The amount of exogenous vitamin B_{12} needed for normal human metabolism is very small. Reported minimum requirements have been from 0.6 to 1.2 μg./day. The ordinary diet easily provides as much and more. For example one cup of milk, one egg, and four ounces of meat provide 2.4 μg. The National Research Council recommends a daily intake of 5 μg. for adults.

Table 6-2. Summary of B complex vitamins

Vitamin	Physiological functions	Clinical applications	Requirement	Food sources
Thiamine (B₁)	Coenzyme in carbohydrate metabolism: TPP—decarboxylation TDP—transketolation	Beriberi (deficiency) GI*: anorexia, gastric atony, indigestion, deficient hydrochloric acid CNS*: fatigue, apathy, neuritis, paralysis CV*: cardiac failure, peripheral vasodilation and edema of extremities	0.4 mg. per 1,000 calories	Pork, beef, liver, whole or enriched grains, legumes
Riboflavin (B₂)	Coenzyme in protein of energy metabolism (flavoproteins) FMN (flavin mononucleotide) FAD (flavin adenine dinucleotide)	Wound aggravation Cheilosis (cracks at corners of mouth) Glossitis Eye irritation; photophobia Seborrheic dermatitis	0.6 mg. per 1,000 calories	Milk, liver, enriched cereals
Niacin (nicotinic acid) (precursor—tryptophan)	Coenzyme in tissue oxidation to produce energy (ATP) NAD (nicotinamide adenine dinucleotide) NADP (nicotinamide adenine dinucleotide phosphate)	Pellagra (deficiency) Weakness, lassitude, anorexia Skin: scaly dermatitis CNS: neuritis, confusion	14-19 mg. (niacin equivalent)	Meat, peanuts, enriched grains
Pyridoxine (B₆)	Coenzyme in amino acid metabolism Decarboxylation Deamination Transamination Transsulfuration Niacin formation from tryptophan Heme formation Amino acid absorption	Anemia (hypochromic microcytic) CNS: hyperirritability, convulsions, neuritis Isoniazid is an antagonist for pyridoxine Pregnancy: anemia	0.2 mg.	Wheat, corn, meat, liver
Pantothenic acid	Coenzyme in formation of active acetate (CoA)—acetylation	Contributes to: Lipogenesis Amino acid activation Formation of cholesterol Formation of steroid hormones Formation of heme Excretion of drugs		Liver, egg, skimmed milk

Name	Function	Clinical use	Dosage	Sources
Lipoic acid (sulfur-containing fatty acid)	Coenzyme (with thiamine) in carbohydrate metabolism to reduce pyruvate to active acetate; Oxidative decarboxylation	Undetermined (see Thiamine)		Liver, yeast
Biotin	Coenzyme in decarboxylation (synthesis of fatty acids, amino acids, purines); deamination	Undetermined		Egg yolk, liver
Folic acid	Coenzyme for single carbon transfer—purines, thymine, hemoglobin; Transmethylation	Blood cell regeneration in pernicious anemia but not control of its neurological problems; Megaloblastic anemia; Macrocytic anemia of pregnancy; Sprue treatment; Aminopterin is folic acid antagonist	0.4 mg. Pregnancy: 0.8 mg. Lactation: 0.5 mg.	Liver, green leafy vegetables, asparagus
PABA (part of folic acid)		Treatment of rickettsial diseases; Anemias (see Folic acid)		Same as folic acid
Cobalamin (B_{12})	Coenzyme in protein synthesis; Formation of nucleic acid and cell proteins—red blood cells; Transmethylation	Extrinsic factor in pernicious anemia—combines with intrinsic factor of gastric secretions for absorption; forms red blood cells (with folic acid); Sprue treatment (with folic acid)	5 µg.	Liver, meats, milk, egg, cheese
Inositol	Lipotropic agent (?)	Undetermined		Citrus fruit, grains, meat, milk
Choline	Lipotropic agent; Forms nerve mediator—acetylcholine	Fatty liver—hepatitis, cirrhosis (undetermined in human nutrition)		Meat, cereals, egg yolk

*GI = gastrointestinal; CNS = central nervous system; CV = cardiovascular.

This amount allows a margin of safety to cover variance in individual needs in absorption and body stores.

■ **What are the main food sources of vitamin B$_{12}$?**

This vitamin is supplied almost entirely by animal foods. The richest sources are liver, kidney, and lean meat, milk, egg, and cheese. A natural dietary deficiency is rare. The only reported manifestations of deficiency (general nervous symptoms, sore mouth and tongue, paresthesia, amenorrhea) have come from a group of true vegetarians, "Vegands," who live in Great Britain, and from other vegetarian groups in India. Because vitamin B$_{12}$ comes from animal foods it is evident that an adequate supply of it is of concern in any vegetarian diet.

Choline

■ **What is the nature of choline?**

Although choline is sometimes classified with the B-vitamin family, in reality it is not a vitamin, because the body can manufacture choline and uses it in quantities larger than the small amounts that form part of the definition of true vitamins. Choline is closely related to protein metabolism. Two essential amino acids are used in the synthesis of choline. Serine serves as a base and methionine donates three methyl groups to complete it. This transfer of key single carbon groups to form vital metabolites is the important process of *transmethylation*. In this process folic acid and vitamin B$_{12}$ are coenzyme factors. Thus adequate dietary protein is essential to supply the building materials. Choline is also a key component of two phospholipids: (1) *lecithin* is a phospholipid important in the metabolism of fat by the liver, and (2) *sphingomyelin* is a phospholipid in brain and nerve tissue.

■ **What is the physiologic function of choline?**

Choline is a lipotropic agent in hepatic fat metabolism. The word "lipotropic" means "having an affinity for fat." To prevent the accumulation of damaging amounts of fat in the liver, fat must be changed from storage forms to transport forms—lipoproteins. Any substance that has an affinity for fat and attaches itself to fat to make a transport form is called a lipotropic substance. This turnover of fat, especially in the liver, is a conversion of fatty acids to lipoproteins, the form in which they may be carried to the fat depots of the body. This lipotropic role of choline thus plays a part in liver disease, such as hepatitis or cirrhosis.

■ **What is acetylcholine?**

Acetylcholine is an important chemical mediator in nerve activity. It is formed from the combination of choline with active acetate. There is also evidence that acetylcholine may have an influence on cell permeability.

■ **Is there a stated requirement for choline in the diet?**

No. Dietary requirements for choline are not stated, because materials required for its synthesis, such as methione and essential fatty acids, are available in the diet. Moreover, choline is widely distributed in foods that are usually associated with proteins. Thus, such sources would include egg yolk, meat, cereals, and legumes. There is very little choline in fruits and vegetables.

A summary of the B vitamins and their functional roles in the body is given in Table 6-2 for review and reference.

Ascorbic acid (vitamin C)

■ **What is the nature of vitamin C?**

Vitamin C was given the name ascorbic acid because the discovery of the vitamin was the result of a search for the answer to the disease *scurvy*, from the Latin word for this disease, "scorbutus." Scurvy is a disease characterized by tissue hemorrhages, caused by fragility of blood capillaries. A hexuronic acid was isolated in lemon juice and was demonstrated to prevent or cure scurvy. Hence, the name ascorbic acid was given to the substance because of its antiscorbutic properties.

Vitamin C is an odorless, white crystalline powder, that is soluble in water but not in fat. It is unstable, easily oxidized, and can be destroyed by oxygen, alkalis, and high temperatures. It also reacts with the metallic ions of iron and copper.

■ **What is the relation of vitamin C to glucose?**

Vitamin C is closely related to glucose in its molecular structure. This relationship indicates an interesting genetic defect in man. Glucose is the natural precursor of vitamin C. Plants make this conversion to produce the vitamin. Also, almost every animal species can make this same conversion and hence do not require a food source of vitamin C. Man is one of the few exceptions, along with monkeys, guinea pigs, a rare Indian fruit bat, and the red-vented bulbul (a bird). These few species lack the enzyme necessary to make the conversion from l-gulonic acid to ascorbic acid. In the last analysis, therefore, scurvy can really be called a disease of genetic origin, an inherited metabolic error. A defect in carbohydrate metabolism results from the lack of an enzyme, an oxidase, which in turn results from the lack of a specific gene.

■ **How is vitamin C absorbed?**

Vitamin C is easily absorbed from the small intestine. Since vitamin C is an acid and is destroyed by alkalis, absorption is hindered by lack of hydrochloric acid or by bleeding from the gastrointestinal tract.

■ **Is vitamin C stored in the body?**

No, not in the sense that fat-soluble vitamins, such as vitamin A, are stored in the liver. However, vitamin C "reserves" are generally distributed throughout the body tissues. This is referred to as the "degree of tissue saturation" of vitamin C. The amount of vitamin C in white blood cells is used as a general indicator of the degree of body tissue saturation. A small amount (from 1.0 to 1.2 mg./100 ml.) circulates in the blood plasma and any excess of this amount is readily excreted. So if large amounts are ingested, more is excreted, depending on the state of tissue stores.

■ **Is there sufficient vitamin C in milk for the needs of infants?**

Not in cow's milk, as it is used in formulas for infant feeding. A child being fed by bottle feeding, therefore, should have his diet supplemented by ascorbic acid. However, sufficient vitamin C for needs in early infancy is present in breast milk.

■ **What is the basic physiologic function of vitamin C?**

The well-established role of vitamin C in human nutrition concerns the provision of an intercellular cementing substance that is necessary to build collagen or supportive tissue. Thus, the presence of vitamin C is required to build and maintain bone matrix, cartilage, dentine, collagen, and connective tissue. The precise mechanism of this function is not known, but when vitamin C is absent this important ground substance does not develop into collagen. When vitamin C is given, the formation of this ground substance follows quickly. *Collagen* is a protein substance that exists in many tissues of the body, such as the white fibers of connective tissue. The term is derived from two Greek words: *kolla*, glue; and *gennan*, to produce. Evidently vitamin C helps provide the glue.

Vascular tissue is particularly weakened, therefore, without the cementing substance of vitamin C to provide firm capillary walls. Deficiency states of vitamin C are characterized by fragile, easily ruptured capillaries with consequent diffuse tissue bleeding. Clinical conditions include easy bruising, pin-point peripheral hemorrhages, bone and joint hemorrhages, easy bone fracture, poor wound healing, and friable bleeding gums with loosened teeth (gingivitis).

■ **Does vitamin C have other functions in general body metabolism?**

Yes, particularly in the formation of hemoglobin and the maturation of red blood cells. Vitamin C influences the removal of iron from ferritin (the protein-iron-phosphorus complex in which iron is stored in the body). This action is present particularly in reticuloendothelial cells of the liver, spleen, and bone marrow where red cells are formed. Because of this reaction, more iron is thus made available in the body fluids for the formation of heme. Also, vitamin C influences the conversion in the liver of folic acid to a related compound, folinic acid, which is a factor that has been used in the treatment of megaloblastic anemia. Folinic acid has been called the "citrovorum factor" (CF) because it supplies an essential growth factor of a lactobacillus, *L. citrovorum*.

■ **Does vitamin C have any relationship to amino acid metabolism that may help also to explain its role in tissue building and wound healing?**

Yes, a relationship of vitamin C to several amino acids has been indicated by certain observations made in the search for protein links:

1. Metabolism of phenylalanine and tyrosine is defective in premature infants who lack adequate vitamin C. In several reactions tyrosine is not converted properly without vitamin C.
2. Vitamin C seems to participate in the synthesis of hydroxyproline from proline. This may be related to its role in collagen formation.

■ **What is the relationship, therefore, of vitamin C to wound healing?**

The significant role of vitamin C in cementing the ground substance of supportive tissue makes it an important agent in wound healing. This has evident implications in clinical practice for vitamin C therapy. For example, in surgery, especially where extensive tissue regeneration is involved, such as in a mastectomy or severe burns, a patient may need from 1 to 2 gm. daily *or more* of vitamin C, an amount ten or more times the usual daily allowance.

■ **Does vitamin C help prevent infections, such as the common cold?**

It is true that infectious processes deplete tissue stores of vitamin C and necessitate additional intake. Apparently this is especially true of infection with bacteria. Optimum tissue stores of vitamin C, therefore, help maintain resistance to infection. Just how large a therapeutic dose may be required to maintain this prevention of in-

fections is not known. There is much controversy concerning the effective use of massive doses of vitamin C in the prevention of the common cold. As yet there is not sufficient evidence to substantiate claims for the validity of such megadoses. The result beyond the level at which tissue saturation is maintained is excreted in the urine; and hence one may only be producing an expensive urine rather than maintaining great therapeutic effectiveness. Fevers also deplete tissue stores of vitamin C, since they accompany infectious processes and have a catabolic effect on tissue.

■ **Is vitamin C related to general physiologic stress?**

Yes. Any body stress, such as injury, fracture, general illness, or shock, calls on vitamin C tissue stores. The reaction to stress by the body is to mobilize its protective forces, especially those chemical messengers, the hormones, which trigger protective homeostatic mechanisms. Large amounts of vitamin C tissue stores have been found concentrated in adrenal tissue, for example. A dose of ACTH has been demonstrated to deplete the adrenal tissue of vitamin C. Thus it is evident that optimum tissue stores of vitamin C are a protection in times of stress.

Normal physiologic stress periods, such as growth, also require additional vitamin C. During pregnancy, therefore, additional vitamin C is needed for fetal growth and maternal tissues. Also, infancy and childhood require additional vitamin C, especially in rapid growth periods, such as during adolescence.

■ **What is the requirement for vitamin C?**

There are a number of difficulties in establishing precise requirements for vitamin C. Questions revolve around individual tissue need, presence of stress situations, and whether minimum or optimum intakes are desired. Although studies indicate that a lower intake (from 20 to 30 mg. daily) will suffice for the average adult, the National Research Council's revised allowances recommend 60 mg. daily for optimum margins to cover variances in tissue de-

Table 6-3. Summary of vitamin C (ascorbic acid)

Physiological functions	Clinical applications	Requirement	Food sources

Intercellular cement substance:
  1. collagen formation
  2. firm capillary walls
General metabolism:
  1. makes iron available for
    hemoglobin and maturation
    of red blood cells
  2. influences conversion of
    folic acid to "citrovorum
    factor" (folinic acid)
	Scurvy (deficiency)
	Megaloblastic anemia
	Wound healing; tissue
	  formation
	Fevers and infections
	Stress reactions
	Growth periods
		60 mg. daily
		(adults)
			Citrus fruits
			Tomatoes
			Cabbage
			Potatoes
			Strawberries
			Melon
			Chili peppers

mands. In considering vitamin C requirements, it seems wise to follow such logical recommendations to provide safety ranges for optimum need. But at the same time it seems wise to avoid extravagant and wasteful excesses in the name of good health when the situation does not demand therapeutic measures.

■ **What are the main food sources of vitamin C?**

Vitamin C can be oxidized easily. Thus the adequacy of any food source must consider the handling, preparation, cooking, and processing of that food source in evaluation of its contribution to the diet of this vitamin. Well-known sources include citrus fruit and tomatoes. Additional good sources include cabbage, sweet potatoes, white potatoes, and green and yellow vegetables. Seasonal or regional foods, such as berries, melons, chili peppers, green peppers, guavas, pineapple, chard, kale, turnip greens, broccoli, and asparagus also provide additional sources.

A summary of vitamin C and its role in metabolism is given in Table 6-3.

■ **What are bioflavonoids?**

Bioflavonoids is a term given to a widely occurring group of natural pigments in flowers, fruits, grains, and vegetables. These substances are called flavonoids because of their basic yellow coloring (L. *flavus*, yellow). Some of these materials are naturally occurring yellow dyes. In the early research for a substance to cure scurvy, these materials were thought to present some hope for isolating the factor involved. However, the hope did not materialize and subsequent tests did not indicate any value in these substances as a treatment for scurvy or related conditions. The name "vitamin P" was originally used for these substances from the name "Permeabilitäts-Vitamin." However, this term has been discontinued and the term "bioflavonoid" has been used instead, although "vitamin P" may still appear occasionally in literature. Although it has been several decades since this work was done, numerous workers have since tried to study the effects of the flavonoids (*citrin*, from citrus rind and *rutin*, from buckwheat) on capillary fragility, infections, the common cold, hypertension, and various hemorrhagic disorders. As yet, however, no therapeutic value has been demonstrated. Although the bioflavonoids may possess mild pharmacologic properties under certain conditions, they have no known nutritional functions, and they cannot be considered essential nutrients.

7 Minerals

Minerals are inorganic elements that are widely distributed in nature, many of which have vital roles in metabolism. Far from being static, inert body materials, the minerals are active participants in the overall metabolic process. They are builders, activators, regulators, transmitters, and controllers. The minerals found in the human body may be grouped as to whether they are found in large amounts (major minerals), are present in small amounts and have a known function (trace minerals), or are present in small amounts but their function is not understood. There are seven minerals in each of these three groups. The major minerals contribute 60% to 80% of all the inorganic material in the body.

Group I: Major minerals

Calcium (Ca)	Magnesium (Mg)
Sodium (Na)	Potassium (K)
Phosphorus (P)	Sulfur (S)
Chlorine (Cl)	

Group II: Trace minerals

Iron (Fe)	Copper (Cu)
Iodine (I)	Manganese (Mn)
Cobalt (Co)	Zinc (Zn)
Molybdenum (Mo)	

Group III: Function unknown

Fluorine (Fl)	Aluminum (Al)
Boron (Br)	Selenium (Se)
Cadmium (Cd)	Chromium (Cr)
Vanadium (V)	

Each of the minerals in Groups I and II above is known to act dynamically in human physiology.

MAJOR MINERALS
Calcium

■ **How much calcium is there in the body and where is it located?**

Calcium is present in by far the largest amounts of all the minerals in the human body. It comprises about 1.5% to 2.0% of the total body weight. For example, a person weighing about 120 pounds has about 2 pounds of calcium in his body. Most of this mineral—99%—is in skeletal tissue (bones and teeth) as deposits of the calcium salts, dahllite or apatite. The remaining 1% of the total body calcium occurs in the plasma and other body fluids and performs highly important metabolic tasks.

■ **In what forms does calcium occur in the body fluids?**

The 1% of total body calcium that appears in the body fluids occurs in three forms: nondiffusible, diffusible, and constituent of an organic complex. These three fractions are normally in equilibrium:

1. *Nondiffusible fraction.* About half of the calcium in the plasma and other body fluids is bound with plasma proteins, albumin, and globulin; thus it is nondiffusible. Since the levels of plasma proteins vary, the size of this fraction varies accordingly.

2. *Diffusible calcium.* Ionized free calcium (Ca^{++}) makes up the other half of the calcium in the plasma. Since it is ionized and thus diffusible, it has the greatest physiologic effect of all three fractions. It exerts a profound influence on metabolism and function of bone, the nervous system. and the heart.

3. *Organic complex form.* About 5% of the plasma calcium occurs as part of organic complexes, such as citrate and other substances. In this form it is diffusible with the complex.

■ **What is meant by the "serum ratio" of calcium to phosphorus—Ca:P?**

The amounts of calcium and phosphorus in the serum are normally maintained in a definite relationship called the *serum calcium-to-phosphorus ratio.* This ratio may be expressed in the following equation: $Ca \times P = K$. The letter "K" stands for the constant product of the two materials, which must be maintained in the serum. This ratio, thus, is the product (solubility product) of calcium times phosphorus, expressed in milligrams of each mineral per 100 ml. of serum. Since the serum level of calcium is normally 10 mg./100 ml., and that of phosphorus is normally 4 mg./100 ml. in adults (5 mg./100 ml. in children), the normal Ca:P ratios are $10 \times 4 = 40$ for adults and $10 \times 5 = 50$ for children. Briefly expressed, the ratios are Ca:P = 40 (adult) and Ca:P = 50 (child). It is evident, then, that a change in the quantity of either mineral would necessitate a subsequent opposite change in the mineral in order that the product (solubility product) of the two minerals could be held at its necessary constant figure. For example, if an excess load of phosphate enters the system, there necessarily follows a consequent drop in the calcium in the serum in order to maintain the solubility product constant.

■ **How may the concept of homeostasis be applied to calcium metabolism?**

Formerly, bone tissue was thought of as an inert site of static deposit of calcium for storage. It has been demonstrated that this is not true. Between the large bone compartment of calcium in the body and the smaller circulating serum calcium there is a constant interchange to maintain a balance between the two. Balance mechanisms are constantly at work to maintain the level of calcium in the circulating plasma within its narrow, normal range. The concepts that have emerged are basic to the understanding of the metabolism of many substances and are highly significant. Using calcium as a model, four interrelated metabolic activities emerge:

General metabolic concept	Application to calcium homeostasis
1. Maintenance of intestinal absorption-excretion balance	1. Intestinal adjustment of calcium absorption and excretion
2. Renal adjustment of excretion (the kidney threshold)	2. Renal adjustment of calcium excretion in the urine
3. Maintenance of a storage compartment	3. Maintenance of calcium stores in bone
4. Hormonal regulation	4. Parathyroid hormone control of calcium homeostasis

Thus, it can be seen that the homeostatic mechanisms involved in calcium balance may be viewed around two basic pairs of balances: (1) absorption-excretion balance, and (2) deposition-mobilization balance.

■ **How is calcium absorbed?**

From 10% to 30% of the calcium in an average diet is absorbed through the intestine. Absorption takes place chiefly in the proximal intestinal tract (the duodenal area), where the pH tends to be lower than in the distant portion of the intestine because the acidity of the gastric juices has not yet been reduced. Since calcium salts are relatively insoluble in a less acid medium, absorption is favored by the greater acidity of the chyme as it immediately enters the duodenum. The necessary agent for this absorption is vitamin D. Vitamin D appears to have some direct effect on the intestinal mucosa, which increases the active transport of calcium across the membrane.

■ **What factors increase calcium absorption?**

Calcium absorption is increased or favored by several factors, including the need of the body, the nature of the diet, and the degree of acidity of the intestinal medium:

1. *Body need.* During periods of greater demand, such as growth or depletion states, more calcium is absorbed. In well-nourished individuals a relatively small percentage of the total calcium ingested is absorbed.

2. *Calcium ion concentration in extracellular fluid.* Even a small change in the

concentration of ionized calcium in the body fluids is reflected in a several-fold rise in the rate of calcium absorption. The maintenance of ionized calcium concentration within this narrow range is controlled by the parathyroid hormone.

3. *Protein intake.* A greater percentage of calcium is absorbed when the diet is high in protein than when it is low in protein. This is probably caused by the influence of the amino acids lysine, arginine, and serine on intestinal pH and on the formation of soluble calcium–amino acid complexes.

4. *Carbohydrate intake.* Lactose especially seems to enhance the absorption of calcium in the ileum, perhaps through action of the lactobacilli to produce lactic acid, which in turn lowers the pH.

5. *Acidity.* Generally the higher the acidity of the solution the greater the solubility of calcium and consequently its absorption. Hence a lower pH favors absorption.

■ **What factors decrease or hinder calcium absorption?**

A number of factors decrease calcium absorption. These include:

1. *Vitamin D deficiency.* Since vitamin D is necessary for the absorption of calcium, the mineral cannot be absorbed without it.

2. *Fats.* Excess fat in the diet or poor absorption of fats results in an excess of free fatty acids in the intestine. The fatty acids and companion glycerides combine with free calcium to form insoluble soaps, a process called *saponification.* These insoluble soaps are then excreted, with consequent loss of the incorporated calcium. This condition occurs, for example, in such intestinal malabsorption diseases as celiac disease and sprue. These conditions are characterized by the passage of multiple, large foamy stools.

3. *Ratio of calcium to phosphorus in the diet.* The optimal *dietary ratio* of calcium to phosphorus is 1:1 in the diet of children and of women during the latter half of pregnancy and during lactation. Other adults require phosphorus in an amount one to one and one-half times the intake of calcium. If either mineral is taken in excess of this ratio, absorption of both is hindered. The lesser mineral is excreted, then, in larger amounts.

4. *Binding agents.* Certain binding agents that occur naturally in foods along with calcium may bind the calcium and prevent its absorption. Oxalic acid, for example, a constituent of some foods, such as spinach, combines with calcium to produce calcium oxalate, a relatively insoluble compound, and thus prevents calcium absorption. Phytic acid, a material found in the outer hulls of many cereal grains, especially wheat, also forms an insoluble compound with calcium, calcium phytate, which binds the calcium and prevents its absorption.

5. *Alkalinity.* Calcium is insoluble in an alkaline medium and therefore is poorly absorbed in this state.

■ **How is calcium excreted and what factors influence this excretion?**

Calcium may be excreted through several channels—the feces, the urine, and in bile. The quantity of calcium excreted tends to balance the quantity absorbed. Amounts that are ingested in excess of need and that remain unabsorbed in the intestine are excreted in the feces. For example, from an average American diet that contains ample amounts of calcium, 70% to 90% of the total calcium ingested is thus excreted.

When the calcium level in serum is high as a result of excess bone destruction or mobilization of calcium from any storage site, the excess calcium is excreted in the urine. Ordinarily, however, about 99% of the ionized calcium filtered by the renal glomeruli is reabsorbed in the renal tubules. Thus a relatively small amount of calcium is excreted by way of the urine.

Calcium is also excreted through the intestinal digestive secretions, especially the bile. The intestinal juices contain about 500 mg. of calcium.

■ **How is the necessary balance of calcium maintained in bone tissue?**

Bone is a dynamic tissue characterized

by a constant turnover of calcium. Balance results from this constant process of laying down of calcium (accretion or deposition) and the breaking down of calcium (resorption or mobilization). Circulating ionized calcium is constantly being deposited in bone, whereas the calcium stored in bone is perpetually being mobilized and withdrawn. There is an actively exchangeable reservoir of about 4 gm. of calcium in equilibrium with the free plasma ionized calcium, and there is a much larger, more stable calcium bone reserve that exchanges more slowly. The agents that control this vital balance of calcium between the bone compartment and the circulating serum calcium are parthyroid hormone and vitamin D.

1. *Parathyroid hormone* (*PH*). The parathyroid gland is particularly sensitive to changes in the circulating plasma level of free ionized calcium. In the typical feedback mechanism involved with endocrine secretions, when serum calcium level drops, the parathyroid releases its hormone, which acts in three ways to restore the normal calcium level:

a. It stimulates the intestinal mucosa to increase the absorption of calcium.

b. It mobilizes calcium rapidly from the bone compartment.

c. It causes renal excretion of phosphate.

These combined activities restore calcium and phosphorus to their correctly balanced ratios in the blood. Then by the feedback mechanism, as this correct blood level is attained, the hormone supply is cut off.

2. *Vitamin D.* Vitamin D not only plays a part in the absorption of calcium but also influences the deposition of calcium in the bone matrix. Studies have shown that vitamin D has a direct influence on the calcification of bone tissue, although not as great an influence as at the point of absorption in the intestine. The effect of the other agent, parathyroid hormone, is greater at the point of bone calcium mobilization. Thus, it is the cooperative action

of these two factors in synergistic behavior that maintains the balance of calcium and phosphorus in the blood. The various factors that influence and control the balance of calcium in the body are shown in the diagram in Fig. 7-1.

■ **How does calcium function in bone and teeth formation?**

The major function of calcium in the body is to build and maintain skeletal tissue. Of the total amount present in the body, 99% is engaged in this purpose. This process is carried on by two types of cells. *Osteoblasts* continually form new bone matrixes, basic protein material, to which calcium phosphate is anchored, and bone crystals develop. *Osteoclasts* continually balance this depositing or mineralizing activity by absorbing bone tissue. The inorganic material of bone consists mainly of phosphate and carbonate salts of calcium anchored to a protein bone matrix. The organic material in bone, the bone matrix, is similar to that of cartilage in that it contains collagen, which can be converted to gelatin. There are also other protein compounds, a glycoprotein named *osseo-mucoid* and an *osseo-albumoid*.

Calcium phosphate deposits are also important in *tooth formation*. As the teeth develop, tooth-forming organs called *ameloblasts* deposit calcium and other constituents. The mineral exchange continues, as in bone, though at a slower rate. This exchange occurs mainly in the dentine and cementum. Very little exchange occurs in the enamel. For proper calcification to proceed, the diet must not only contain adequate calcium and phosphorus but also vitamins A, C, and D. When the diet is low in calcium and phosphorus, the demineralization of bone exceeds that of teeth. In fact, the teeth may actually calcify during the restricted period but at a slower than normal rate. This suggests that the mineral metabolism of teeth and that of bone is not necessarily parallel.

■ **What relation does calcium have to blood clotting?**

The remaining 1% of the body's calcium performs several vital physiologic func-

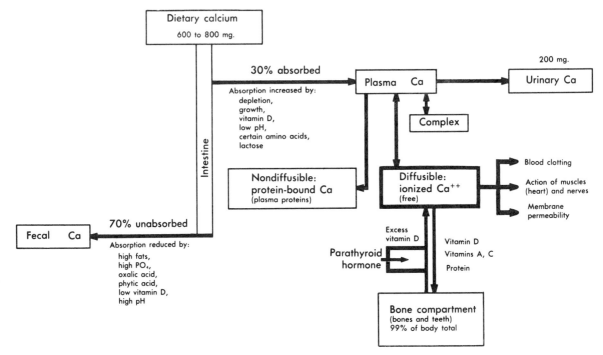

Fig. 7-1. Calcium metabolism. Note the relative distribution of calcium in the body.

tions. It participates in the blood-clotting mechanism through its ionized portion of diffusible free calcium. In blood clotting these calcium ions enhance bonding between fibrin molecules and give stability to the fibrin threads required for conversion of prothrombin to thrombin (see Fig. 6-1, p. 50).

■ **How does calcium function in muscle contraction and relaxation?**

Ionized serum calcium, the free diffusible fraction, plays an important role in the initiation of muscle contraction. Each muscle fiber contains hundreds of small contractile units called *myofibrils*, which are composed of the muscle protein filaments, *myosin* and *actin*. Alongside each myofibril is a fine system of tubes—the *tubular reticulum*. Calcium is firmly bound to this reticulum. When the signal for contraction comes, the calcium ions activate the chemical reaction between myosin and actin filaments that releases a large amount of energy from ATP and brings about the contraction. The calcium ions

are then immediately bound back on the reticulum, causing relaxation. Other elements, such as ionized magnesium and potassium, are also involved in this process. The catalyzing action of calcium ions on the muscle protein filaments myosin and actin, which allows the sliding contraction between them to occur, is particularly vital in the contraction-relaxation cycle of the heart muscle.

■ **Does calcium also have a role in nerve transmission?**

Yes. Calcium is required for normal transmission of nerve impulses. Calcium ions in the extracellular fluid at the neuromuscular junction apparently cause the excitatory transmitting substance *acetylcholine* to rupture through the separating membranes at the tips of the many nerve branches and thus excite the muscle fiber. Acetylcholine is the chemical transmitter substance that carries the nerve impulse from the nerve to the muscle.

■ **Does calcium have an effect on cell wall permeability?**

Yes. Ionized calcium controls the passage of fluid through cell walls by affecting cell wall permeability. This is apparently the result of calcium's influence on the integrity of the intercellular cement substance to which vitamin C contributes (see p. 67).

■ **What relation does calcium have to enzyme action?**

Calcium ions are important activators of certain enzymes, such as adenosine triphosphatase (ATPase). This enzyme plays an important role in the energy release for muscle contraction by catalyzing the breaking off of a phosphate bond on ATP. Calcium ions play a similar role with other enzymes, including lipase and some members of the protein-splitting enzyme system.

■ **What disease conditions result from disorders in calcium balance in metabolism?**

A number of clinical situations are related to calcium metabolism:

1. *Tetany.* A decrease in ionized serum calcium causes tetany, a state marked by severe, intermittent spastic contractions of the muscle and by muscular pain. It is manifested by a characteristic carpopedal spasm of the muscles in the upper extremity, which causes flexion of wrist and thumb with extension of the fingers. This characteristic spasm is called *Trousseau's sign* and is a diagnostic observation for the presence of tetany.

Tetanylike responses may be caused by an increase in the serum phosphorus fraction in the calcium-to-phosphorus ratio (see p. 71), which causes a decrease in the calcium level to maintain the solubility product of calcium × phosphorus. Two examples of this response are: (1) A so-called *milk tetany* may occur in newborn infants fed undiluted cow's milk. Cow's milk contains a greater phosphorus-to-calcium ratio than does breast milk, and the kidneys of the newborn human infant may not clear this phosphate load. Phosphorus, therefore, accumulates in the serum. This rise in serum phosphorus causes a compensatory decrease in serum calcium in order to maintain the necessary calcium × phosphorus solubility product in the serum. The calcium decrease in turn causes the typical tetanylike muscular spasms. (2) Occasional leg cramps of pregnancy have been attributed by some observers to a similar rise in phosphorus intake, although other factors may cause this phenomenon. If the pregnant woman drinks an excess of the recommended amount of milk (three to four cups daily), she may be consuming a greater amount of phosphorus in relation to calcium than is wise for her.

2. *Rickets.* When adequate calcium and phosphorus are not absorbed because sufficient vitamin D is not present to control this absorption, proper bone formation cannot take place. Thus the inadequately mineralized bones respond to various pressures of weight bearing and cause symptoms such as bowed legs or beaded ribs (see p. 175).

3. *Renal calculi.* The great majority of renal stones are composed of calcium compounds. A predisposing factor to the formation of these calculi may be an increase in the amount of calcium that must be excreted in the urine as calcium is mobilized or withdrawn from the bone compartment. Immobilization of the body is one condition that causes such resorption of calcium from bone stores into the blood. This has definite clinical implications. When a full body cast or some other orthopedic device immobilizes the body for a long period, dietary calcium intake should be adequate but should not exceed the usual daily allowance. If renal stones have already occurred, the amount of calcium in the diet should be somewhat reduced.

4. *Hyperparathyroidism and hypoparathyroidism.* Calcium and phosphorus metabolism are directly controlled by parathyroid hormone. Therefore conditions of the parathyroid gland that increase or decrease the secretion of its hormone will immediately be reflected in abnormal metabolism of these two minerals.

■ **What is the dietary requirement for calcium?**

The National Research Council recommends allowances for calcium of 800 mg. daily for men or women, with increases to 1.3 gm. during pregnancy and lactation. Infants younger than 1 year should have 400 to 600 mg., and children of older ages should have 0.7 to 1.4 gm. daily.

■ **What are the main food sources of calcium?**

Dairy products supply the bulk of dietary calcium. One quart of milk contains about 1 gm. of calcium and cheese contains a comparable amount. Secondary sources include egg yolk, green leafy vegetables, legumes, nuts, and whole grains.

Phosphorus

■ **How much phosphorus is there in the body and where is it located?**

Phosphorus comprises 0.8% to 1.1% of the total body weight. For example, a person weighing 120 pounds would have about 1.2 pounds of phosphorus in his body. From 80% to 90% of this phosphorus is in the skeleton, including the teeth, compounded with calcium. The remaining 20% is in the serum and distributed throughout the cells. In the cells it has essential relationships with proteins, lipids, and carbohydrates to produce energy to build and repair tissues and to act as a buffer.

The serum phosphorus level normally ranges from 3 to 4.5 mg./100 ml. in adults and is somewhat higher, 4 to 7 mg./100 ml., in children. The serum phosphorus is maintained in a definite relationship with serum calcium (see p. 71). The higher range of serum phosphorus for children during the growth years is a significant clue to the role of this mineral in cell metabolism. The total inorganic serum phosphorus exists in the form of the two balancing buffer anions: $HPO_4^=$ (phosphate), 2.1 mEq./liter; and $H_2PO_4^-$ (phosphoric acid), 0.26 mEq./liter. Other phosphorus in the body occurs as a constituent of organic compounds.

■ **How is phosphorus absorbed?**

The absorption of phosphorus is closely related to that of calcium (see p. 71). Equal amounts of the two minerals in the diet is an optimal ratio. Excess of either causes increased fecal excretion of the other. Apparently phosphorus is more efficiently absorbed than calcium, however, since only 30% of the ingested phosphorus (bound to calcium) is excreted in the feces and about 70% is absorbed, compared with only 10% to 30% of dietary calcium that is absorbed.

The mechanism of absorption is related to vitamin D as is calcium. This relation to vitamin D is not a direct one, apparently, as it is with calcium, but an indirect one in that as calcium is absorbed under the influence of vitamin D the absorption of phosphorus follows. Factors that influence the absorption of calcium also affect phosphorus.

■ **How is phosphorus excreted and what factors influence this excretion?**

The main avenue of phosphorus excretion is through the kidneys. The *renal threshold for phosphate* means that the amount of phosphate excreted by the kidney is relative to the serum phosphorus level. If the serum phosphorus level falls, the renal tubules respond by returning more phosphorus to the blood. If the serum phosphorus level rises, the renal tubules respond by excreting more. When the diet lacks sufficient phosphorus, the renal tubules conserve phosphorus by returning it to the blood. By this means, normal serum phosphorus levels are maintained through the work of the kidney. The amount of phosphorus excreted in the urine of a person ingesting an average diet is 0.6 to 1.0 gm. every 24 hours. The normal excretion balance may be influenced abnormally by excessive secretions of parathyroid hormone.

■ **What is the role of parathyroid hormone in phosphorus metabolism?**

The homeostatic mechanism by which the kidneys maintain the serum phosphorus level is controlled by the parathyroid hormone. This action is usually interdependent with calcium balance (see p. 73). When

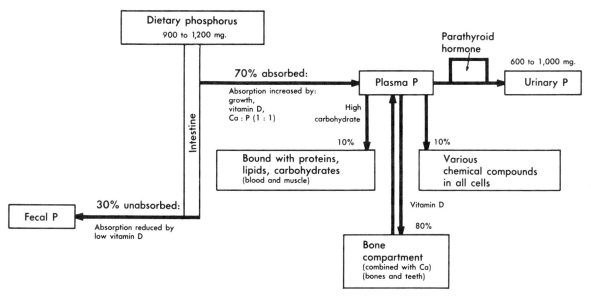

Fig. 7-2. Relative distribution and interchange of phosphorus in the body.

the serum phosphorus level rises, the parathyroid hormone blocks renal tubular resorption of phosphorus so that more phosphorus is excreted in the urine. The serum phosphorus level and the calcium-to-phosphorus ratio are returned, therefore, to normal. The balance concept is applied to the equilibrium existing between the phosphorus in the bone compartment and the phosphorus in the circulating serum. These various relationships are shown in Fig. 7-2.

■ **How does phosphorus function in the formation of bones and teeth?**

Eighty percent of body phosphorus contributes to mineralization of bones and teeth. As a component of calcium phosphate, it is constantly being deposited and reabsorbed in the dynamic process of bone formation (see p. 73).

■ **How does phosphorus function in overall body metabolism?**

Far out of proportion in importance to the relatively small amount of the remainder, 20% of the body phosphorus is intimately involved in overall human metabolism. This vital role is indicated by its presence in every living cell. There are a number of relationships with other nutrients:

1. *Absorption of glucose and glycerol.*

By the process of phosphorylation, phosphorus combines with glucose and glycerol from fat to promote the absorption of these substances from the intestine. Phosphorylation also promotes the renal tubular reabsorption of glucose by which this sugar is conserved and returned to the blood.

2. *Transport of fatty acids.* By combination with fat as phospholipids, phosphorus helps to provide a vehicular form for fat.

3. *Energy metabolism.* Phosphorus is an essential part of such key cellular nucleoprotein substances as DNA and phosphatides, which also participate in the formation of numerous enzymes in the pathway for glucose oxidation and final energy production. These nucleoprotein substances are a key power source in the high-energy phosphate bonds of such compounds as ATP.

4. *Buffer system.* The phosphate buffer system of phosphoric acid and phosphate contributes additional control of acidotic and alkalotic states in the blood.

■ **Does normal growth affect serum phosphorus levels?**

Yes. Growing children usually have high serum phosphate levels, probably resulting from high levels of growth hormone. Also, the need for phosphorus is increased in the growth process because of the vital relationship of phosphorus to bone growth and metabolism, and hence to overall tissue growth.

■ **What clinical conditions are related to changes in serum phosphorus levels?**

Several clinical conditions affect the serum phosphorus level:

1. *Recovery from diabetic acidosis.* Active carbohydrate absorption and metabolism use much phosphorus, depositing it with glycogen, thus causing temporary hypophosphatemia.

2. *Hypophosphatemia.* Intestinal diseases, such as sprue and celiac disease, in which phosphorus absorption is hindered, or bone diseases, such as rickets or osteomalacia, in which the calcium-to-phosphorus balance is upset, are characterized by low serum phosphorus levels. The serum phosphorus level is also low in primary hyperparathyroidism. The excess quantity of parathyroid hormone secreted results in excessive renal tubular excretion of phosphorus. Symptoms of hypophosphatemia include muscle weakness, because the muscle cells are deprived of phosphorus essential for energy metabolism.

3. *Hyperphosphatemia.* Renal insufficiency or hypoparathyroidism cause excessive accumulation of serum phosphorus. As a result the calcium side of the calcium-to-phosphorus serum ratio is low. This causes tetanylike response.

■ **What is the dietary requirement of phosphorus?**

The National Research Council recommends a phosphorus allowance equal to that for calcium for all ages except the young infant. For the infant the proportion of phosphorus is *lower* than calcium. During growth, pregnancy, and lactation, the ratio of phosphorus to calcium in the diet is ideally 1:1. In ordinary adult life the intake of phosphorus is about one to one and one-half times that of calcium. A specific quantitative requirement is not stated because the two minerals are generally found in the same food sources, and if calcium needs are met adequate phosphorus will be assured.

■ **What are the main food sources of phosphorus?**

Milk and milk products are the most significant sources of phosphorus, just as they are for calcium. However, because of the role of phosphorus in cell metabolism and hence the presence of phosphorus in muscle cells, lean meats are also a good source.

Magnesium

■ **How much magnesium is there in the body and where is it located?**

There are about 25 gm. of magnesium in an adult, and 70% of this is combined with calcium and phosphorus in the bone salts complex. The remaining 30% is distributed in various soft tissues and body fluids. Plasma magnesium values range from 1.4 to 2.5 mg./100 ml. Unlike calcium, magnesium occurs predominantly in the red blood cells and there is relatively little in the serum. About 80% of the blood magnesium is ionized and diffusible. The remainder is bound with serum protein as is the nondiffusible calcium. Muscle tissue contains more magnesium than calcium, whereas blood contains more calcium than magnesium.

■ **How is magnesium absorbed?**

On an average diet only about 45% of the ingested magnesium is absorbed. The remaining 55% is excreted in the feces. Absorption occurs in the upper small intestine. Factors that inhibit calcium absorption also hinder magnesium absorption. These include the presence of excess fat, phosphate, calcium, or alkalis. Parathyroid hormone also increases magnesium absorption from the intestine. Vitamin D, however, apparently does not affect magnesium absorption. Urinary excretion is relatively low, since the kidney conserves magnesium efficiently. Aldosterone increases the renal clearance of magnesium, as it does that of potassium, in exchange for sodium conservation.

■ **What are the metabolic functions of magnesium?**

Ionized magnesium is essential to cellular metabolism of both carbohydrate and protein because it is a significant cation of the intracellular fluid. These metabolic functions of magnesium include the following:

1. *Carbohydrate metabolism.* Ionized magnesium serves as an activator of many enzymes in the reactions of the initial Embden-Meyerhof glycolytic pathway for glucose oxidation (oxidative phosphorylation).

2. *Protein metabolism.* Ionized magnesium is a coenzyme in protein synthesis in the cell ribosomes.

3. *Decreased ionized magnesium concentration.* This causes vasodilation and inhibits smooth muscle action. Normally ionized magnesium, like potassium, is concentrated in the intracellular fluid. Any changes in this concentration produce neuromuscular irritability.

■ **What clinical conditions are related to magnesium deficiency?**

Magnesium deficiency may be related to gastrointestinal disorders. In prolonged diarrhea or vomiting, as in diseases characterized by intestinal malabsorption, excessive amounts of magnesium are lost. Dehydration must be accompanied by adequate magnesium replacement. Otherwise the resulting low-serum magnesium level may give rise to general neuromuscular irritability, manifested by tremor, spasm, and increased startle response to sound and touch. A tetanylike syndrome has also been observed in persons with chronic alcoholism in whom magnesium deficiency has developed.

■ **What is the requirement for magnesium?**

The National Research Council has set adult recommendations at 350 mg. daily for men and 300 mg. for women. A natural magnesium deficiency in man, however, is unlikely. Any deficiency would probably be long term and cumulative and may have a role in chronic cardiovascular, neuromuscular, and renal diseases.

■ **What are the main food sources of magnesium?**

Magnesium is relatively widespread in nature. Its main sources include nuts, soybeans, cocoa, seafood, whole grains, dried beans, and peas.

Sodium

■ **How much sodium is there in the body and where is it located?**

Sodium is crucial to many important metabolic activities, and as such is one of the most plentiful of the minerals in the body. Of the 4 ounces or so in the body of a person weighing 154 pounds about one third is present in the skeleton as inorganic bound material. The remaining two thirds—the majority—is found in the extracellular fluids, where it functions as the major cation. This extracellular ionized sodium (Na^+) is largely distributed in plasma and in nerve and muscle tissue. Normal blood serum values range from 136 to 145 mEq./liter or from 310 to 340 mg./100 ml.

■ **How is the absorption and excretion of sodium regulated?**

Sodium is readily absorbed from the intestine. Normally only about 5% of all the sodium ingested is lost in the feces. Larger amounts are passed by this route in abnormal states, such as diarrhea, when the intestinal contents leave the body in large volumes. Almost all of the sodium that leaves the body—95%—is excreted in the urine. This renal control of sodium excretion is regulated largely by hormones of the adrenal gland, especially the powerful mineralocorticoid *aldosterone* (see p. 112). The aldosterone mechanism for sodium conservation is one of the major homeostatic controls of the body sodium and hence of body water.

■ **What are the metabolic functions of sodium?**

Since sodium ions largely relate to water in the body, the major metabolic functions concern fluid balance and acid-base balance. Other functions relate to cell permeability and normal muscle irritability.

1. *Fluid balance.* Since ionized sodium

is the major cation of the water outside the cells, variations in the concentration of ionized sodium largely determine the shift of water by osmosis from one body area to another. These shifts of water from one part of the body to another are the means whereby substances in solution in the body water can circulate between the cells and the fluid that surrounds them. Such shifts also protect the body against large fluid losses. The role of sodium in the maintenance of fluid balance is vital to body metabolism.

2. *Acid-base balance.* Through its association with chloride and bicarbonate ions, ionized sodium is an important factor in the regulation of the acid-base balance of the body. The carbonic acid-sodium bicarbonate buffer system is the main system used by the body to maintain acid-base balance.

3. *Cell permeability.* The sodium pump associated with glucose metabolism and the cellular exchange of ionized sodium affects cell permeability (see p. 9). By this active mode of transport sodium appears to be essential to the passage of glucose and potassium through cell walls.

4. *Normal muscle irritability.* Sodium ions transmit electrochemical impulses along nerve and muscle membranes and therefore maintain normal muscle irritability or excitability. Potassium and sodium ions balance the response of nerves to stimulation, the travel of nerve impulses to muscles, and the resulting contraction of the muscle fibers.

■ **What is the requirement for sodium?**

A specific dietary requirement for sodium is not stated. Apparently the body can function on a rather wide range of exogenous sodium through the operation of mechanisms designed to conserve or excrete this mineral. The amount of sodium in the American diet is 4 gm. of sodium in the average 10 gm. of table salt consumed daily. This is about ten times the quantity that the body requires for the maintenance of adequate balance. Thus, it is a learned taste level, not a physiologic necessity. An intake of about 5 gm. of table

salt, or 2 gm. of sodium, has been recommended for adults. For those with a family history of hypertension, however, the recommended quantity in food is even less—from 1 to 2 gm. of salt daily.

■ **What are the main food sources of sodium?**

Common salt (NaCl) used in cooking and for seasoning is the main dietary source of sodium. Other food sources include milk, meat, egg, and certain vegetables, such as carrots, beets, spinach and other leafy greens, celery, artichokes, and asparagus.

Potassium

■ **How much potassium is in the body and where is it located?**

Potassium is about twice as plentiful as sodium in the body. The body of an average man weighing 154 pounds contains about 9 ounces (4,000 mEq.) of potassium. By far the larger portion is found inside the cells. Potassium is the major cation (K^+) of the water inside the cell (see p. 104). However, the relatively small amount in extracellular fluid has a significant effect on muscle activity, especially the heart muscle. The normal blood serum values for potassium range from 3.5 to 5.0 mEq./liter or 14 to 20 mg./100 ml. In comparison, the cell concentration of potassium is about 115 mEq./liter of cell water.

■ **How is the absorption and excretion of potassium regulated?**

Potassium ingested in food is easily absorbed from the small intestine. Since potassium is a component of the digestive juices, a considerable amount of potassium is also secreted into the intestine. However, this potassium in the digestive juices is later reabsorbed during the continuous cycle of gastrointestinal circulation of water and electrolytes. Little potassium is lost in the feces.

Urinary excretion is the principal route of loss. Since maintenance of serum potassium within the narrow normal range is vital to heart muscle action and is an indicator of electrolyte balance, the kidneys guard potassium carefully. The renal glomeruli and tubules filter, reabsorb, secrete, and excrete potassium to maintain normal serum levels even in the face of relatively large injections of potassium. Changes in acid-base balance are reflected in compensatory changes in the amount of potassium excreted in the urine. Hormones of the adrenal cortex, especially aldosterone, also influence potassium excretion. As a part of the aldosterone mechanism that conserves sodium, ionized potassium is excreted in an ion exchange for sodium in the distal renal tubule (see p. 112).

■ **What are the metabolic functions of potassium?**

Potassium serves a number of vital metabolic functions. These include:

1. *Fluid-electrolyte balance.* As a major cation of the intracellular fluid, ionized potassium functions in balance with the extracellular ionized sodium to maintain the normal osmotic pressures and water balance, which guard the integrity of the cellular fluid.

2. *Acid-base balance.* Ionized potassium also exerts an influence on acid-base balance through its operation with ionized sodium and ionized hydrogen.

3. *Muscle activity.* Ionized potassium functions with ionized sodium and calcium to regulate neuromuscular excitability and stimulation, transmission of electrochemical impulses, and contraction of muscle fibers. This effect of ionized potassium is particularly notable in the action of heart muscle. Even small variations in serum potassium concentration are reflected in electrocardiographic changes. Excess serum potassium (hyperkalemia), a common and life-threatening complication of renal failure, severe dehydration, or shock, causes the heart to dilate and become flaccid, which slows its rate. Eventually transmission of the electrochemical impulse that mediates the flow of the beat through the heart may be blocked between the atrium and the ventricles. This is called *atrioventricular block.* An increase in serum potassium concentration to only two or three times the normal level may weaken cardiac

contractions sufficiently to cause death. Low serum potassium concentrations (hypokalemia) may cause muscle irritability and paralysis. The heart may develop gallop rhythm, tachycardia, and finally cardiac arrest.

4. *Carbohydrate metabolism.* When blood glucose is converted to glycogen for storage, potassium is stored with the glycogen. It has been calculated that for every 1 gm. of glycogen stored, 0.36 mM. of potassium is also retained. When a patient in diabetic acidosis is treated by the administration of insulin and glucose, glycogen is rapidly produced and stored. The potassium that is to be stored with the glycogen is quickly withdrawn from the serum. The resulting hypokalemia may be fatal. For this reason the treatment of diabetic acidosis includes replacement of serum potassium.

5. *Protein synthesis.* Potassium is required for the storage of nitrogen as muscle protein. When muscle tissue is broken down, both potassium and nitrogen are lost. Replacement therapy includes amino acids for resynthesis of muscle protein and potassium to ensure nitrogen retention.

■ **What clinical conditions result from elevated serum potassium?**

Any condition that results in renal failure precludes the normal adjustment and clearance of ionized potassium. Serum potassium then rises to toxic levels (hyperkalemia). The too-rapid intravenous administration of potassium may also cause hyperkalemia. Hyperkalemia from either cause results in characteristic weakening of heart action, mental confusion, poor respiration caused by weakening of the respiratory muscles, and numbness of extremities.

■ **What clinical conditions may result from low serum potassium?**

Hypokalemia of dangerous degree may be caused by prolonged wasting disease with tissue destruction and malnutrition. It may also be caused by prolonged gastrointestinal loss of potassium as in diarrhea, vomiting, or gastric suction. The continuous use of certain diuretic drugs, such as chlorothiazide (Diuril) or acetozolamide (Diamox), increases ionized potassium excretion and may leave the serum potassium level abnormally low. Thus, the administration of such drugs is usually accompanied by some source of potassium to replace the loss, and the dose schedule is an intermittent one.

Heart failure and subsequent depletion of ionized potassium in the heart muscle makes the myocardial tissue more sensitive to digitalis toxicity and arrhythmia (irregular contractions). Potassium should be given in such cases to prevent these complications of cardiac failure, especially when potassium-depleting diuretics are also used. Diabetic acidosis requires replacement of potassium for incorporation with glycogen storage.

■ **What is the requirement for potassium?**

No dietary requirement is specified for potassium. The usual diet contains 2 to 4 gm. daily, which seems ample for common need. No deficiency is likely, except in the clinical situations described in the preceding answer.

■ **What are the main food sources of potassium?**

Potassium is widely distributed in natural foods. Meats, legumes, leafy vegetables, whole grains, and certain fruits, such as oranges, bananas, and prunes supply considerable amounts. Many other foods are supplementary sources.

Chlorine

■ **How much chlorine is in the body and where is it located?**

Chlorine accounts for about 3% of the body's total mineral content. It occurs in the body as the chloride ion (Cl^-). Ionized chlorine is the major anion of the extracellular fluid. The cerebrospinal fluid has the highest concentration of chloride (124 mEq./liter or 440 mg./100 ml.). The normal range for plasma level is from 95 to 105 mEq./liter or 340 to 370 mg./100 ml. A relatively large amount of ionized chloride is found in the gastrointestinal secretions as a component of gastric hydrochloric acid. As such it plays a part in acid-base balance.

■ **How is chlorine absorbed and excreted?**

Chloride is almost completely absorbed in the intestine with only a functional fecal loss. Excretion is mainly accomplished through the kidneys. Like sodium, chloride is a threshold substance. It is largely conserved by reabsorption in the renal tubules where it is returned to the circulating plasma. This reabsorption is enhanced by the adrenal hormone aldosterone. The resorption of chloride is secondary to aldosterone's control over the renal absorption of sodium. Since ionized chlorine is a major component of the gastrointestinal circulation, relatively large losses may occur in prolonged vomiting or diarrhea. Such prolonged loss accompanies acid loss as hydrochloric acid, and hence contributes to a state of hypochloremic alkalosis.

■ **What are the metabolic functions of chlorine?**

Chlorine functions mainly in relationship to fluid and electrolyte balance, acid-base balance, and gastric acidity:

1. *Fluid-electrolyte balance.* Together with ionized sodium, ionized chlorine in the extracellular fluid helps to maintain water balance and to regulate osmotic pressure.

2. *Acid-base balance.* Ionized chlorine plays a special role in maintaining a constant pH in the blood through its participation in the *chloride-bicarbonate shift mechanism.* This mechanism operates between the plasma and the red blood cell; ionized chlorine goes into the cell in exchange for HCO_3 (the chloride-bicarbonate shift). This provides constant bicarbonate buffering for the rapidly formed carbonic acid (H_2CO_3) from water and carbon dioxide. These reactions are then reversed in the lungs as carbon dioxide is expired.

3. *Gastric acidity.* Chloride is secreted by the mucosa of the stomach as gastric hydrochloric acid. In this form it provides the necessary acid medium for digestion in the stomach. It also is necessary for the ac-

tivation of enzymes, such as conversion of the pepsinogen to active pepsin in the stomach for initial protein splitting.

■ **What clinical conditions may result from chlorine imbalances?**

Clinical problems resulting from imbalances in chlorine levels in the body include:

1. *Gastrointestinal disorders.* Large amounts of chlorine may be lost during continued vomiting, diarrhea, or tube drainage. Such loss would contribute the complications of hypochloremic alkalosis to the clinical state produced by dehydration. Hence prompt replacement of chloride is essential in rehydration.

2. *Alkalosis.* Gastric secretions such as hydrochloric acid are low in sodium but high in chlorine. Thus, when such secretions are lost, bicarbonate replaces the depleted chloride ions. This produces a type of metabolic alkalosis called hypochloremic alkalosis. Potassium deficiency is a frequent accompaniment.

3. *Endocrine disorders.* Cushing's disease, which is caused by hyperactivity of the adrenal cortex, or excessive quantities of ACTH or cortisone given as therapy, may produce hypokalemia and hypochloremic alkalosis may result.

■ **Is there a specific requirement for chlorine?**

No. A quantitative statement of human requirements of chloride has not been established.

■ **What are the main food sources of chlorine?**

Almost the sole dietary source of chlorine is in table salt (NaCl). When sodium intake is adequate chloride will be amply supplied.

Sulfur

■ **Where does sulfur occur in the body?**

Sulfur occurs in some form throughout the body and is present in all cells. It is usually an essential constituent of cell protein. The plasma sulfur level ranges from 0.7 to 1.5 mEq./liter.

Organic sulfur is divided into nonprotein sulfur and protein sulfur. Nonprotein forms include sulfalipids and sulfatides. Protein forms include sulfur-containing amino acids (methionine and cystine), glycoproteins (conjugates of sulfate and sulfuric acid with carbohydrate derivatives, such as material found in cartilage, tendon, and bone matrix), detoxification products (conjugates that are products formed in part from bacterial putrefaction activity in the intestine), other organic compounds, such as heparin, insulin, thiamine, biotin, lipoic acid, and coenzyme A. Organic sulfur is also found in keratin, the protein of hair and skin. Inorganic forms of sulfur are the sulfates combined with sodium, potassium, and magnesium.

■ **How is sulfur absorbed and excreted?**

Inorganic sulfate compounds are absorbed in the intestine as such and go directly into the portal blood circulation. The sulfur-containing amino acids, methionine and cystine, are split off from protein during digestion and are also absorbed into the portal circulation. These two amino acids are the most important sources of sulfur in the body.

Excretion of sulfur occurs by way of the urine. Since sulfur enters the body chiefly with protein, the amount excreted varies directly with the amount of protein ingested and with the extent of tissue protein breakdown.

■ **What are the metabolic functions of sulfur?**

Sulfur functions in several important metabolic processes:

1. *Maintenance of protein structure.* Disulfide linkages (—S—S—) form an important secondary structure between parallel peptide chains to maintain the stability of proteins.

2. *Activation of enzymes.* Many enzymes depend on a free sulfhydryl group (—SH) to maintain their activity. In this capacity sulfur participates in tissue respiration or biologic oxidation.

3. *Energy metabolism.* The sulfhydryl group (—SH) also forms a high-energy sulfur bond similar to the high-energy phosphate bond (see p. 38). This is an impor-

Table 7-1. Summary of major minerals

Mineral	Metabolism	Physiologic functions	Clinical application	Requirement	Food sources
Calcium (Ca)	Absorption according to body need, aided by vitamin D; favored by protein, lactose, acidity; hindered by excess fats and binding agents (phosphates, oxylates, phytate) Excretion chiefly in feces, 70 to 90% of amount ingested Deposition-mobilization in bone compartment constant; deposition aided by vitamin D Parathyroid hormone controls absorption and mobilization	Bone formation Teeth Blood clotting Muscle contraction and relaxation Heart action Nerve transmission Cell wall permeability Enzyme activation (ATPase)	Tetany—decrease in ionized serum calcium Rickets Renal calculi Hyperparathyroidism Hypoparathyroidism	Adults: .8 gm. Pregnancy and lactation: 1.3 gm. Infants: .7 gm. Children: 0.8 to 1.4 gm.	Milk Cheese Green leafy vegetables Whole grains Egg yolk Legumes, nuts
Phosphorus (P)	Absorption with calcium aided by vitamin D; hindered by excess binding agents (calcium, aluminum and iron) Excretion chiefly by kidney according to renal threshold blood level Parathyroid hormone controls renal excretion balance with blood level Deposition-mobilization in bone compartment constant	Bone formation Overall metabolism: Absorption of glucose and glycerol (phosphorylation) Transport of fatty acids Energy metabolism (enzymes, ATP) Buffer system	Growth Hypophosphatemia: Recovery state from diabetic acidosis Sprue, celiac disease (malabsorption) Bone diseases (upset Ca : P balance) Hyperphosphatemia: Renal insufficiency Hypoparathyroidism Tetany	Adults: 1½ times calcium intake Pregnancy and lactation: 1.3 gm. Infants: 0.2 to 0.5 mg. Children: 0.8 to 1.4 gm.	Milk Cheese Meat Egg yolk Whole grains Legumes, nuts
Magnesium (Mg)	Absorption increased by parathyroid hormone; hindered by excess fat, phosphate, calcium Excretion regulated by kidney	Constituent of bones and teeth Activator and coenzyme in carbohydrate and protein metabolism Essential intracellular fluid (ICF) cation Muscle and nerve irritability	Tremor, spasm; low serum level following gastrointestinal losses	300 to 350 mg. Deficiency in man unlikely	Whole grains Nuts Meat Milk Legumes

Mineral	Metabolism	Physiologic functions	Clinical applications	Daily requirement	Food sources
Sodium (Na)	Readily absorbed. Excretion chiefly by kidney, controlled by aldosterone, acid-base balance	Major extracellular fluid (ECF) cation. Water balance; osmotic pressure. Acid-base balance. Cell permeability; absorption of glucose. Muscle irritability; transmission of electrochemical impulse and resulting contraction	Fluid shifts and control. Buffer system. Losses in gastrointestinal disorders	About 0.5 gm. Diet usually has more: 2 to 6 gm.	Table salt (NaCl). Milk. Meat. Egg. Baking soda. Baking powder. Carrots, beets, spinach, celery
Potassium (K)	Secreted and reabsorbed in digestive juices. Excretion guarded by kidney according to blood levels; increased by aldosterone	Major ICF cation. Acid-base balance. Regulates neuromuscular excitability and muscle contraction. Glycogen formation. Protein synthesis	Fluid shifts. Losses in: Starvation, Diabetic acidosis, Adrenal tumors. Heart action—low serum potassium (tachycardia, cardiac arrest). Treatment of diabetic acidosis (rapid glycogen production reduces serum potassium). Tissue catabolism—potassium loss	About 2 to 4 gm. Diet adequate in protein, calcium, and iron contains adequate potassium	Whole grains. Meat. Legumes. Fruits. Vegetables
Chlorine (Cl)	Absorbed readily. Excretion controlled by kidney	Major ECF anion. Acid-base balance—chloride-bicarbonate shift. Water balance. Gastric hydrochloric acid—digestion	Hypochloremic alkalosis in prolonged vomiting, diarrhea, tube drainage	About 0.5 gm. Diet usually has more: 2 to 6 gm.	Table salt
Sulfur (S)	Absorbed as such and as constituent of sulfur-containing amino acid, methionine. Excreted by kidney in relation to protein intake and tissue catabolism	Essential constituent of cell protein. Activates enzymes. High-energy sulfur bonds in energy metabolism. Detoxification reactions	Cystine renal calculi. Cystinuria	Diet adequate in protein contains adequate sulfur	Meat. Egg. Cheese. Milk. Nuts, legumes

tant aspect of the metabolic activity of acetyl coenzyme A (CoA.SH) or active acetate.

4. *Detoxification.* Sulfur participates in several important detoxification reactions by which toxic materials are conjugated with active sulfate and converted to a nontoxic form for excretion in the urine.

■ **What is the relation of sulfur to cystine renal calculi?**

Cystine renal stones are the result of a relatively rare hereditary defect in renal tubular reabsorption of the amino acid cystine. This defect causes excessive urinary excretion of cystine (cystinuria) and consequently repeated production of kidney stones formed of cystine crystals. These stones are yellowish in color because of the high sulfur content. A low-methionine diet (methionine is the precursor of cystine) is given to reduce the intake and synthesis of these sulfur-containing amino acids.

■ **What is the requirement for sulfur?**

No quantitative dietary requirement has been specified for sulfur, because its major dietary source is in the sulfur-containing amino acids, methionine and cystine. Cystine may be synthesized in the body from the precursor amino acid, methionine. Hence the major food sources are protein foods.

A summary of the major minerals is given in Table 7-1 for review and reference.

TRACE MINERALS
Iron

■ **How small an amount of iron is there in the body? Where is it located?**

The body contains about 45 mg. of iron per kg. of body weight. Thus, a person weighing 55 kg. (121 pounds) would have about 2.5 gm. of iron. This iron is distributed in the body in four main forms, which point to its basic metabolic functions: (1) a transport form of iron called *transferrin;* (2) hemoglobin, about 75% of the body's iron; (3) storage iron, a protein-iron compound called *ferritin,* mainly found in liver, spleen, and bone marrow; and (4) cellular tissue iron, a remaining 5% of total body iron distributed throughout all cells as a

major component of oxidative enzyme systems for the production of energy.

■ **How is the absorption of iron controlled?**

Iron enters the body usually as ferric iron (Fe^{+++}) in food. In the acid medium of the stomach ferric iron is reduced to ferrous (Fe^{++}), the form necessary for absorption. Of the total amount of iron ingested, only about 10% to 30% is absorbed and this absorption occurs mostly in the stomach and the duodenum. The remaining 70% to 90% is eliminated in the feces.

An interesting mechanism, sometimes called the "ironstat," controls the absorption of iron. This mechanism involves the compound storage form of iron called *ferritin.* Iron enters the mucosal cells of the intestine in a complex with amino acids. Here it combines with a protein, *apoferritin,* to form ferritin. The ferritin then controls the absorption or rejection of ingested iron according to the amount of the compound present in the intestinal mucosa. When all available apoferritin has been bound to iron to form ferritin, any additional iron that arrives at the binding site is rejected, returned to the lumen of the intestine, and passed on for excretion in the feces.

■ **What factors facilitate iron absorption?**

Several factors facilitate iron absorption. These include:

1. The amount of reserve ferritin present in mucosal cells correlates with the body's need for iron. Thus, in deficiency states or in periods of extra demand as in growth or pregnancy, mucosal ferritin is lower and greater absorption of iron is facilitated. When tissue reserves are ample or saturated, there is more ferritin present in the mucosal tissues and iron is rejected or excreted.

2. Ascorbic acid (vitamin C) facilitates the absorption of iron by its reducing action and effect on acidity, changing dietary iron (ferric iron, Fe^{+++}) to the ferrous form (Fe^{++}), in which it can be absorbed. Other metabolic reducing agents have similar effects.

3. The amount of hydrochloric acid present influences iron absorption. The optimum acid medium of the gastric secretions prepares the iron for absorption and utilization.

4. An adequate amount of calcium helps to bind and remove agents such as phosphate and phytate, which if not removed would combine with iron and inhibit its absorption.

■ **What factors hinder iron absorption?**

Several factors hinder iron absorption. These include:

1. Surgical removal of stomach tissue (gastrectomy) reduces the number of cells that secrete hydrochloric acid. This acid medium necessary for iron reduction is therefore not provided adequately.

2. Malabsorption syndromes or any disturbance that causes diarrhea or steatorrhea will hinder iron absorption.

3. Severe infection hinders iron absorption.

4. The presence of binding agents such as phosphate, phytate, and oxalate remove iron from the body.

■ **What is the transport form of iron?**

Transferrin is the transport form of iron. Mucosal ferritin delivers ferrous iron to the portal blood system. Here the iron is converted back to the ferric state by oxidation, then as ferric iron it combines with a plasma beta-globulin, transferrin (or siderophilin), to form a ferric-protein complex, which is the plasma transport form of iron. Transferrin is about 30% to 40% saturated with iron and the remaining 60% to 70% forms an unsaturated, unbound, latent reserve in the plasma for handling iron as needed.

■ **How is iron stored?**

The plasma transport form, transferrin, conveys iron to the various body cells for storage and utilization. The main storage organs are the liver, spleen, and bone marrow, which participate in the forming of red blood cells. In these sites the iron is stored as ferritin and as *hemosiderin.* Hemosiderin is a secondary, less soluble compound. It is a protein-bound ferric oxide with 35% iron. Hemosiderin formation increases as excess iron accumulates, such as during rapid destruction of red blood cells in hemolytic anemia. From these storage compounds, iron is mobilized for hemoglobin synthesis as needed. In the average adult 20 to 25 mg. of iron is involved daily in hemoglobin synthesis.

■ **When red blood cells are destroyed, is the iron content then excreted?**

No. The body avidly conserves its iron stores. As red cells are destroyed after their average life span of about 120 days, approximately 90% of the iron that is released is conserved and used over and over and over again.

Careful study of the diagram in Fig. 7-3 shows these important relationships in the absorption, transport, and storage of iron.

■ **How is iron excreted?**

Since the main mechanism controlling iron intake into the body system is at the point of absorption—the "ironstat" mechanism involving *ferritin*—the main excretion route for this unabsorbed iron is in the feces, about 0.2 to 0.5 mg. daily. Additional trace amounts are lost through the urine (0.1 mg.) and through sweat (0.05 to 1.0 mg.). In girls and women monthly menstrual losses are about 20 mg.

■ **What is the metabolic function of iron?**

The major metabolic function of iron is its participation in hemoglobin formation. Iron is the core of the *heme* molecule, the fundamental protein of hemoglobin. Hemoglobin in the red blood cell is the oxygen transport unit of the blood that conveys oxygen to the cells for respiration and metabolism.

Smaller amounts of iron also function in the cells as a vital component of enzyme systems for oxidation of glucose to produce energy. In the Krebs cycle, for example, iron is a constituent of the *cytochrome* compounds that are used in the oxidative chains producing high-energy ATP bond (see p. 13).

■ **Why does a newborn infant need other food in addition to his milk diet by the time he is 3 to 6 months old?**

The newborn infant has, at birth, about

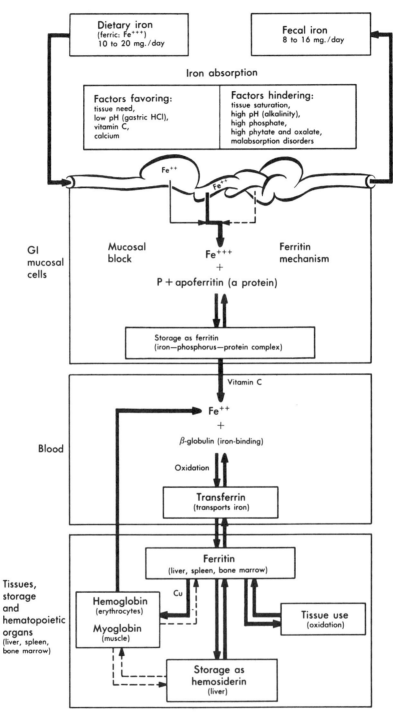

Fig. 7-3. Summary of iron metabolism, showing its absorption, transport, main use in hemoglobin formation, and its storage forms (ferritin and hemosiderin).

a 3- to 6-months supply of iron, which was stored in the liver during fetal development. Since milk does not supply iron, supplementary iron-rich foods must be added. Unless iron sources are made available by the time the fetal supply runs out, a condition will develop called "milk anemia." Iron is needed for continued growth as the child develops to build up reserves for the physiologic stress of adolescence, especially the onset of menses in girls. These food sources of iron, which should be added to the infant's diet by the middle of the first year at the latest, include such items as enriched cereal, green vegetables, and smooth forms of meat.

■ **What is the iron cost of pregnancy?**

The following calculation clearly indicates the demand for iron during pregnancy:

Extra iron in:
Products of conception		370 mg.
Maternal blood		290 mg.
	Total	660 mg.

Minus: Iron "saved" by cessation of menstruation		120 mg.
	Total demand	540 mg.

About 400 to as much as 900 mg. of iron may be involved in a usual pregnancy and delivery. Hence the National Research Council recommends that all women receive 30 to 60 mg. of iron as a daily supplement during the second and third trimesters. Additional iron, therefore, will supply the need for increased total number of red blood cells in the expanding circulating blood volume, and will supply the iron for storage in the developing fetal liver. Finally, it will cover normal blood loss during delivery.

■ **What types of anemia may result from an iron deficiency?**

A deficiency of iron results in a hypochromic microcytic anemia. This lack of iron or inability to use it may be the result of one of several causes:

1. An inadequate supply of iron in the diet—nutritional anemia.

2. Excessive blood-iron loss—hemorrhagic anemia.

3. Inability to form hemoglobin in the absence of other necessary factors, such as vitamin B_{12}—pernicious anemia (see p. 63), or folic acid—megaloblastic anemia.

4. Lack of gastric hydrochloric acid necessary to liberate iron for absorption—postgastrectomy anemia.

5. Presence of iron inhibitors of absorption, such as phosphate or phytate, or mucosal lesions that affect the absorbing surface, leading to malabsorption anemia.

■ **What clinical problems may result from excessive amounts of iron?**

Excessive amounts of iron may accumulate in the body because of inefficient excretory mechanism, and saturated iron storage capacities. This buildup of iron may be the result of one of several causes:

1. Excess iron intake or excess red blood cell destruction, as in malaria or hemolytic anemias, produces a condition known as *hemosiderosis.* Hemosiderosis has been reported among the Bantu natives of Africa from their unusually high iron intake of about 200 mg./day. The main grain in their diet, corn, is low in phosphates to bind iron, and they cook their food in heavy iron pots. Thus, the continuous high iron intake with little phosphate to hinder its absorption results in excessive liver storage and liver damage. This condition has been called *Bantu siderosis.*

2. Excess intravenous iron or repeated transfusions may cause an accumulation of iron. This is associated with long-standing aplastic or hemolytic anemias with excess breakdown of red blood cells.

3. *Hemochromatosis* is a rare disease that occurs chiefly in males. It is believed by some investigators to be genetically transmitted. Saturation of the body tissues with iron causes a bronze coloration, liver damage, and severe diabetes. Recently a potent iron-chelating agent, *desferrioxamine,* has been developed for use in treating this condition.

■ **What is a chelate?**

The word "chelate" comes from the Greek word *chele* meaning "claw." Thus, a chelating agent is a substance that can grasp and incorporate a metallic ion in its molecular structure; it then binds and removes the ion from the tissue or from the circulating blood. In this instance, therefore, the iron chelating agent, desferrioxamine, would grasp and incorporate iron into its molecular structure, binding it and removing it from the body, thus reducing the excessive amount.

■ **What is the daily requirement for iron?**

The National Research Council recommends a general daily adult dietary intake of iron at 10 mg. for men and 18 mg. for women during the childbearing years. This greater amount for women is needed to cover menstrual losses and the demands of pregnancy. It is doubtful that the woman's ordinary diet can supply this larger quantity of iron needed during pregnancy, and fortification with iron supplements is indicated. Infant allowances are 6 to 15 mg. Recommendations for children start at 15 mg. for children ages 1 to 3, and decrease to 10 mg. for children ages 3 to 12. The daily need is 18 mg. for boys 12 to 18 and for girls from age 10 on through the reproductive years. Iron needs vary, of course, with age and situation, and these allowances are designed to provide margins for safety.

■ **What are the main food sources of iron?**

Organ meats, especially liver, are by far the best sources of iron. For example, a 3 ounce portion of roast beef contains about 2.2 mg. of iron, whereas a similar 3 ounce portion of beef liver contains 7.5 mg. of iron, approximately three times as much or better. Other food sources include meats, egg yolk, whole wheat, seafood, green leafy vegetables, nuts, and legumes.

Copper

■ **Why is copper called the "iron twin"?**

Copper has frequently been given the name "iron twin" because it behaves in the body as a companion to iron. The two

are metabolized in much the same way and share some functions:

1. Copper, like iron, is involved in the cyotchrome oxidation system of tissue cells for energy production, as well as being a constituent of several other oxidative enzymes for amino acids.
2. Copper is essential, together with iron, in the formation of hemoglobin. A copper-containing protein, *erythrocuprein,* is found in red blood cells.
3. Copper promotes the absorption of iron from the gastrointestinal tract and is also involved in transporting iron from the tissues into the plasma.

■ **How small an amount of copper is in the body, and where is it located?**

The adult human body contains only about 100 to 150 mg. of copper. This amount is distributed mainly in the muscle, bone, liver, heart, kidneys, and central nervous system. A small quantity is bound to plasma protein. The serum values are highly variable but usually range from 130 to 230 μg./100 ml. In the serum about 5% of the copper is bound with albumin, and about 95% is bound with an α-globulin as the copper-binding protein *ceruloplasmin.*

■ **What is the absorption-transport-storage-excretion route of copper in the body?**

Copper is absorbed in the proximal portion of the small intestine, although the exact mechanism is not understood. The absorbed copper is first taken up by the plasma albumin and initially transported in this bound form. Within 24 hours, however, the copper is bound by the α-globulin to form ceruloplasmin. From 50% to 75% of the total body copper is then stored in the muscle mass and bones, and higher concentrations are stored in liver, heart, kidney, and central nervous system. The main route of excretion is the intestine. Some additional copper is lost in urine, sweat, and menstrual flow.

■ **Does copper have additional metabolic functions apart from those of iron?**

Yes. In addition to its iron-related functions, copper is involved in two other areas of metabolism: (1) bone formation, and (2) brain tissue formation and maintenance of myelin in the nervous system.

■ **Are there any clinical conditions associated with copper deficiency?**

A primary deficiency of copper is unknown. However, secondary deficiency states of low-plasma copper levels (*hypocupremia*) may occur because of urinary loss of ceruloplasmin in nephrosis. Also, because of the malabsorption of copper in diseases such as sprue, low plasma levels may result.

An excess accumulation of copper occurs in a rare inherited condition known as Wilson's disease, which is characterized by degenerative changes in brain tissue (basal ganglia) and in the liver. Large amounts of copper are absorbed in this condition and storage is increased in the liver, brain, kidneys, and cornea. A copper-chelating agent, *penicillamine*, is used to bind the excess copper and cause it to be excreted.

■ **What is the requirement for copper?**

Balance studies indicate that adults require about 2.5 mg. of copper daily. Infants and children require about 0.05 mg. per kg. of body weight. However, because primary deficiency states in man are unknown, there is no stated dietary requirement.

■ **What are the main food sources of copper?**

Copper is widely distributed in natural foods. This accounts for a lack of deficiency states. The average daily diet contains about 2.5 to 5.0 mg. Therefore, with a sufficient caloric intake, copper will be amply supplied.

Iodine

■ **How small an amount of iodine is in the body and where is it located?**

Iodine is a trace element associated mainly with the thyroid gland. The total iodine in the body is from 20 to 50 mg. Of this amount, approximately 20% is in the thyroid gland, 50% is in the muscles, 10% is in the skin, and 6% is in the skeleton. The remaining 14% is scattered in other endocrine tissue, in the central nervous system, and in plasma transport. By far the greatest concentration of iodine in tissue, however, is in the thyroid.

■ **How is the absorption and excretion of iodine controlled?**

After ingestion with food, iodine is absorbed in the small intestine as iodides. These are loosely bound in the intestinal wall with proteins and are then conveyed by the blood to the thyroid gland. About one third of it is selectively absorbed by the thyroid cells and removed from circulation. The remaining two thirds is usually excreted in the urine within 2 to 3 days after ingestion.

The absorption and uptake by the thyroid gland of iodine in iodide form is under the control of a pituitary hormone, TSH (thyroid stimulating hormone, or thyrotropic hormone). The amount of TSH that is released by the pituitary is, in turn, governed by the level of thyroid hormone in the circulating blood. This typical feedback mechanism normally maintains a healthy balance between supply and demand.

■ **How is iodide selectively absorbed by the thyroid gland?**

The cell membranes of the thyroid gland have a tremendous specific capacity to take up or trap iodides by an active transport mechanism. This mechanism has been called the "iodine pump." The concentration of iodides in these structures is normally about 25 times that of their concentration in the blood plasma. Highly active thyroid cells can accomplish an iodide concentration of 350 times that in blood.

■ **How does iodine participate in the synthesis of the thyroid hormone, thyroxine?**

A neutral protein of large molecular weight, *thyroglobulin*, which is secreted into the thyroid follicle, forms both the working base for synthesizing the hormone and the molecular storage complex for holding it until needed. This complex is

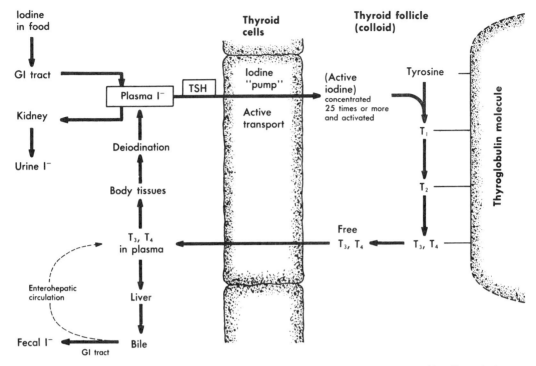

Fig. 7-4. Summary of iodine metabolism, showing active iodine pump in the thyroid cells and the synthesis of thyroxine in the colloid tissue of the thyroid follicles. (TSH = thyroid stimulating hormone; T_1 = monoiodotyronine; T_2 = diiodotyrosine; T_3 = triiodothyronine; T_4 = tetraiodothyronine.)

called *colloid*. The amino acid tyrosine, a part of the thyroglobulin molecule, forms the base structure which, through successive stages of iodination, finally builds the hormone *thyroxine*. The successive stages of this synthesis of thyroxine involving iodine and protein, especially the amino acid thyrosine, are shown in the diagram in Fig. 7-4.

■ **What is the metabolic function of thyroid hormone (thyroxine) and in turn that of iodine?**

The thyroid hormone stimulates cell oxidation, apparently by increasing oxygen uptake, and reaction rates of enzyme systems handling glucose. Therefore, iodine indirectly exerts tremendous influence on overall body metabolism.

■ **What is the transport form of iodine?**

The free thyroxine with its associated iodine is secreted into the bloodstream and bound to plasma protein for transport to body cells as needed. This transport form of iodine is called serum *protein-bound io-*

dine (PBI). The serum level of PBI normally ranges from 4 to 8 μg./100 ml. After being used to stimulate oxidation in the cell, thyroxine is then degraded in the liver, and the iodine is excreted in bile as inorganic iodine.

■ **What clinical problems result from imbalances in thyroid hormone production?**

Clinical problems result from excessive production of thyroxine, hyperthyroidism, as well as from deficient production of thyroid production, hypothyroidism.

1. *Hyperthyroidism.* Excessive production of thyroid hormone produces a generally diffuse or nodular enlargement of the thyroid gland. Increased body metabolism is the result. Symptoms of this increased metabolism include: (1) abnormal tolerance of cold or intolerance of heat; (2) activation of the heat-loss mechanism, with cutaneous vasodilation and sweating (hot, moist palms are characteristic); (3) increased appetite despite which weight loss may be severe; (4) tremor of the hands; and (5) irritable behavior and emotional lability. Also present may be a classic change in the eyes creating a "pop-eyed" expression caused by lid retraction, exophthalmos, and supraorbital swelling. These typical eye changes are characteristic of the classic Graves' disease.

2. *Hypothyroidism.* An insufficient secretion of thyroid hormone may also cause clinical problems. Primary hypothyroidism is caused by insufficient thyroid hormone and secondary hypothyroidism is related to problems of pituitary origin and the secretion of TSH to stimulate thyroid production of thyroxine. Hypothyroidism usually has a gradual onset: (1) a progressive lethargy and disinterest, slurred speech, and often deafness; (2) loss of appetite but a moderate increase in weight caused largely by water retention; and (3) increasing intolerance to cold. In addition, the general appearance is characterized by a thickening of the skin of the lips and fingers and edema below the eyes. The hair is usually brittle and scanty. Mental changes may occur, ranking from mild depression to the stage of psychosis. Myxedema, the deposition of an excess of mucoprotein in the skin, usually occurs in the forearms and often in the legs and feet, although these changes are present only in severe cases.

■ **What is endemic colloid goiter?**

Endemic colloid goiter is a classic condition characterized by great enlargement of the thyroid gland. Endemic colloid goiter occurs in residents of areas where the water and soil (and therefore locally grown foods) contain little iodine. The thyroid gland is starved for iodine and cannot produce a normal quantity of thyroxine. The amount of thyroxine that is secreted into the bloodstream is, therefore, too low to shut off TSH secretion by the pituitary in the normal feedback mechanism. The pituitary persists in putting out TSH, and these large quantities of TSH continue to stimulate the thyroid gland, calling upon it to produce the thyroxine

that it cannot supply because of the lack of iodine. The only response that the iodine-starved gland can make is to increase the amount of thyroglobulin (colloid), which then acculates in the thyroid follicles and causes enlargement of the gland. Such a gland becomes increasingly engorged and may attain a tremendous size, weighing 500 to 700 gm. (1 to 1½ pounds or more). This greatly enlarged size of the thyroid gland may be compared with the normal shape and size of the thyroid gland —about that of a lima bean.

■ **What is cretinism?**

Cretinism is a severe form of mental retardation. In areas where the soil is poor in iodine and goiter has affected a number of generations, severe iodine deficiency in mothers produces an endemic form of cretinism in successive generations of offspring. The condition is characterized by stunted growth, dwarfism, and various degrees of mental retardation.

■ **What tests are used to measure iodine metabolism?**

The *PBI test* measures the amount of iodine that is bound to thyroxine and in transit in the plasma. A small amount of free inorganic iodide may also be present. The normal range is from 4 to 8 μg./100 ml. of serum. Values below 4 indicate hypothyroidism. Values above 8 indicate hyperthyroidism. Unfortunately, falsely high readings may result from the presence in the system of other iodine compounds, such as certain iodine-containing radiopaque substances that may have been administered in conjunction with x-ray studies or iodine-containing therapeutic agents. Mercurial diuretics may cause falsely low readings. The I^{131} *test* uses radioactive iodine to measure the uptake and utilization of iodine by the thyroid gland.

■ **What is the daily requirement for iodine?**

The National Research Council has recommended daily adult allowances of 140 μg. for young men and 100 μg. for young women. These needs normally decrease with age. The demand is increased during periods of accelerated growth, such as adolescence and pregnancy.

■ **What are the food sources of iodine?**

Seafood provides a considerable amount of iodine. However, the quantity in natural sources varies broadly, depending on the iodine content of the soil. The average diet falls somewhat below the requirement. The commercial iodizing of table salt, therefore, in the proportions of 1 mg. to every 10 gm. of salt, provides the main dietary source of iodine. Sometimes a noniodized form of salt may be suggested by some practitioners for conditions of acne in adolescents. This practice, however, has no basis in scientific fact. The demands of iodine for adolescent growth are great, hence, the practice should be avoided.

Manganese

■ **How small an amount of manganese is there in the body and where is it located?**

Only about 10 mg. of manganese is present in the adult body, chiefly in the liver and kidneys, with small amounts in other tissues such as the retina, bones, and salivary glands. Blood values are very low—4 to 20 μg./100 ml. have been reported.

■ **What is the metabolic function of manganese?**

Manganese functions mainly as an essential activating agent that strengthens and stimulates a number of vital metabolic reactions. Some of these reactions include:

1. *Urea formation.* Activates an enzyme in the formation of urea, may help prevent ammonia toxicity.
2. *Protein metabolism.* Activates amino acid interconversions; activates peptidases for splitting specific amino acids such as leucine.
3. *Carbohydrate metabolism.* Activates several conversion reactions of the glycolytic pathway and Krebs cycle in glucose oxidation.
4. *Fat metabolism.* Activates the serum fat-clearing factor, lipoprotein lipase, and operates as a cofactor in the synthesis of long-chain fatty acids.

■ **What clinical problems are associated with manganese?**

Although many clinical evidences of manganese deficiency have been established in animals, none have been observed in humans. However, an industrial disease syndrome, representing *inhalation toxicity,* occurs in miners and other workers who undergo prolonged exposure to manganese dust. The excessive manganese accumulates in the liver and central nervous system and eventually produces severe neuromuscular manifestations that resemble those of Parkinson's disease.

■ **What is the requirement for manganese?**

Whether there is a specific human requirement for manganese is unknown. The average diet provides from 3 to 9 μg. daily, which apparently is highly adequate.

■ **What are the main food sources of manganese?**

The best food sources of manganese are of plant origin. These include cereal bran, soybeans, legumes, nuts, tea, and coffee. Animal foods are relatively poor sources.

Cobalt

■ **How small an amount of cobalt is in the body, and where is it located?**

Cobalt occurs in only minute traces in the body tissues. The main storage area is the liver. The normal blood level, representing the amount in transit and in the red blood cells, is about 1 μg./100 ml. Variable amounts of cobalt are absorbed and apparently quickly excreted in the urine. Unabsorbed cobalt is lost in the feces. The main form in which it is absorbed and used is as a constituent of vitamin B_{12}.

■ **What is the metabolic function of cobalt?**

The basic function of cobalt in human nutrition that has been demonstrated is that of a constituent of vitamin B_{12}, an essential factor in the formation of red blood cells. However, the widespread distribution of cobalt in nature, and its ready uptake by plants, lead one to speculate about possible broader functions. As yet such have not been established. With its position as the brilliant red atom at the core of vitamin B_{12}, however, cobalt plays a vital role in red blood cell formation.

■ **What clinical problems are associated with cobalt?**

A deficiency of cobalt per se is well known to have deleterious effects in animals. In man, however, a deficiency of cobalt is associated only with a deficiency of vitamin B_{12} and the consequent development of pernicious anemia (see p. 63). An excess of cobalt has led to *polycythemia*. This is a condition characterized by the formation of an excess number of red blood cells that contain a relatively high concentration of hemoglobin.

■ **What is the requirement of cobalt?**

The quantitative human requirement of cobalt is unknown but is evidently minute. For example, as small an amount as .045 to .09 μg. daily maintains bone marrow function in patients with pernicious anemia.

■ **What are the food sources of cobalt?**

Cobalt is widely distributed in nature. However, for man's chief need—as a constituent of vitamin B_{12}—cobalt is best obtained in the preformed vitamin. This vitamin is synthesized in animals by gastrointestinal bacteria. Vitamin B_{12} is supplied almost entirely by animal foods: the richest sources are liver and kidney; and lean meat, milk, eggs, and cheese supply additional amounts. Natural dietary deficiency of cobalt is rare.

Zinc

■ **How small an amount of zinc is present in the body and where is it located?**

Zinc occurs in the human body in amounts larger than those of other trace elements except iron. The body's total zinc content ranges from 1.3 to 2.3 gm. It is distributed in many tissues, including the pancreas, liver, kidney, lung, muscles, bones, eye (cornea, iris, retina, and lens), endocrine glands, prostate secretions and spermatozoa. The normal human prostate gland contains 850 ppm. of zinc and its secretions contain three to four times that amount. The concentration of zinc in sper-

matozoa is roughly 2,000 ppm. The plasma zinc level is about 120 μg./100 ml.

■ **What is the metabolic function of zinc?**

Zinc functions mainly as an essential constituent of several important enzymes. These include carbonic anhydrase, carboxypeptidase, and lactic dehydrogenase.

1. Zinc is an integral part of *carbonic anhydrase*, which acts as a carbon dioxide carrier especially in red blood cells. It takes up carbon dioxide from the cells, combines it with water to form carbonic acid (H_2CO_3), and then releases carbon dioxide from the capillaries into the alveoli of the lung. This enzyme also functions in the renal tubules cells in the maintenance of acid-base balance, in mucosal cells, and in glands of the body.

2. Zinc is a cofactor of the protein-splitting enzyme, *carboxypeptidase*, which removes the carboxyl group (COOH) from peptides to produce amino acids. Zinc, therefore, has a key role in protein digestion.

3. Zinc is a part of *lactic dehydrogenase*. This enzyme is essential for the interconversion of pyruvic acid and lactic acid in the glycolytic pathway for glucose oxidation. Thus, zinc also plays a part in carbohydrate digestion.

■ **What is the role of zinc in normal growth and development?**

Zinc is associated with iron in a characteristic clinical syndrome in children. Without sufficient zinc, longitudinal growth slows, producing dwarfism; and sexual development is arrested.

■ **What is the relation of zinc to insulin?**

Zinc readily combines with insulin in the pancreas. This compound of zinc-insulin serves perhaps as the storage form of the hormone. The diabetic pancreas contains about half the normal amount of zinc. Prepared forms of insulin used to treat diabetes include a protamine zinc form (PZI) in which zinc is combined with the insulin to produce a long-acting form of insulin.

■ **Is zinc related in any way to cirrhosis?**

A possible relation of zinc metabolism with liver disease has aroused the interest

Table 7-2. Summary of trace minerals

Mineral	Metabolism	Physiologic function	Clinical application	Requirement	Food source
Iron (Fe)	Absorption according to body need controlled by mucosal block—ferritin mechanism; aided by vitamin C, gastric hydrochloric acid. Transport—transferrin. Storage—ferritin, hemosiderin. Excretion from tissue in minute quantities; body conserves and re-uses	Hemoglobin formation. Cellular oxidation (cytochrome system producing ATP)	Growth (milk anemia). Pregnancy demands. Deficiency—anemia. Excess—hemosiderosis; hemochromatosis	Men: 10 mg. Women: 18 mg. Pregnancy: 18 mg. Lactation: 18 mg. Children: 10 to 18 mg.	Liver. Meats. Egg yolk. Whole grains. Enriched bread and cereal. Dark green vegetables. Legumes, nuts
Copper (Cu)	Transported bound to an α-globulin as ceruloplasmin. Stored in muscle, bone, liver, heart, kidney and central nervous system	Associated with iron in: Enzyme systems. Hemoglobin synthesis. Absorption and transport of iron. Involved in bone formation and maintenance of brain tissue and myelin sheath in nervous system	Hypocupremia: Nephrosis. Malabsorption. Wilson's disease—excess copper storage	2 to 2.5 mg. Diet provides 2 to 5 mg.	Liver. Meat. Seafood. Whole grains. Legumes, nuts
Iodine (I)	Absorbed as iodides, taken up by thyroid gland under control of thyroid-stimulating hormone (TSH). Excretion by kidney	Synthesis of thyroxine, the thyroid hormone, which regulates cell oxidation	Deficiency—endemic colloid goiter; cretinism	Men: 140 μg. Women: 100 μg. Infants: 25 to 45 μg. Children: 55 to 140 μg.	Iodized salt. Seafoods
Manganese (Mn)	Absorption limited. Excretion mainly by intestine	Activates reactions in: Urea formation. Protein metabolism. Glucose oxidation. Lipoprotein clearance and synthesis of fatty acids	No clinical deficiency observed in humans. Inhalation toxicity in miners	Unknown. Diet provides 3 to 9 μg.	Cereals. Soybeans. Legumes, nuts. Tea, coffee

Cobalt (Co)	Absorbed chiefly as constituent of vitamin B_{12}	Constituent of vitamin B_{12}, essential factor in red blood cell formation	Deficiency associated with deficiency of vitamin B_{12}—pernicious anemia	Unknown	Supplied by preformed vitamin B_{12}
Zinc (Zn)	Transported with plasma proteins Excretion largely intestinal Stored in liver, muscle, bone, and organs	Essential enzyme constituent: Carbonic anhydrase Carboxypeptidase Lactic dehydrogenase Combines with insulin for storage of the hormone	Possible relation to liver disease	Unknown Average diet supplies 10 to 15 mg.	Widely distributed Liver Seafood
Molybdenum (Mo)	Minute traces in the body	Constituent of specific enzymes involved in: Purine conversion to uric acid Aldehyde oxidation		Unknown	Organ meats Milk Whole grains Leafy vegetables Legumes
Fluorine (Fl)	Deposited in bones and teeth Excreted in urine	Associated with dental health	Small amount prevents dental caries Excess causes endemic dental fluorosis		Water (1 ppm. Fl)
Selenium (Se)		Associated with fat metabolism	Constituent of "factor 3" which acts with vitamin E to prevent fatty liver		
Chromium (Cr)		Associated with glucose metabolism	Infants unable to metabolize sugar and adult diabetics showed definite improvement when small amounts of chromium added to diet Possible link with cardiovascular disorders and diabetes		

of investigators. In cirrhosis of the liver, serum zinc levels are low; urinary excretion is increased. Postmortem studies have revealed reduced zinc concentrations in the liver. It is speculated that the disease may increase the need for zinc and therefore deficiency results from the usual intake.

■ **What is the requirement for zinc?**

No specific quantitative requirement for zinc has been established in man. Balance studies indicate that a daily intake of 0.3 mg./kg. of body weight is adequate. Since the usual intake on the average diet is from 10 to 15 mg daily, a deficiency is highly unlikely.

■ **What are the food sources of zinc?**

Zinc is easily obtained in widespread natural sources. Zinc in natural sources approximates that of iron.

Molybdenum

■ **What is the metabolic function of molybdenum?**

Amounts of molybdenum in the body are very minute. This trace mineral is present in bound form as an integral part of various enzyme molecules and thus functions in facilitating the action of the specific enzyme involved. Examples of molybdenum-containing enzymes are *xanthine oxidase* and *liver aldehyde oxidase*. In purine catabolism xanthine oxidase catalyzes the oxidation of xanthine to uric acid. It has been isolated from milk and liver. Liver aldehyde oxidase is a flavoprotein. It catalyzes the oxidation of aldehydes to corresponding carboxylic acid.

■ **What are the food sources of molybdenum?**

Food sources of molybdenum include legumes, whole grains, milk, leafy vegetables, and organ meats. There is no known requirement.

TRACE MINERALS WITH UNKNOWN FUNCTION
Fluorine

■ **What is the relation of fluorine to dental health?**

The only relationship thus far established for fluorine in human metabolism is its association with dental health. Basic observations have centered around the results of an excess intake of fluorine and of a small intake.

1. *Excess intake. Endemic dental fluorosis* has been observed in communities where the natural fluorine content of the water supply is high. The largest known such region in the United States is the West Texas Panhandle. Apparently fluorine excesses act on teeth in the budding stage of formation, so that by the time they erupt their enamel is mottled, pitted, and discolored. Adults who habitually eat excessive quantities of fluoride may suffer from osteosclerosis. Osteosclerosis is abnormal density of the skeletal bone, which in some cases is so mild that it can barely be detected by x-rays but in other instances is so severe as to be called crippling fluorosis. These conditions, however, are rare.

2. *Small intake. Dental caries* have been demonstrated to be largely preventable by the addition of a small amount of fluorine to fluorine-poor drinking water or by the topical application of fluoride solutions to young developing teeth.

■ **How much fluorine does water fluoridation involve?**

Public health authorities advocate the fluoridation of public drinking water in the amount of 1 ppm. in areas where the drinking water is low in fluoride content. The mechanism by which fluorine prevents dental caries is unknown.

Selenium

■ **Is selenium related to liver disease?**

Interest in selenium has recently centered about the discovery of a potent, metabolically active, selenium-containing compound called "factor 3." This factor has been observed to protect the liver against fatty infiltration and necrosis. The action of selenium in this factor may be related to that of vitamin E, since the two substances appear to act synergistically in curing the hepatic disease and certain muscle disorders induced in animals.

The function of selenium involved is probably that of a cofactor for enzyme systems related to cell oxidation.

Aluminum

■ **How much aluminum is there in the body?**

The total aluminum content of the adult human body is from 50 to 150 mg. The amount ingested in the average diet ranges widely from about 10 mg. to more than 100 mg. daily. Aluminum is found in many plant and animal foods.

■ **What clue might there be to the metabolic function of aluminum?**

Despite its wide intake and distribution, no clear function for aluminum in human nutrition has been established. A clue may be present in model systems studies of certain transaminase reactions with amino acids. The mechanism and significance of these reactions is not clear, however.

Boron

■ **What possible metabolic functions for boron in human nutrition have been found?**

Minute traces of boron are found in body tissues. No clues to its purpose have been discovered. Boron has been found to be essential, however, for plant nutrition and growth. Experiments in animals have not demonstrated any evidences of deficiency after boron deprivation.

Cadmium

■ **What possible function may develop for cadmium in human nutrition?**

That traces of cadmium are present in body tissues has been known for some time. Not until recently, however, was cadmium isolated as a definite component of a metal-containing protein. This protein, *metallothionein,* found in the renal cortex of the horse, contains cadmium, zinc, and sulfur. The significance of this cadmium-containing protein in animals is not yet clear, but it points to the possibility that the mineral functions in some basic biologic system in human nutrition.

Chromium

■ **What clues are there to the possible function of chromium?**

The minute traces of chromium present in the body were not recognized until two decades ago, when analytic methods were developed that were sufficiently sensitive to detect them. There are about twenty parts of chromium in one billion parts of blood. However, certain cell proteins can achieve much higher concentrations of chromium than this. These greater concentrations in cells indicate a probable role in glucose metabolism. In animals made chromium deficient by deprivation, fasting blood sugar levels were elevated and glycosuria followed. In man, recent studies showed the ability of chromium to raise abnormally low fasting blood sugar levels and to improve faulty intake of sugar by body tissues. Physicians working in Jerusalem with refugee infants suffering from severe malnutrition and an inability to use sugar found that when small amounts of chromium were added to their diet the infants made rapid recovery.

A summary of the trace minerals is presented in Table 7-2 for review and reference.

8 Water and electrolytes

Water is the most basic nutrient to man's survival. Several basic concepts are essential to understanding the uses of water in the human body. First, there is the concept of a *unified whole;* man is one continuous body of water. The "sea within" is held in shape by a protective envelope of skin. Water diffuses freely to all parts and is controlled only by the water's own chemical potential. In this warm, fluid, chemical environment, life processes are sustained.

Second, there is the concept of *compartments of water* within the whole separated by membranes. The quantities of water contained in each compartment are balanced by forces that maintain an equilibrium among the parts.

Third, there is the concept of *particles* (charged electrolytes and other solutes) *in the water solution.* It is the concentration and distribution of these particles that determines internal shifts and balances in body water.

Involved throughout is the unifying concept of homeostasis. The body has a tremendous resilience through its capacity to employ numerous finely balanced homeostatic mechanisms that protect its vital fluid supply.

BODY WATER AND ITS DISTRIBUTION

■ **What proportion of body weight is water?**

The body of the adult male is 55% to 65% water; that of a woman is 50% to 55% water. The higher water content in men is generally because of the greater muscle mass.

Striated muscle contains more water than any body tissue other than blood. The remaining 40% of a man's weight is about 18% protein and related substances, 15% fat, and 7% minerals.

■ **What functions does body water perform?**

Body water performs three functions that are essential to life: (1) it helps give structure and form to the body through the turgor it provides for tissue, (2) it provides the aqueous environment that is necessary for cell metabolism and all the life processes it sustains, and (3) it provides the means for maintaining a stable body temperature.

■ **How is body water distributed?**

Body water is distributed in cells and in spaces outside of cells. Thus the concept of water compartments is useful. The extracellular fluid compartment (ECF) is made up of all the water outside the cells. The intracellular fluid compartment (ICF) is made up of all the water inside the cells.

1. *Extracellular fluid compartment (ECF).* The collective water outside the cells makes up about 20% of the total body weight. About one fourth of this, 5% of the body weight, is contained in the blood plasma. The plasma includes the total fluid within the heart and the blood vessels. The remaining three fourths, 15% of the body weight, is made up of water surrounding the cells: (1) the *interstitial fluid and lymph,* which make up the fluid environment in which the cells are bathed; (2) the water in *dense tissue,* such as connective tissue, cartilage, and bone; and (3) the water in *transit secretions,* including

cerebrospinal fluid and secretions, such as those of the salivary gland, thyroid gland, liver, pancreas, gallbladder, gastrointestinal tract, gonads, various mucous membranes, skin, kidneys, and eye spaces.

2. *Intracellular fluid compartment (ICF).* The total water inside the body cells amounts to about twice that outside the cells. This is not surprising, since the cell is the basic unit of structure of the entire body; and the cells are the sites of the vast metabolic activity of the body. This intracellular fluid compartment makes up about 40% to 45% of the total body weight. The relative sizes of these body water compartments may be compared in the diagram in Fig. 8-1.

■ **In the overall water balance between intake and output, how much water does the average adult metabolize daily?**

The average adult metabolizes from 2½ to 3 liters of water per day in a constant turnover balanced between intake and output. Normally water enters and leaves the body by various routes under the control of such basic mechanisms as thirst and hormonal control of renal excretion.

■ **What are the routes of water intake or replacement?**

Water enters the body in three main forms:

1. *Preformed water in liquids.* Water and other beverages are the main source of ingested fluid. From 1,200 to 1,500 ml. of liquid is ingested daily in this form.

2. *Preformed water in foods.* Foods vary in their water content. Some foods, such as tomatoes, oranges, and watermelon, contain much water. Others, such as dried fruit and legumes, contain less. The total water ingested with foods that are eaten, rather than as liquid that is drunk, contributes from 700 to 1,000 ml. daily.

3. *Water of oxidation.* When nutrients are burned or oxidized in the body, one of the end products is water. The amount of metabolic water produced varies with different nutrients. For example, 100 gm. of fat produces 107 gm. of water; 100 gm. of carbohydrate produces 55 gm. of water; and 100 gm. of protein produces 41 gm. of water. On the whole, 200 to 300 ml. of water is contributed daily from the body's metabolic activity.

These three sources, preformed water in

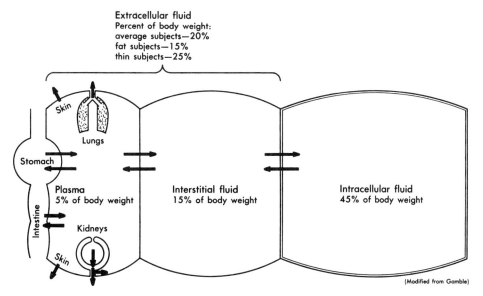

(Modified from Gamble)

Fig. 8-1. Body fluid compartments. Note the relative total quantities of water in the intracellular compartment and in the extracellular compartment.

Table 8-1. Approximate daily adult intake and output of water

Intake (replacement) ml. per day		Output (loss)	
		Obligatory (insensible) ml. per day	Additional (according to need) ml. per day
Preformed		Lungs 350	
Liquids	1,200 to 1,500	Skin	
In foods	700 to 1,000	Diffusion 350	
		Sweat 100	±250
Metabolism (oxidation		Kidneys 900	±500
of food)	200 to 300	Feces 150	
Total	2,100 to 2,800	1,850	750
	(approx. 2,600 ml. per day)	(approx. 2,600 ml. per day)	

liquids, preformed water in foods, and water of oxidation, bring the daily water intake to 2,100 to 2,800 ml.

■ **What are the routes of water output or loss?**

Water leaves the body through four main routes:

1. *Kidneys.* The kidneys of an adult normally excrete from 1 to 2 liters of urine daily. The water in this total amount is made up of two portions, the obligatory water excretion and the facultative water excretion. *Obligatory water excretion* is the amount of water that the kidney is "obligated" to excrete in order to rid the body of its daily load of urinary solutes. Since about 15 ml. of water is required to dissolve 1 gm. of solute, the quantity of obligatory water excretion depends on how large a load of metabolic end products (solutes such as urea and other metabolites) is seeking excretion, and also on the concentrative power of the kidney. The average obligatory water excretion of an adult is approximately 900 ml. daily. *Facultative water excretion* occurs in addition to obligatory water loss. An additional 500 ml. more or less may be excreted according to fluctuating body need and the renal tubular reabsorption rate.

2. *Skin.* About 350 ml. of water is lost daily through the skin by diffusion. Be-

cause man is unaware of this loss it is called insensible water loss. An additional 100 ml. may be lost in normal perspiration. Heavier sweating, caused by heat or increased activity, may cause the loss of 250 ml. of water, more or less according to body need. Therefore, under usual circumstances 450 to 700 ml. of water is lost daily through the skin. Excessive sweating or loss of skin as in extensive burns further increases the water output.

3. *Lungs.* An insensible water loss of about 350 ml. occurs daily through normal respiration vapor. This amount varies with climate, being least in hot humid weather and greatest in very cold temperatures.

4. *Feces.* A small amount of water, 150 to 200 ml., is usually lost daily through intestinal elimination. In abnormal conditions, such as diarrhea or dysentery, much greater losses will occur.

On the average, thus, daily water output from the adult body totals about 2,600 ml. This comparative intake and output balance is summarized in Table 8-1 for review and reference.

FORCES INFLUENCING WATER DISTRIBUTION AND BALANCE

Forces that influence and control the distribution and balance of water in the body revolve around two basic concepts:

(1) the *solutes*, the particles in solution in body water, including electrolytes, plasma protein, and other smaller organic compounds; (2) the *separating membranes* between the water compartments, the cell wall, and the capillary wall. The resulting forces and mechanisms that move water and solutes across membranes according to need form the basis for an understanding of the vital balance that must prevail to maintain life.

Solutes

■ What are electrolytes?

Certain inorganic compounds, usually an acid, an alkali, or a salt, partly dissociate into their constituent ions when they are dissolved in water. An *ion* is an atom or a group of atoms that carries an electrical charge. This charge is positive if the atom has *lost* one of the negatively charged electrons that orbit around its nucleus. The charge is negative if the atom has gained a negatively charged orbiting electron. The word ion is derived from the Greek word meaning "wanderer." Thus such an atom wanders freely in a solution, dissociated from the compound of which it was a part. A compound that dissociates into ions when in solution is called an *electrolyte.* This term refers to the fact that a solution containing one of these substances can transmit an electric current.

The two forms of ions are cations and anions. A *cation* is an ion that carries a positive charge (Na^+, K^+, Ca^{++}, Mg^{++}). An *anion* is an ion that carries a negative charge (Cl^-, HCO_3^-, $HPO_4^=$, $SO_4^=$). Electrolytes constitute a major force controlling fluid balances within the body.

■ How are electrolytes in body fluids measured?

The chemical activity of a solution is determined by the concentration of electrolytes (charged solutes) in a given volume of the solution. Concentration is a function of volume, since the degree of concentration indicates the number of particles or charges in a unit volume. It is the *number* of particles in the solution, not the *weights* of the various particles, that is the important factor in determining chemical combining power. Electrolytes are dynamically active chemicals. The ions that are released when the electrolyte enters into solution carry charges of electrical energy, and each particle contributes chemical combining power to the whole according to its *valence*, not its weight. Therefore electrolytes are measured according to the total number of particles in solution rather than the total weight.

■ What is a milliequivalent?

The unit of measure commonly used is an *equivalent*, with hydrogen as a reference point. One equivalent of a substance is equal to the combining power of 1 gm. of hydrogen. Since small amounts are usually in question, most physiologic measurements are expressed in terms of *milliequivalents*. One milliequivalent (mEq.) is equal to the chemical combining power of 1 mg. of hydrogen. The term milliequivalents refers to the number of ions (cations and anions) in solution, as determined by their concentration in a given volume. This measure is expressed in the number of milliequivalents per liter (mEq./L.)

■ What is the relation of milliequivalents to milligrams of an ionized substance in solution?

Equivalents of an ionized substance in solution are calculated in terms of the molecular weight and valence of that substance. One equivalent (Eq.) is one mol (the gram molecular weight of a substance, that is, the molecular weight of the substance in grams) divided by its valence. The milliequivalent is one one-thousandth of an equivalent. Thus:

$$1 \text{ Eq. } Na^+ = \text{(23 gm. [molecular weight of sodium]} \div 1) = 23 \text{ gm.}$$
$$1 \text{ mEq. } Na^+ = 23 \text{ mg.}$$
$$1 \text{ Eq. } Ca^{++} = \text{(40 gms. [molecular weight of calcium]} \div 2) = 20 \text{ gm.}$$
$$1 \text{ mEq. } Ca^{++} = 20 \text{ mg.}$$

Thus the milliequivalents per liter equals the milligrams per liter divided by the equivalent weight.

Equivalent weight equals gram molecular weight (atomic weight) divided by valence.

■ What is the electrolyte composition of the extracellular fluid?

Ionized sodium (Na^+) is the main cation in extracellular fluid. Sodium provides about 90% of the total base concentration, or about 45% of the total electrolyte concentration, in the body water outside the cells. Its concentration here is much greater than inside the cell. The sodium in the extracellular fluid provides the primary osmotic force that maintains the water volume necessary for the cell environment. The amounts of the other cations (K^+, Ca^{++}, Mg^{++}) in the extracellular fluid are relatively small.

Ionized chlorine (Cl^-) is the main anion in extracellular fluid. Chloride provides the main balancing anion in the extracellular fluid. It is present in particularly high concentrations in gastric secretions as a constituent of hydrochloric acid and in interstitial lymph.

The variable anion bicarbonate (HCO_3^-), the fixed anions phosphate ($HPO_4^=$), sulfate ($SO_4^=$), and protein, together with various organic acids, such as lactic acid and pyruvic acid, comprise the remaining materials in the extracellular fluid. The protein portion of the extracellular fluid is in the plasma portion. If the electrolyte profiles of interstitial and plasma portions of the extracellular fluid are compared, it will be noted that they are the same except for this one important difference, the presence of protein in the plasma portion only. These are the plasma proteins present in the blood vessels that provide the colloidal osmotic pressure necessary to maintain the integrity of blood volume.

■ What is the electrolyte composition of the intracellular fluid?

Ionized potassium (K^+) is the main cation in the intracellular fluid. The relative concentrations of ionized sodium and potassium in the intracellular fluid are the reverse of those in the extracellular fluid. Ionized potassium concentrated within the cells provides a major osmotic force for main-

taining the necessary water volume inside the cell. Most of the cellular potassium is free. However, a significant amount—about one third—is bound with the cell protein. Therefore, when cell protein is broken down, as in tissue oxidation or extensive tissue destruction, more potassium is freed and influences fluid shifts.

Phosphate ($HPO_4^=$) is the main anion in the intracellular fluid. Because of the significant role of phosphate in cell metabolism in the various energy-producing chains and pathways for glucose oxidation, a much greater concentration of this anion is found inside the cells than outside.

The quantity of protein in the cell fluid is three or four times greater than that in the extracellular plasma. Again, this is not surprising because of the greater protoplasmic mass in tissue cells, and the important work of protein synthesis constantly going on in each cell. Together with phosphate, then, protein constitutes a major cellular anion.

■ What is the significance of the balance between anions and cations within a fluid compartment?

Biochemical and electrophysical laws demand that in a stable solution the number of positively charged particles must equal the number of negatively charged particles. In other words the solution must be electrically neutral. When shifts and losses occur, compensating shifts and gains follow to maintain electroneutrality. Such a balance does indeed exist in body fluids. A comparison of these respective balances is shown in Table 8-2.

■ How does electrolyte balance control body hydration?

Ionized sodium is the chief cation of extracellular fluid, and ionized potassium is the chief cation of intracellular fluid. These two electrolytes, with the others present in smaller amounts, exercise control over the amount of water to be retained in any given compartment. The usual bases for these shifts in water from one compartment to another are changes occurring in the *extracellular* concentrations of these elec-

Table 8-2. Balance of cation and anion concentrations in extracellular fluid (ECF) and intracellular fluid (ICF), which maintains electroneutrality within each compartment

		ECF		ICF	
Cation	Anion	Cation (mEq./L.)	Anion (mEq./L.)	Cation (mEq./L.)	Anion (mEq./L.)
Na^+		142		35	
K^+		5		123	
Ca^{++}		5		15	
Mg^{++}		3		2	
	Cl^-		104		5
	$HPO_4^=$		2		80
	$SO_4^=$		1		10
	Org. acids		5		
	Protein		16		70
	HCO_3^-		27		10
Totals		155	155	175	175

trolytes. The terms *hypertonic dehydration* and *hypotonic dehydration* refer to the electrolyte concentration of the *water outside the cell*, which in turn causes a shift of water into or out of the cell.

■ **What is hypertonic dehydration?**

In the extracellular fluid, when water loss exceeds electrolyte loss, the extracellular fluid becomes hypertonic to the intracellular fluid (the osmotic pressure of the extracellular fluid is higher than that of the intracellular fluid). This imbalance in osmotic pressures causes water to shift from the cell into the extracellular fluid spaces. This situation could occur either from excess water loss or from water restriction. Clinical manifestations include severe thirst, hot, dry body (especially the tongue), vomiting, disorientation, and scanty and concentrated urine.

■ **What is hypotonic dehydration?**

When large amounts of water are added to the extracellular fluid without the addition of sufficient electrolytes to maintain the normal density of the solutions, the extracellular fluid becomes hypotonic to the intracellular fluid. This type of imbalance in osmotic pressures causes a compensatory shift of water from the extracellular fluid into the cell. The result is a dangerous shrinking of the extracellular fluid, especially the blood volume. Renal blood flow is impaired, and swelling of cells (cellular edema) occurs. This serious situation could result either from over-zealous hydration of patients (giving too much plain water without accompanying electrolytes) or from losses of both water and electrolytes and replacement with water only. Clinical manifestations include progressive weakness without thirst or decreased urine ouput. Also, the hematocrit reading and the red blood cell count are elevated because of concentration of the blood.

■ **How do plasma proteins influence internal fluid shifts?**

The plasma proteins exert a tremendous colloidal osmotic pressure within the capillaries, which pulls fluid and solutes from the interstitial spaces into the blood. This action maintains the necessary plasma volume. About 70% of this total colloidal osmotic pressure comes from the albumin that is present in a greater quantity than any other plasma protein. The remaining 30% is from the presence of globulins and fibrinogen.

Because the molecules of the plasma

proteins are for the most part too large to pass through the capillary wall, they exert a constant osmotic pull on the interstitial fluid. However, this osmotic pull is balanced by an opposite outward thrust (hydrostatic pressure) of the blood within the capillary. This blood pressure tends to push fluid out of the capillary lumen into the interstitial fluid. Throughout the length of the capillary, from the end at which it emerges from the arteriole to the end at which it merges into the venule, these two forces play against one another in a dynamic balance. At the arteriole end of the capillary the hydrostatic pressure predominates just enough to filter some water and solutes, including salts and a small amount of protein, out into the tissue fluids. By the time the blood has reached the venous end of the capillary it has lost so much water that the relative osmotic pull of the plasma proteins within its lumen has risen considerably. Meanwhile the opposing hydrostatic outward thrust has diminished because the fluid is just that much farther from the heart. The balance topples to the other side; water and solutes are drawn through the wall of the capillary into its lumen to continue in circulation.

The statement of this equilibrium of pressure was first proposed in 1895 by E. H. Starling and is now called *Starling's law of the capillaries,* or the *capillary fluid shift mechanism.* The equilibrium shift is one of the body's most important homeostatic mechanisms to maintain fluid balance. The diagram illustrating this fluid shift is shown in Fig. 8-2.

The constant operation of this mechanism maintains the plasma volume and provides the transfer fluid environment necessary to serve the cells' needs.

■ **How does cell protein protect cell water?**

In much the same way that the plasma proteins provide colloidal osmotic pressure to maintain the integrity of plasma volume, the cell protein (protoplasm) provides the osmotic pressure that maintains the integrity of cell water. Added to the osmotic pressure from the cell protein is the osmotic pressure provided by the intracellular ionized potassium. Balanced against the total intracellular pressure from these two sources is the osmotic pressure outside the cell, which is maintained by ionized sodium. As a result of the balance between the intracellular and the extracellular osmotic pressures, water and nutrients flow in and water and metabolic wastes flow out through the cell membrane.

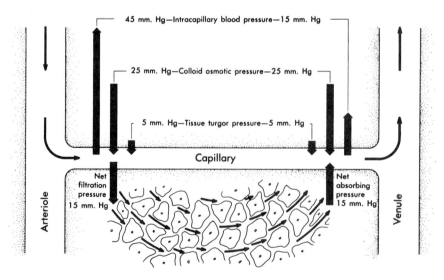

Fig. 8-2. The fluid shift mechanism. Note the balance of pressures that controls the flow of fluid.

■ **How does the lymphatic system help control body water?**

Protein in the lymphatic fluid provides a further means of removing excess water from the tissue spaces. During periods of relative inactivity of tissue the capillaries are adequate to drain away the water that remains after exchanges. In an active organ, however, such as a contracting muscle, more water is produced. Here the lymphatic vessels help to carry off the excess water, averting the accumulation of fluid (edema) in the interstitial spaces. The severe leg edema seen in elephantiasis, for example, is the result of a cutting off of this lymph circulation. A parasitic worm lodges in the lymph vessel and obstructs it, causing these fluids to accumulate, and the leg swells.

■ **Do other organic compounds smaller than protein also influence water balance?**

Yes, if they occur in sufficient quantity. These organic compounds of small molecular size include such substances as glucose, urea, and amino acids. Because of their small size they diffuse freely. They affect water balance only if they occur in unusually large amounts. For example, the large amount of glucose in the urine of a patient with uncontrolled diabetes causes an abnormal osmotic diuresis or excess water output.

Separating membranes

■ **What is the nature of the membranes separating the various body water compartments?**

Two basic types of separating membranes are involved in the movements of water and solutes within the body. These are the capillary wall and the cell wall. The capillary wall is a relatively free or rapid membrane, across which electrolytes pass readily. The cell wall is a slow membrane and is more difficult to penetrate. It is composed essentially of a lipid matrix, covered on either surface by a layer of protein. The metabolic processes within the cell usually govern the passage of electrolytes, and therefore water, across this barrier.

■ **What are the mechanisms that move water and solutes across membranes in the body?**

According to the type of membrane and the number of particles in the involved solution (the size and solubility of the material), water and solutes move across membranes by one or more of five mechanisms:

1. Osmosis. Osmosis is the process by which water molecules pass through a semipermeable membrane separating two solutions. The molecules pass from the more dilute solution (water concentration is higher, the solute concentration is lower) to the more dense solution (water concentration is lower, the solute concentration is higher). Osmotic pressure is created by the difference in molecular pressure on either side of the membrane. It tends to equalize the concentration of solutes and the fluid pressure on each side of a membrane. Thus, it effectively controls the movement of water from place to place in the body.

2. Diffusion. Diffusion is the process by which particles in solution spread throughout the solution and across separating membranes from the place of highest solute concentration to all spaces of lesser solute concentration. There are two types of diffusion: (1) *passive diffusion*, which is simple diffusion without assistance; and (2) *carrier-mediated or facilitated diffusion* in which the particles are moved with the assistance of another substance. Carrier-mediated diffusion and passive diffusion both go with the pressure gradient, not against it. The carrier-mediated form is apparently needed in instances in which the size of the molecule or the solubility factor involved requires the carrier aid. A comparison of the movement of molecules in osmosis and simple diffusion is shown in Fig. 8-3.

3. Active transport. Active transport is the process by which particles in solution are moved *against* a pressure gradient. Many times this movement across a mem-

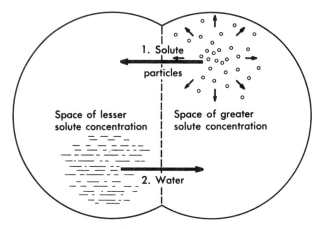

Fig. 8-3. Movement of molecules, water, and solutes by osmosis and diffusion.

brane is necessary despite the opposing pressure and hence some form of active process is needed. This may be compared to a person swimming upstream or walking uphill against gravity's pull. Obviously such movement against pressure requires energy. In the case of substances moving across membranes in the body, the required energy comes from metabolism in the cells. Usually some vehicle or mechanism of transport is needed in addition. An example of such active transport is the operation of the sodium pump by which glucose is absorbed from the intestinal lumen and into the individual cells (see p. 9). Other molecules, such as amino acids and fatty acids, enter and leave cells by a similar means of active transport.

4. *Filtration.* Fluid is forced or filtered through membranes when there is a difference in pressures on the two sides. For example, filtration occurs across the capillary walls because the hydrostatic pressure within the capillary is greater than that of the surrounding interstitial fluid area. Small molecules pass with the fluid out of the capillary lumen, but the large molecules of plasma protein remain. These pressures are diagrammed in Fig. 8-2, p. 106.

5. *Pinocytosis.* Proteins and fats sometimes enter the cells by the interesting process of pinocytosis. The word means "cell drinking." As these large molecules become attached to the cell's outer surface the cell membrane forms a pocket and encircles them. This creates an invagination, or incupping, on the cell's surface from which engulfed material is eventually released into the cell cytoplasm. Apparently this is the mechanism by which fat, for example, is absorbed into the small intestine.

ROLE OF THE GASTROINTESTINAL TRACT IN WATER BALANCE

■ **What is the "gastrointestinal circulation"?**

In considering total fluid and electrolyte balance in the body it is easy to lose sight of the vast importance of the gastrointestinal secretions in maintaining that balance. Water from the plasma, containing ions in various patterns, is converted by the appropriate sections of the gastrointestinal tract into the digestive secretions. These secretions, which are produced daily, function progressively throughout the alimentary system in the processes of digestion and absorption. They circulate constantly between plasma and the secreting cells. Finally in the distal portion of the intestine, most of the water and electrolytes are reabsorbed into the plasma to circulate again. This constant cycling of water and electrolytes as part of the digestive secretions is called the "gastrointestinal circulation."

■ **What electrolytes are contained in the gastrointestinal fluids?**

The cations sodium and potassium and

Table 8-3. Approximate concentration of certain electrolytes in digestive fluids (mEq./L.)

	Na$^+$	K$^+$	Cl$^-$	HCO$_3^-$
Saliva	10	25	10	15
Gastric	40	10	145	0
Pancreatic	140	5	40	110
Jejunal	135	5	110	30
Bile	140	10	110	40

the anions chloride and bicarbonate are the major electrolytes in the digestive fluids. The relative concentrations of these electrolytes in the saliva, the gastric and pancreatic juices, in the jejunal secretions and in the bile are indicated in Table 8-3. It is evident that with upper and lower gastrointestinal losses large amounts of electrolytes can also be lost.

■ **How does the law of isotonicity apply to gastrointestinal fluids?**

The gastrointestinal fluids are held in *isotonicity* (equality of osmotic pressure caused by ion equilibrium) with the extracellular fluid compartment. When water is drunk without solutes or accompanying food, electrolytes and salts are drawn into the intestines from the extracellular fluid. However, if a hypertonic solution of food is ingested, water is drawn into the intestine from the extracellular fluid. In each instance water and electrolytes shift from compartment to compartment to maintain solutions in the alimentary tract isotonic with the extracellular fluid.

This law of isotonicity has many clinical implications. For example, if a patient on gastric suction drank water, the water would cause the stomach to produce more secretions containing electrolytes. The electrolytes would, in turn, be lost in the suctioning. The plasma from which the electrolytes are supplied would be gradually depleted of them and would be unable to supply these essential nutrients to tissue cells. If a patient being maintained on a tube feeding were given his formula too rapidly,

the hypertonic solution being given by tube would cause a shift of water into the intestine, which would rapidly shrink the vascular volume of the extracellular fluid.

■ **What clinical problems result from gastrointestinal losses?**

The loss of gastrointestinal secretion is the most common cause of clinical fluid and electrolyte problems. The biochemical problem differs according to whether the upper or the lower portion of the alimentary tract is involved. For example, in persistent vomiting much fluid and hydrochloric acid is eliminated and dehydration, a potassium deficit, and alkalosis result.

■ **Why does potassium depletion occur in prolonged diarrhea?**

In prolonged diarrhea, large amounts of water, sodium, chloride, and bicarbonate are lost. As sodium losses continue in the stools, sodium is shifted from the plasma and interstitial fluid to replace it, and potassium then moves out of the cells to replace the lost extracellular sodium. The loss of potassium is further compounded by the triggering of the aldosterone mechanism, a hormonal device for the conservation of sodium, and more potassium is eliminated in the process.

ROLE OF THE KIDNEYS IN WATER AND ELECTROLYTE BALANCE

■ **What is the functional unit of the kidney?**

The functional unit of the kidney is the nephron. In the cortex of each kidney there are about one million of these minute, finely structured units. Their tremendous capacity to select, reject, conserve, and eliminate is demonstrated over and over again, as they cleanse the blood fifteen to eighteen times every day.

■ **How do the nephrons control water and electrolyte balance?**

The nephrons control overall water and electrolyte balance through three basic functions: filtration, tubular reabsorption, and secretion.

■ **How is the nephron adapted to perform its filtration function?**

Filtration is one of the mechanisms by which water and certain solutes move across capillary walls as the result of pressure differences on either side. Because the intracapillary fluid pressure is greater than the interstitial fluid pressure, water and small, freely diffusible molecules pass out of the capillary through its wall into the surrounding interstitial fluid and thence into the absorbing capsule of the renal tubule. In the nephron several structures are especially adapted to facilitate this initial filtration process:

1. *Afferent and efferent arterioles.* The head of the nephron consists of a cuplike structure called Bowman's capsule, which holds the glomerulus (a tuft of branching capillaries). The afferent (entering) arteriole is relatively large. As it breaks up into its many branching capillaries it offers a narrowing stream bed that effectively slows down the renal blood flow to promote filtration. The loops of the capillary tuft join again to form a single vessel, the efferent (leaving) arteriole, which is of smaller diameter than the afferent arteriole. This smaller diameter offers resistance to flow and produces additional backward pressure to favor filtration.

Further control is added by the ability of the uniquely muscular afferent and efferent arterioles to constrict or dilate independently of one another, according to blood pressure requirements. For example, when the blood pressure is lower, the afferent arteriole may dilate and the efferent arteriole may constrict to provide additional pressure favoring filtration. If the blood pressure is high, this reaction is reversed.

2. *Cells in walls of glomerulus and capsule.* The glomerulus and the receiving tubular capsule are lined with long, thin, flat cells, especially structured to provide optimum filtration and absorbing surfaces. Resistance to flow here is therefore minimized and filtration occurs readily.

■ **What is the function of the tubules?**

Reabsorption on a selective basis takes place in the tubules of the nephron. After water and filterable solutes are filtered from the blood via the glomerulus into the receiving capsule, they pass in turn through the three portions of the tubule in which this selective absorption takes place. These three areas are the proximal tubule, the loop of Henle, which is a narrowing of the tubule and a turning upward, and the distal tubule. It is in these areas that the nephron carries on its highly selective process of reabsorbing needed materials and rejecting others for eventual elimination. In this process the nephron controls the amount of water in the body and the electrolyte level, excretes various electrolytes as waste products, and excretes excess metabolic materials.

1. *Amount of water in the body.* The control of water is largely regulated by certain hormones, such as the antidiuretic hormone (ADH, vasopressin) from the pituitary. Indirect control is also exerted by aldosterone. Thus by varying the amount of water retained or eliminated under the control of these hormones, the nephrons effectively guard the total fluid volume. As the result of this renal tubular control of hydration, 99% of the water filtered is recovered and returned to the bloodstream to be reused.

2. *Levels of electrolytes in the body.* The integrity of the concentration of certain electrolytes, especially of sodium and potassium, is necessary for delicate fluid-electrolyte and acid-base balances throughout the body. The control of sodium concentration illustrates the adaptation of the

nephron structure and function to the maintenance of the proper supply of electrolytes. Two mechanisms are involved. One is the aldosterone mechanism, which is periodically triggered by a threatened loss of sodium. The other is a continuous active transport process that involves a countercurrent system against the usual osmotic pressure gradient. This system makes use of the sodium pump (see Fig. 8-4).

3. *Excretion of various metabolites as waste products.* The waste products excreted by the nephrons include such materials as urea and excess ketones, which the nephrons selectively reject and discard, thus preventing their harmful accumulation in the blood.

4. *Excretion of excess metabolic materials.* The nephrons excrete harmful excess loads of otherwise beneficial metabolic products. Glucose, for example, is a beneficial product of the metabolism of carbohydrates. Normally it is not excreted but is conserved for use. However, in uncontrolled diabetes, the glucose accumulates in the blood to harmful levels, and the kidney then begins to excrete these excesses, to maintain normal blood levels.

■ **How does the secretion function of the nephron help to control fluid and electrolyte balances?**

A third major function of the nephron involved in control of fluid and electrolytes is secretion. This process is especially related to acid-base balance. Control of acidity is maintained by secretion of hydrogen ions and ammonia from the blood.

■ **How does the nephron conserve water and thus concentrate urine?**

The nephron conserves water and makes urine through a continuous reabsorption of sodium. This reabsorption of sodium occurs between the two limbs of the loop of Henle and involves a *countercurrent system* of active transport. As the fluid that has passed through the distal convoluted tubule flows through the portion of the loop of Henle that descends into the inner zone of the renal medulla, much of its

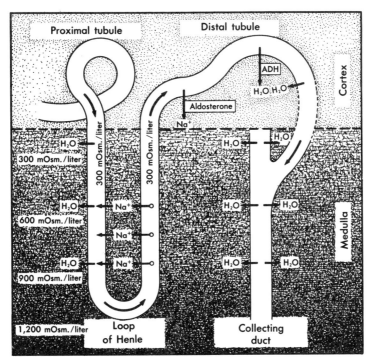

Fig. 8-4. Countercurrent system of sodium (Na) and water exchange operating between the two limbs of the loop of Henle.

water passes out into the interstitial fluid, whereas the sodium moves on into the ascending limb of the loop of Henle. From this site the sodium is actively transported out of the ascending limb into the interstitial fluid of the medulla, then back into the descending limb by means of a series of sodium pumps. The result is a progressive increase in sodium concentration (and therefore in the osmolarity) of the urine in all structures from the inner to outer portions of the renal medulla. The net effect is to conserve water and concentrate the urine in the distal collecting duct as it passes through this hyperosmolar section of the medulla on its way to the renal pelvis. The total system that controls levels of osmolarity has come to be known as the *countercurrent multiplier of concentration*. These relationships are shown in Fig. 8-4.

■ **What is the ADH mechanism?**

The antidiuretic hormone (ADH) secreted by the posterior lobe of the pituitary gland acts mainly in the distal collecting tubule. It stimulates the reabsorption of water according to need. Excess secretion of the hormone may be triggered by a real or apparent loss of body water. The actual loss of body water, as in a hemorrhage, engages the ADH mechanism

in an effort to conserve water. In certain situations, however, such as congestive heart failure, the body water is not actually diminished but is shifted from the circulating plasma into the interstitial extracellular fluid spaces by the diminished action of the heart. Included in this general reduction of plasma flow to all organs is reduction of plasma flow to the kidney. The kidney interprets this diminished plasma flow to mean that the body is deprived of water, and the ADH mechanism is set in motion in an effort to conserve water for the total body. The mechanism by which ADH is released from the pituitary is believed to be mediated by changes of the osmotic pressure in the plasma that bathes the hypothalamus. It is further believed that in the hypothalamus there are pressure-sensitive centers called osmoreceptors (volume receptors). Their precise location within the hypothalmus is not known. Various stress reactions, including shock, stimulate release of the hormone to guard water and electrolytes.

■ **How is the aldosterone mechanism related to the renin-angiotensin cycle?**

A second important hormone that governs the renal control of water and electrolyte balance is the aldosterone mechanism (Fig. 8-5). This mechanism is pri-

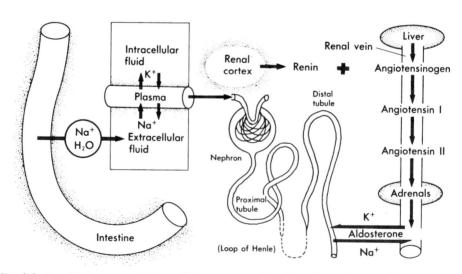

Fig. 8-5. The aldosterone mechanism, which conserves sodium in exchange for potassium and causes increased reabsorption of water.

marily a sodium-conserving device, but in carrying out this function it also exerts a secondary control over the diuresis of water. Therefore it essentially restores the volume of extracellular fluid and of circulating blood in times of stress and threatened loss. The operation of the aldosterone mechanism involves a specific cycle of events:

1. When sodium intake is decreased, or sodium is lost, or body fluid volume is contracted, the renal cortex forms the enzyme *renin* and secretes it into the blood via the renal vein. In the blood renin acts on its specific substrate from the liver, *angiotensinogen,* to form angiotensin I, which in turn is converted to angiotensin II. The latter is an active pressor substance that increases the force of the heartbeat, constricts the arterioles, and diminishes renal blood flow.

2. Angiotensin II stimulates secretion of aldosterone by the adrenals. Aldosterone then causes retention and reabsorption of

sodium and, therefore, of water. Improved renal circulation follows. A secondary result, however, of aldosterone activity is a potassium loss in the tubular ion exchange for sodium. Aldosterone is operative chiefly in the distal renal tubule. It can increase reabsorption up to 98% as in shock, because of lowered blood volume. Shock shrinks the total fluid compartment. Less fluid, therefore, circulates through the kidneys and reabsorption of greater quantity is needed to supply the deficit.

■ **How does stress affect renal function?**

Aldosterone release may also be stimulated by ACTH, a hormone secreted by the anterior pituitary in response to body stress. Both ADH and aldosterone mechanisms may be activated by stress situations, such as bodily injury or surgery. The relationship of these hormones to stress is illustrated in the diagram in Fig. 8-6.

■ **What are some clinical problems that result from imbalances in water and electrolytes?**

Clinical applications center around such problems as postgastrectomy "dumping syndrome," edema in congestive heart failure, ascites in advanced liver disease, renal disease, such as the nephrotic syndrome, edema of starvation, and others.

ACID-BASE BUFFER SYSTEM

■ **What is the difference between an acid and a base?**

A substance is *more* or *less* acid, according to the degree of its concentration of ionized hydrogen. An acid may be defined as a compound that has enough hydrogen ions to give some away. When in aqueous solution, an acid releases hydrogen ion. The following are some examples of acids and their donation of ionized hydrogen when in aqueous solution:

$$H_2CO_3 \longrightarrow H^+ + HCO_3$$
$$HCl \longrightarrow H^+ + Cl$$
$$H_2SO_4 \longrightarrow 2H^+ + SO_4$$
$$H_3PO_4 \longrightarrow 2H^+ + HPO_4$$

A base possesses few hydrogen ions. It therefore takes up ionized hydrogen. The following are examples of bases:

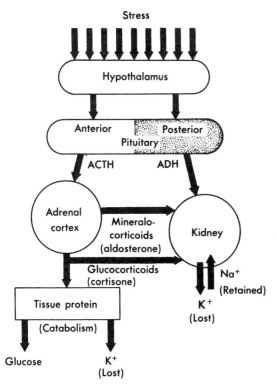

Fig. 8-6. Hormonal response to stress.

$$OH^- + H^+ \longrightarrow H_2O$$
$$HCO_3 + H^+ \longrightarrow H_2CO_3$$
$$OH^- + H_2CO_3 \longrightarrow H_2O + HCO_3$$

■ **What is the meaning of the symbol pH?**

The degree of acidity of a solution is expressed in terms of pH. The symbol pH is derived from a mathematical term. It is the negative logarithm expressed as an exponential *power* of the *H*ydrogen ion concentration. If the pH of a solution is 5, its hydrogen ion concentration is 10^{-5}. The hydrogen ion concentration in pure water is 10^{-7}. Therefore, the pH of pure water is 7. A pH of 7 is the neutral point between an acid and an alkaline (base). Substances with a pH lower than 7 are acid, since the pH is the negative logarithm. The higher the hydrogen ion concentration, the lower the pH. Substances with a pH above 7 are alkaline.

■ **What is a buffer?**

In chemistry a buffer is a mixture of acidic and alkaline components, which protects a solution against wide variations in its pH, even when strong bases or acids are added to it. A solution containing such a protective mixture is called a "buffered solution." A buffer protects the acid-base balance of a solution by rapidly offsetting changes in its ionized hydrogen concentration. It works by protecting against either added acid or base.

If a strong acid is added to a buffered solution, the base partner of the acid-base buffer reacts with the added acid to form a weaker acid. The acidity of the total solution is effectively lowered toward or to the starting point. The formula below shows the reaction when hydrochloric acid is taken up by the bicarbonate to form a weaker acid:

(strong acid)		(base-buffer)	
HCl	+	NaHCO$_3$	$\longrightarrow$
hydrochloric acid		sodium bicarbonate	

(weaker acid)		(salt)
H$_2$CO$_3$	+	NaCl
carbonic acid		table salt

If a strong base is added to a buffered solution, the acid partner of the buffer do-

nates ionized hydrogen, which combines with the intruder to form a weaker base and restores the pH to the starting point. The formula below shows the reaction that occurs if sodium hydroxide is added to a buffered solution:

(strong base)		(acid-buffer)	
NaOH	+	H$_2$CO$_3$	$\longrightarrow$
sodium hydroxide		carbonic acid	

(weaker base)		(water)
NaHCO$_3$	+	H$_2$O
sodium bicarbonate		water

■ **What is the body's main buffer system?**

The human body contains many buffered solutions, including those that involve hemoglobin, oxyhemoglobin, protein, and the disodium hydrogen phosphate-sodium dihydrogen phosphate system (Na_2HPO_4-NaH_2PO_4). Its main buffer system, however, is the relatively weak carbonic acid-sodium bicarbonate system (H_2CO_3-$NaHCO_3$). The body selects this as its principal buffer system for two reasons: (1) the raw materials for the production of carbonic acid ($CO_2 + H_2O = H_2CO_3$) are readily available, and (2) the lungs and kidneys can easily adjust to ratio alterations between carbonic acid and the base bicarbonate, sodium bicarbonate.

The normal pH of the extracellular fluid is 7.4, with a normal range from 7.35 to 7.45. Maintenance of the pH within this narrow range is necessary to sustain the life of the cells. The carbonic acid-sodium bicarbonate buffer system is able to stabilize the extracellular fluid at this pH because the base bicarbonate partner in this buffer system is about twenty times as abundant as the carbonic acid. This 20:1 ratio of base to acid is normally maintained even though the absolute amounts may fluctuate during compensation periods from the normal concentrations of 27 mEq./L. of base bicarbonate and 1.35 mEq./L. of carbonic acid. However, as long as the 20:1 ratio is maintained, the extracellular fluid acid-base balance is held constant. This important 20:1 ratio is shown at various levels in Fig. 8-7.

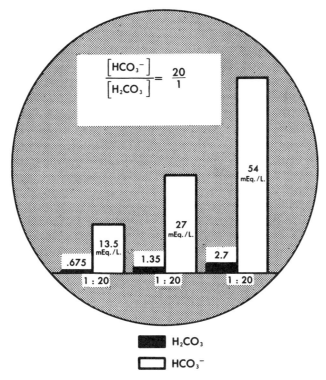

$$\frac{[\text{HCO}_3^-]}{[\text{H}_2\text{CO}_3]} = \frac{20}{1}$$

.675   13.5 mEq./L.   1.35   27 mEq./L.   2.7   54 mEq./L.

1 : 20   1 : 20   1 : 20

■ H_2CO_3

☐ HCO_3^-

Fig. 8-7. The base-to-acid ratio of 20:1 maintains a constant normal blood pH of 7.4.

■ **What is the role of the lungs in maintaining this buffer system?**

The lungs ultimately control the body supply of carbonic acid. Carbonic acid is formed from carbon dioxide and water:

$$CO_2 + H_2O \longrightarrow H_2CO_3$$

Changes in rate and depth of breathing alter the amounts of carbon dioxide that enter the body, thus effectively controlling the level of carbonic acid in blood and tissues. When the blood level of sodium bicarbonate goes down, the lungs expel excess carbon dioxide. This decreases the quantity of raw material available for the production of carbonic acid, and the ratio of base to acid in the buffer system is restored to 20:1.

■ **What is the role of the kidneys in maintaining this buffer system?**

The kidneys maintain the base bicarbonate component of this buffer system. They do this in several ways. In the renal tubule hydrogen ions are secreted. In an ion exchange with hydrogen, sodium is re-captured and returned to the bloodstream. The sodium then is combined with HCO_3^- to form sodium bicarbonate ($NaHCO_3$). The kidney also conserves base by eliminating extra hydrogen ions through the production and excretion of ammonia (NH_4):

$$NH_3 + H^+ \longrightarrow NH_4$$
$$\updownarrow$$
from
deamination of
amino acids

The kidney secures the NH_3 for this process from the deamination of amino acids.

■ **What is the meaning of acidosis and alkalosis?**

The key concept to an understanding of the clinical states of acidosis and alkalosis is ionized hydrogen *concentration.* Formerly these states were thought of as merely conditions in which the blood was "more acid" or "more alkaline." *In acidosis, the ionized hydrogen concentration is above normal. In alkalosis, ionized hydro-*

gen concentration is below normal. Either of these abnormal states initiates compensatory responses in the buffer system, lungs, and kidneys, which cause body fluids to accept, to release, or to excrete ionized hydrogen. Increases and decreases in ionized hydrogen concentration are therefore modified so that the pH is not significantly changed from its normal range of 7.35 to 7.45. Failure of either the lungs or the kidneys to carry out their functions results in acidosis or alkalosis. If the failure is predominantly related to the pulmonary system, the clinical result is called respiratory acidosis or respiratory alkalosis. If the failure is chiefly related to the renal system, the resultant clinical state is called metabolic acidosis or metabolic alkalosis.

■ **What causes** *respiratory acidosis?*

Any condition that interferes with normal breathing may cause respiratory acidosis by impeding the release of carbon dioxide from the lung. The retained carbon dioxide combines with water and forms carbonic acid. In such conditions the carbonic acid level may rise to twice the normal level. In addition, the carbon dioxide combining power in the serum is increased by the presence of the carbon dioxide that was retained by the lungs.

This exchange of gases, oxygen, and carbon dioxide, occurs at the alveolo-capillary membrane. A variety of diseases may affect the lung and involve this membrane and therefore contribute to the development of respiratory acidosis. These diseases include emphysema, bronchiectasis, asthma, pulmonary edema, bronchial pneumonia, and congestive heart failure. A similar effect may follow inhalation anesthesia in a patient whose pulmonary function is marginal or weak. Respiratory acidosis may also occur because of paralysis of respiratory muscles as in poliomyelitis.

■ **How do the lungs and kidneys compensate in response to respiratory acidosis?**

The lung attempts to increase ventilation in order to expel the excess carbon dioxide. However, this is often unsuccessful because the same disease that initiated the problem does not allow adequate increased ventilation. The kidney makes two compensatory responses: (1) Increased ionized hydrogen is secreted by the renal tubule and exchanged for sodium. The sodium is then combined with bicarbonate (HCO_3) to form sodium bicarbonate ($NaHCO_3$), and is returned to the bloodstream. This action elevates the base bicarbonate component of the buffer system. (2) A second compensatory response is the production of increased quantities of ammonia so that more ionized hydrogen is excreted.

■ **What causes** *respiratory alkalosis?*

The primary cause of respiratory alkalosis is excess carbon dioxide output, which in turn is caused by hyperventilation. The resulting decrease in available carbon dioxide lowers the production of carbonic acid and the ionized hydrogen concentration therefore falls (pH rises). In addition, because less carbon dioxide is available, the carbon dioxide combining power is diminished. Common causes of respiratory alkalosis are the hyperventilation syndrome brought about by hysteria or acute anxiety, hyperpnea (labored breathing) in response to hot weather, high altitude, or fever. Excessive breathing may also be forced on a patient by a poorly adjusted mechanical respirator. Respiratory alkalosis may also result from overstimulation of the respiratory center in the brain, which may be brought about by salicylate (aspirin) poisoning, a frequent occurrence in children, or by meningitis or encephalitis.

■ **How do the lungs and the kidneys compensate in response to respiratory alkalosis?**

The lung cannot initiate efforts to compensate for respiratory alkalosis because it is directly involved in the cause. However, the decreased carbonic acid level in the extracellular fluid tends to gradually depress respiration. Therefore the major task of compensation falls to the kidneys, where tubular ionized hydrogen formation is suppressed so that sodium bicarbonate is excreted. Ammonia formation is also diminished so that further sodium can be excreted.

■ **What causes *metabolic acidosis?***

Metabolic acidosis results in certain disorders in which the blood may contain an excess of specific metabolic organic acids, such as ketones or lactic acid. Part of the bicarbonate in the buffer system is displaced by these acids, and the ionized hydrogen concentration rises.

A major clinical example of metabolic acidosis is the condition resulting from an imbalance in diabetes. This potentially dangerous consequence is brought about because in situations of uncontrolled diabetes the body cannot properly metabolize blood glucose and turns for its energy to catabolism of protein and of fat. A similar metabolic situation exists in starvation, when the body turns to its own body stores of protein and fat to supply its needs. Another such metabolic situation exists in states of accelerated metabolism, such as thyrotoxicosis, when increased metabolic demands rapidly deplete carbohydrate stores. In all these situations the body burns protein and fat stores, producing ketosis.

Gastrointestinal problems may also produce metabolic acidosis. For example, although initial vomiting may cause metabolic acidosis as the result of a loss of gastric hydrochloric acid, prolonged vomiting frequently causes metabolic acidosis, because the inability to eat results in decreased carbohydrate intake, glycogen depletion, burning of body protein and fat, and finally ketosis. Severe diarrhea may also induce acidosis because large amounts of bicarbonate and sodium as intestinal contents are swept away. Chronic and acute renal diseases may contribute to metabolic acidosis, since the kidney becomes unable to compensate in the face of excess ionized hydrogen concentrations.

■ **How do the lungs and kidney compensate in response to metabolic acidosis?**

In order to reduce the carbonic acid level, the lungs attempt to expel carbon dioxide by deep, pauseless breathing. This is called air hunger or Kussmaul breathing. Kussmaul breathing is characteristic of diabetic acidosis. The renal tubule increases its secretion of hydrogen ions, which are exchanged for sodium. The sodium is then returned to the blood as sodium bicarbonate. The kidney also compensates by increasing ammonia production and taking up ionized hydrogen and excreting it in the urine.

■ **What causes *metabolic alkalosis?***

Metabolic alkalosis is characterized by a fall in ionized hydrogen concentration (rise in pH), caused primarily by an increase in bicarbonate. Such an excess of bicarbonate may be caused by excretion or loss of large amounts of ionized hydrogen, by excess intake of bicarbonate, or by decrease in potassium stores. As ionized hydrogen and sodium move into the cell to replace lost potassium, the extracellular fluid concentration of ionized hydrogen is reduced.

Clinical problems, such as initial vomiting with loss of ionized hydrogen and chlorine, induce metabolic alkalosis. Gastric suction may have the same effect, causing loss of these ions. Also, any obstruction of the proximal intestine, such as pyloric stenosis, will have similar responses. Conditions that involve potassium depletion also increase alkalosis, as ionized hydrogen and sodium move into the cells to replace loss of potassium. This reduces the extracellular fluid hydrogen concentration. Such conditions include lack of potassium intake, gastrointestinal loss of potassium, or ACTH therapy. ACTH induces renal tubular reabsorption of sodium in an ion exchange for potassium, and therefore potassium is excreted. An excess intake of alkali powders or sodium bicarbonate, as in long-term ulcer therapy, may also contribute to metabolic alkalosis.

■ **How do the lungs and kidneys compensate in response to metabolic alkalosis?**

The decreased ionized hydrogen concentration, (increased pH), gradually suppresses ventilation. The lungs tend to conserve carbon dioxide, which gradually increases the production of carbonic acid.

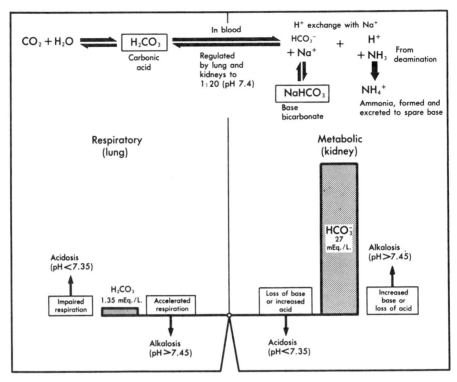

Fig. 8-8. Carbonic acid to sodium (base) bicarbonate buffer system. Note the types of clinical situations that lead to respiratory acidosis and alkalosis and to metabolic acidosis and alkalosis.

The renal tubule suppresses secretion of ionized hydrogen, which allows sodium bicarbonate to be excreted rather than reabsorbed. The kidney also reduces ammonia production so that more base is excreted. The excretion of various acid metabolites is also reduced.

In all states of acid base imbalance, two basic rules of treatment apply: (1) the primary cause of the acidosis or alkalosis is treated, and (2) efforts are made to aid the various compensatory responses of the lungs and kidneys. Each of these therapeutic attempts must be accompanied by careful and continuous evaluation and adjustment. The diagram in Fig. 8-8 summarizes the balances that are involved in the overall buffer system.

9 Digestion, absorption, and metabolism

The digestion-absorption-metabolism continuum is a dynamic unit—a highly integrated overall physiologic process made up of a vast array of interrelated processes involving all of the nutrients. This concept of the *interrelatedness of the nutrients* is basic to an understanding of the wholeness or physical integrity of man and the role of nutrition in maintaining that integrity.

The many processes that comprise the whole digestion-absorption-metabolism spectrum proceed in orderly design through uniquely adapted structures and functions in the successive parts of the system. Why is this intricate complex of biochemical and physiologic activities necessary? Two reasons are apparent, both based on the concept of *change*. First, food as it naturally occurs and as man consumes it is not a single component but a mixture of substances. If energy is to be obtained from these substances, they must be separated into their components so that each component may be handled by the body as a separate unit. Second, because in most instances the still simpler chemical units that make up these nutrient components are still unavailable to the body, some additional means of changing their form must follow. The intermediate unit must be broken down, simplified, regrouped, and rerouted. This exceedingly complex chemical work must take place because man is the most highly organized and intricately balanced of all organisms whose life is developed and sustained in an internal chemical environment.

DIGESTION

■ **What is the purpose of the digestive process?**

Digestion is necessary to produce the initial preparatory changes in ingested foods to render them into forms that the cell can use. This purpose is accomplished through mechanical and chemical processes.

■ **What types of muscles contribute gastrointestinal motility and hence aid mechanical digestion?**

Four types of muscles in the stomach and intestine contribute to gastrointestinal motility:

1. A layer of circular contractile rings that break up, mix, and churn the food particles
2. Longitudinal muscles that help to propel the food mass along
3. Sphincter muscles that act as valves (the pyloric ileocecal, and anal valves) to control passage of material to the next segment of the intestine
4. A thin mucosal layer of smooth muscle that can raise intestinal folds to increase the absorbing surface

These four types of muscles interact to produce two general types of movement: (1) a general muscle tone or tonic contraction that ensures continuous passage and valve control, and (2) periodic, rhythmic contractions that mix and propel the food mass along. These alternating muscular contractions and relaxations that force the contents forward are known by the term *peristalsis*.

■ **How are these muscular actions regulated?**

Specific nerves regulate these muscular actions. A complex, interrelated network of nerves within the gastrointestinal wall, the *intramural nerve plexus*, extends from the esophagus to the anus. The intramural plexus controls muscle tone of the gastro-intestinal wall, regulates the rate and intensity of periodic muscle contractions, and coordinates the various movements. This complex of nerves includes those of the sympathetic and the parasympathetic systems.

■ **What types of secretions provide the basis for chemical digestion?**

Four types of secretions make the necessary chemical changes in food:

1. *Enzymes*—specific in kind and quantity for the degradation of a given nutrient
2. *Hydrochloric acid and buffer ions*—to produce the pH necessary for the activity of given enzymes
3. *Mucus*—for lubrication and protection of the gastrointestinal tract
4. *Water and electrolytes*—in sufficient quantities to carry or circulate the organic substances produced

■ **Where are these secretions produced?**

There are several kinds of cells and glands that produce these secretions. There are single mucous cells on the epithelial surface, called goblet cells, which act alone. In the small intestine there are *multicellular tubular glands,* such as the simple pits lined with goblet mucous cells (crypts of Lieberkühn). Enzymes and hydrochloric acid are secreted by the deeper, branched gastric glands. In addition, there are *complicated glands outside the gastrointestinal tract,* such as the salivary glands, the pancreas, and the liver. These organs secrete enzymes and bile from organized secretory cell structures called *acini,* which feed into ducts that empty into the gastrointestinal lumen. The secretory action of these various special cells or glands may be stimulated locally by the presence of food, by sensory nerve stimuli, or by hormones specific for certain foods.

■ **What mechanical digestive processes occur in the mouth?**

Mastication, (biting and chewing) begins the breaking up of food into smaller particles. The teeth and other oral structures are particularly suited for this function. The incisors cut; the molars grind.

Tremendous force is supplied by the jaw muscles—55 pounds of muscular pressure is applied through incisors and 200 pounds is applied through the molars. Mastication makes it possible for the enlarged surface area of food to be exposed constantly to enzyme action. Also, the fineness of the food particles eases the continued passage of material through the gastrointestinal tract.

■ **How is the swallowing of food accomplished?**

Swallowing of the mixed mass of food particles and its passage down the esophagus are accomplished by peristaltic waves controlled by nerve reflexes. In the usual upright eating position, gravity aids this movement down the esophagus. At the point of entry into the stomach the gastro-esophageal constrictor muscle relaxes to allow food to enter, than constricts again to prevent regurgitation of stomach contents back up into the esophagus. When regurgitation does occur through failure of this mechanism, the patient feels it as "heartburn." Clinical conditions, such as cardiospasm, caused by the failure of the constrictor muscle to relax properly, or hiatus hernia, which is a protrusion of the stomach into the thorax through an abnormal opening in the diaphragm, may also cause problems. In the presence of a hiatus hernia food is held in the out-pouched area and is not allowed to pass normally at this point.

■ **Does any chemical digestion begin in the mouth?**

Very little chemical digestion begins in the mouth. Starch digestion is initiated by ptylin, an enzyme in the salivary juices. However, food is not held long enough in the mouth, usually, for much of this chemical breakdown to occur.

■ **What types of muscle activity aid mechanical digestion in the stomach?**

Muscles in the stomach wall provide three basic motor functions of the stomach: storage, mixing, and slow, controlled emptying. As the food mass enters the stomach it lies against the stomach walls, which can stretch outward to store as much as one liter. Gradually local tonic muscle waves increase their kneading and mixing action as the mass of food and secretions moves on toward the region of the pyloric antrum at the distal end of the stomach. Here waves of peristaltic contractions reduce the mass to a semifluid chyme. Finally, with each peristaltic wave, small amounts of chyme are forced through the pyloric valve. This pyloric pump controls the emptying of the stomach contents into the duodenum by constrictive action of the sphincter muscle (the pyloric valve), and by controlling the rate of propulsive peristaltic activity in the antrum. This control releases the acid chyme slowly enough so that it can be buffered by the alkaline intestinal secretions.

■ **What secretions in the stomach provide agents for chemical digestion?**

About 2,000 ml. of gastric secretions are produced daily. Two basic types of glands in the stomach wall secrete materials that act on specific nutrients:

1. *Gastric gland secretions.* Special secreting cells lining the tubular gastric glands, which are located in the upper portion of the stomach and the wall of the body and fundus, secrete special materials

for digestion. The *chief cells,* also called the *adelomorphous cells,* secrete pepsinogen, which is activated by previously formed pepsin and hydrochloric acid to form the active enzyme pepsin. A highly acid medium (pH approximately 2.0) is required for this enzyme activation. Pepsin begins the enzymatic breakdown of proteins into small polypeptides. The *parietal cells* secrete the necessary hydrochloric acid. *Mucous cells* secrete mucous, which helps to protect the gastric mucosa and to give body and cohesiveness to the food mass. Other enzyme-secreting cells produce small amounts of a specific gastric lipase, tributyrinase, which acts on the tributyrin in butterfat. This is a relatively minor activity.

2. *Pyloric glands.* These glands secrete additional thin mucus. Surface *goblet cells* produce a thicker, more viscous mucus, which coats and protects the stomach wall. When irritation occurs, a still greater quantity of mucus is produced.

■ **How are these gastric secretory processes stimulated?**

Stimuli for these secretions are from nerves and hormones:

1. *Nerve stimulus* is produced in re-

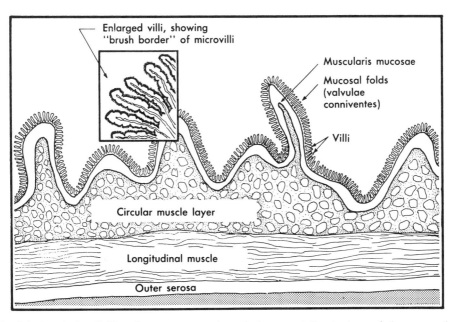

Fig. 9-1. Intestinal wall. Note the arrangement of muscle layers and the structures of the mucosa that increase the surface area for absorption—mucosal folds, villi, and microvilli.

sponse to sensation, to food taken in, and to emotions. For example, in response to anger and hostility, secretions increase. Fear and depression decrease secretions and inhibit blood flow and motility as well.

2. *Hormonal stimulus* is produced in response to the entrance of food into the stomach. Certain stimulants, especially coffee, alcohol, and meat extractives, cause the release of *gastrin* from mucosal glands in the antrum, which in turn stimulates the parietal cells to secrete more hydrochloric acid. When the pH reaches 2.0, a feedback mechanism stops secretion of the hormone to prevent excess acid formation. Another hormone, *enterogastrone*, produced by glands in the duodenal mucosa, counteracts excessive gastric activity by inhibiting acid and pepsin secretion and gastric motility.

■ **What types of muscles and muscle movements aid mechanical digestion in the small intestine?**

The muscles in the small intestine are illustrated in Fig. 9-1. These include three basic layers of muscle: (1) the thin layer of smooth muscle in the mucosa (muscularis mucosa), with fibers extending up into the villi, (2) the circular muscular layer, and (3) the longitudinal muscle next to the outer serosa.

Under the control of the nerve plexus, of wall stretch pressure from food present, or hormonal stimuli, these muscles produce several different types of movement that aid mechanical digestion:

1. *Segmentation rings* from alternate contractions of circular muscle progressively chop the food mass into successive boluses. This action constantly mixes the food materials with secretions.

2. *Longitudinal rotations* by the long muscle running the length of the intestine rolls the slowly moving food mass in a spiral motion, mixing it and exposing new surfaces for absorption.

3. *Pendular movements* from small local muscle contractions sweep back and forth and stir chyme at the mucosal surface.

4. *Peristaltic waves* produced by the contraction of deep circular muscle, propel the food mass slowly forward. The intensity of the waves may be increased by food intake or by the presence of irritants. In some cases this may cause long, sweeping waves over the entire length of the intestine.

5. *Motion of the villi* also aids mechanical digestion. Alternating contractions and extensions of the mucosal muscle fibers constantly agitate the mucosal surface. This action stirs and mixes chyme that is in contact with the intestinal wall and exposes additional nutrient material for absorption. A specific hormone, *villikinin*, is released from the upper intestinal mucosa when it is bathed by chyme entering from the proximal gastrointestinal tract. Villikinin stimulates these contractions, which in turn constantly shorten and lengthen the intestinal villi.

These muscle movements are illustrated in Fig. 9-2.

■ **What secretions of intestinal enzymes aid chemical digestion of fat, protein, and carbohydrate?**

Intestinal glands in the mucosa (crypts of Lieberkühn) secrete enzymes specific for each of the major nutrients:

1. Fat—intestinal lipase converts fat to glycerides and fatty acids.

2. Protein
   a. Enterokinase converts the inactive precursor trypsinogen to active trypsin.
   b. Amino peptidase removes from polypeptides the terminal amino acids that contain a free amino (NH_4) group, by attacking the peptide bond.
   c. Dipeptidase converts dipeptides to amino acids.
   d. Nucleosidase converts nucleosides to a purine or a pyrimidine base and pentose sugar.

3. Carbohydrate—disaccharidases (maltase, lactase, sucrase) convert maltose, lactose, and sucrose to their constituent monosaccharides (glucose, fructose, and galactose).

■ What secretions of pancreatic enzymes aid chemical digestion in the small intestine?

Enzymes from the pancreas also act on all three basic nutrients:

1. Fat—pancreatic lipase converts fats to glycerides and fatty acids.
2. Protein
a. Trypsin causes initial breakdown of proteins and polypeptides to smaller peptides. It also activates chymotrypsinogen to chymotrypsin.
b. Chymotrypsin breaks down proteins and polypeptides to small polypeptides.
c. Carboxypeptidase removes carboxyl (COOH) terminal amino acid from polypeptidases.
d. Nucleases convert nucleic acids (RNA and DNA) to nucleotides.

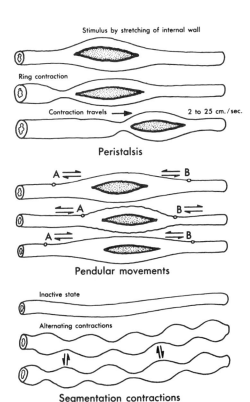

Fig. 9-2. Types of movement produced by muscles of the intestine: peristaltic waves from contractions of deep circular muscle; pendular movements from small local muscles; and segmentation rings formed by alternate contraction and relaxation of circular muscle.

3. Carbohydrate—pancreatic amylase converts starch to disaccharides.

■ How is the mucosal surface of the duodenum protected from the highly acid gastric juices entering at this point?

Large quantities of mucus are secreted by intestinal glands (Brunner's glands) located immediately inside the duodenum. This secretion protects the mucosa from acid irritation and digestion by the gastric juices entering here. Emotions, however, inhibit these mucous secretions and thus are an important factor in the production of duodenal ulcers. Additional mucous cells on the mucosal surface or in intestinal glands continue to secrete mucus as they are touched by the food mass. These additional secretions provide lubrication and protection of tissues. The combined secretions of the mucous glands of the intestine and pancreas total about 4,200 ml. daily (3,000 ml. from intestinal glands and 1,200 ml. from the pancreas).

■ What is the significance of bile in the chemical digestive process?

Bile is produced in the liver and is concentrated and stored by the gallbladder. It serves as an emulsifying agent for fats. When fat enters the duodenum the hormone *cholecystokinin* is secreted by intestinal mucosa glands and stimulates the gallbladder to contract and release bile. From 600 to 700 ml. of bile is produced daily and provides for the repeated circulation of bile salts in the enterohepatic circulation (see p. 19).

■ How are these intestinal secretions stimulated?

Digestive secretions in the intestine are stimulated by hormones. The hormone *secretin*, produced by the mucosa of the upper part of the small intestine, stimulates the pancreatic secretions and regulates their pH so that they are maintained at the alkalinity that is necessary to stop the acidic enzyme activity of chyme entering from the stomach. The unprotected intestinal mucosa alone could not withstand this high degree of acidity. The resultant alkalinity of the medium also provides the

Table 9-1. Summary of digestive processes

Nutrient	Mouth	Stomach	Small Intestine
Carbo-hydrate	Starch $\xrightarrow{\text{Ptyalin}}$ Dextrins		*Pancreas* Starch $\xrightarrow{\text{Amylase}}$ (Disaccharides) Maltose and sucrose *Intestine* Lactose $\xrightarrow{\text{Lactase}}$ (Monosaccharides) Glucose and galactose Sucrose $\xrightarrow{\text{Sucrase}}$ Glucose and fructose Maltose $\xrightarrow{\text{Maltase}}$ Glucose and glucose
Protein		Pepsin Hydrochloric acid Protein $\longrightarrow$ Polypeptides	*Pancreas* Proteins, polypeptides $\xrightarrow{\text{Trypsin}}$ Dipeptides Proteins, polypeptides $\xrightarrow{\text{Chymotrypsin}}$ Dipeptides Polypeptides, dipeptides $\xrightarrow{\text{Carboxypeptidase}}$ Amino acids *Intestine* Polypeptides, dipeptides $\xrightarrow{\text{Aminopeptidase}}$ Amino acids Dipeptides $\xrightarrow{\text{Dipeptidase}}$ Amino acids
Fat		Tributyrin (butterfat) $\xrightarrow{\text{Tributyrinase}}$ Glycerol Fatty acids	*Pancreas* Fats $\xrightarrow{\text{Lipase}}$ Glycerol Glycerides (di-, mono-) Fatty acids *Intestine* Fats $\xrightarrow{\text{Lipase}}$ Glycerol Glycerides (di-, mono-) Fatty acids *Liver and gallbladder* Fats $\xrightarrow{\text{Bile}}$ Emulsified fat

pH (8.0) that is optimum for pancreatic enzyme activity.

A summary of the chemical processes involved in digestion in the mouth, the stomach, and the small intestine, is given in Table 9-1 for review and reference.

ABSORPTION

■ **What are the end products of digestion that are now in forms that can be absorbed?**

After digestion of the food nutrients is complete, the simplified end products are ready to be absorbed. These end products include monosaccharides, such as glucose, fructose and galactose from carbohydrates, fatty acids and glycerides from fats, and amino acids from proteins. Also liberated are vitamins and minerals. Finally, with a water base for solution and transport, plus necessary electrolytes, the total fluid food mass is absorbed. The volume of this in-

Table 9-2. Daily absorption volume in human gastrointestinal system

	Intake (liters)	Intestinal absorption (liters)	Elimination (liters)
Food ingested	1.5		
Gastrointestinal secretions	8.5		
Total	10.0		
Fluid absorbed in small intestine		9.5	
Fluid absorbed in colon		.4	
Total		9.9	
Feces			.1

testinal absorption and the efficiency of this daily process can be seen in Table 9-2.

■ **How is the small intestine structured to provide maximum absorptive surface?**

Three basic structures of the small intestine make or provide maximum absorbing surface to facilitate the absorption of the nutrients:

1. *Mucosal folds.* Easily seen by the naked eye are heaped-up folds along the mucosal surface, like so many hills and valleys in a mountain range.

2. *Villi.* Closer examination by light microscope reveals small, fingerlike projections, the villi, covering these convoluted folds of mucosa. These villi further increase the area of the exposed surface. To receive the absorbed nutrients, each villus has an ample vascular network that involves venous and arterial capillaries and central *lacteals.* Lacteal is the special name given to a lymphatic vessel in the small intestine. It is like any other lymphatic vessel in structure and function. It receives this special name because the chyle that fills it during digestion looks like milk.

3. *Microvilli.* An electron microscope focused on the surface of a single villus brings into view extremely numerous minute surface projections. This vast array of microvilli covering the edge of each villus is called the "brush border," because it looks like bristles on a brush. At the base of the brush border is the basement membrane.

These three types of convolutions and projections, mucosal folds, villi, and microvilli, increase the inner surface of the intestine some 600 times over that of the outer serosa! These special structures of the mucosal surface, plus the contracted links of the live organ (20 to 22 feet) combine to produce a tremendously large absorbing surface area, as large or larger than half a basketball court. The relationship of these structures may be visualized in Fig. 9-1 (see page 121).

■ **What mechanisms facilitate absorption across the intestinal wall?**

Absorption is accomplished by the small intestine by means of a number of processes:

1. *Passive diffusion through epithelial membrane pores.* Where no opposing pressure exists, molecules small enough to pass through the capillary membranes diffuse easily into the capillaries of the villi in the direction of pressure flow in quantities that represent their concentration or electrochemical gradient. For example, electrolytes diffuse in and out of the intestinal lumen as electrochemical need demands.

2. *Osmosis.* Water molecules flow back and forth as osmotic pressures vary (see p. 107).

3. *Carrier-mediated diffusion.* Ferry systems carry molecules across the epithelial cells and basement membrane of the microvilli into the capillary circulation of the villi. This system is used for molecules too large to traverse membrane pores and

hence must be helped through the barrier of the cell wall. Since the pressure gradient is from greater to lesser, the molecule of another nutrient combines with the large molecule to provide a vehicle that carries the large molecule through the barrier. This mechanism operates with a pressure gradient. The need for a carrier is usually based on the size of the molecule or its solubility in the transport medium. For example, the stomach secretes the highly specialized ferry called intrinsic factor (IF), which is required to carry the very large molecule of vitamin B_{12} out of the intestinal lumen into the circulating blood. If the stomach fails to secrete IF, the large vitamin B_{12} molecule lacks the ferrying molecule and cannot enter the blood. Lacking vitamin B_{12}, the red blood cells cannot mature normally and pernicious anemia results (see p. 63).

4. *Energy-dependent active transport.* Even against a pressure gradient, nutrient molecules must cross the intestinal epithelial membrane to feed hungry tissue cells. Such work requires extra machinery and energy. This need is supplied by a mechanism that physiologists have come to call a pump that continuously picks up the waiting molecules and carries them across the membrane. Energy to operate the pump is supplied by the cell's metabolism. The sodium pump that transports glucose molecules is an example of this mechanism.

5. *Engulfing (pinocytosis).* Some even larger macromolecules require still another means of reaching the tissue circulation outposts in the villi. In these instances epithelial cells of the villi act like amebae or leukocytes and ingest the particles. A small portion of the edge of the cell, on coming in contact with the material to be transported, dips inward (invaginates), engulfs the particle, and opens to swallow the particle into the interior of the cell. The particle is then conveyed through the cytoplasm to the opposite side of the epithelial cell, which borders on the capillary lumen. Here the particle is discharged into the intracapillary blood. Occasionally

whole proteins are absorbed by pinocytosis. This mechanism is also involved in the absorption of neutral fat droplets (chylomicrons) and their transportation into the lacteals of the villi.

■ **What is the significance of the word "pump" as used to designate active transport mechanisms?**

The use of the word *pump* for this type of mechanism may be confusing at first. It must be remembered that what makes a pump *pump* is the threat of *vacuum*. A pump pulls material from one place to another by the exercise of negative pressure. The pump is able to suck material from one place to another because the new site *cannot endure the absence of material.* It is from this characteristic that biochemists and physiologists have adopted the name *pump.* The avidity of the empty site for something to fill its space provides the power to move the molecules across membranes. A biochemical "pumping mechanism" is one that works by pulling a fresh molecule in, to fill a place that has been emptied by the removal of a molecule that was formerly present.

■ **By what routes are the absorbed nutrient components transported to the tissues?**

After their absorption by any of these processes, each of the nutrient components from carbohydrates and proteins enters the portal blood system and travels to the body tissues by way of the liver. Only fat is unique in its route. After enzymatic processing in the cells of the intestinal lumen, the fat is largely converted into esterified lipids. These molecules are small enough to pass between the cells of the intestinal mucosa and into the lymph vessels (the lacteals) in the center of the villi. From these they flow into the larger lymph vessels of the mesentery and finally enter the common portal blood flow at the thoracic duct through the left subclavian vein. Exceptions are the medium- and short-chain fatty acids, which, being more soluble in water, are absorbed directly into villi blood circulation. However, most com-

Table 9-3. Intestinal absorption of some major nutrients

Nutrient	Form	Means of absorption	Control agent or required cofactor	Route
Carbohydrate	Monosaccharides (glucose and galactose)	Competitive Selective Active transport via sodium pump	— — Sodium	Blood
Protein	Amino acids	Selective	—	Blood
	Some dipeptides	Carrier transport systems	Pyridoxine (pyridoxal phosphate)	Blood
	Whole protein (rare)	Pinocytosis	—	Blood
Fat	Fatty acids	Fatty acid-bile complex (micelles)	Bile	Lymph
	Glycerides (mono-, di-)		—	Lymph
	Few triglycerides (neutral fat)	Pinocytosis	—	Lymph
Vitamins	B_{12}	Carrier transport	Intrinsic factor (IF)	Blood
	A	Bile complex	Bile	Blood
	K	Bile complex	Bile	From large intestine to blood
Minerals	Sodium	Active transport via sodium pump	—	Blood
	Calcium	Active transport	Vitamin D	Blood
	Iron	Active transport	Ferritin mechanism	Blood (as transferritin)
Water	Water	Osmosis		Blood, lymph, interstitial fluid

monly consumed fats, because they are insoluble in water and made up of long-chain fatty acids, travel the lacteal route.

■ **What absorption occurs in the large intestine?**

There are no digestive enzymes secreted by the colon. The only absorption process occurring here is water absorption. Within a 24-hour period, of the approximate 500 ml. of remaining food mass leaving the ileum (the last portion of the small intestine) and entering the cecum (the pouch at the start of the large intestine), about 350 to 400 ml. of water in this mass is absorbed in the proximal half of the colon. Thus only about 100 to 150 ml. of water remains to form an aid in elimination of the feces.

■ **What is the usual time rate for passage of food material through the gastrointestinal tract?**

Studies with test meals indicate that the food residue mass moves through the large intestine at a gradually slowing pace. Usually the test meal, having traversed the 21 to 22 feet of small intestine, starts to enter the cecum about 4 hours after it was consumed. About 8 hours later it reaches the sigmoid colon, having traveled through the large intestine for a distance of about 3 feet. In the sigmoid colon, the mass descends still more slowly toward the anus. Even 72 hours after the meal has been eaten as much as 25% of it may still remain in the rectum!

■ **What bacterial action occurs in the large intestine?**

Bacteria in the colon are closely associated with a number of vitamins. At birth the colon is sterile but very shortly thereafter intestinal bacterial flora is well established. The adult colon contains large numbers of bacteria, the prominent species being *Escherichia coli*. Great masses of the bacteria are passed in the stool. The colon bacteria synthesize vitamin K and some vitamins of the B complex (especially biotin and folic acid). These vitamins are then absorbed from the colon in sufficient amounts to meet the daily requirements. Although vitamin B_{12} is also synthesized by intestinal bacteria, it is not absorbed from the large intestine. Since the intestine lacks the necessary cofactor (IF), the vitamin cannot be transported through the wall of the colon and is eliminated in the feces.

Intestinal bacteria also affect the color and odor of the stool. The brown color represents bile pigments that are formed by the colon bacteria from bilirubin. Thus in conditions where bile flow is hindered the stools may become clay colored or white. The characteristic odor results from amines, especially indole and skatole, formed by bacterial enzymes from amino acids.

Gas, or flatus, formed in the large intestine contains hydrogen sulfide or methane produced by the bacteria. Gas formation, however, is attributable not so much to specific foods per se as to the state of the body that receives them. Many foods have been labeled gas formers, but in reality such classifications have little or no scientific basis.

Since man, unlike herbivorous animals and some insects, such as the termite, has no microorganisms or enzymes to break down cellulose, this plant product remains after digestion and absorption as residue. Cellulose contributes important bulk to the diet and helps form the feces. The feces contain about 75% water and 25% solids. The solids include cellulose, bacteria, inorganic matter (mostly calcium and phosphates) a small amount of fat and its derivatives, some mucus, and sloughed-off mucosal cells.

A summary of the intestinal absorption

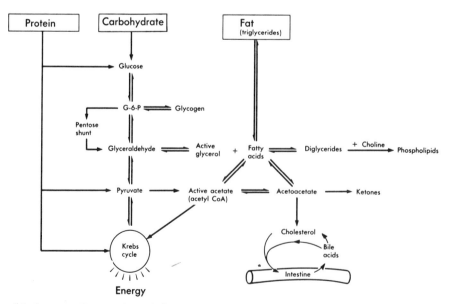

Fig. 9-3. Summary diagram of metabolism of the nutrients. Note metabolic interrelationships of carbohydrate, protein, and fat.

of some major nutrients is given in Table 9-3 for review and reference.

METABOLISM

■ What basic problems of physical survival are solved by cell metabolism?

Two basic problems necessary for survival are accomplished by cell metabolism: (1) energy production, and (2) the maintenance of a dynamic equilibrium between building up and breaking down of tissue.

■ How are these solutions accomplished?

Solutions to the basic problems of energy and tissue synthesis are accomplished through an interrelated series of chemical changes that determines the final use of the individual nutrients. The controlling agents in the cells are the cellular enzymes, their coenzymes (many of which are B vitamins), other cofactors, and hormones. A summary diagram showing the interrelationship of these various processes that sustain life can be seen in Fig. 9-3.

II
Community nutrition

10 The food environment

The scientific principles of human nutrition have meaning only in terms of people—people in every conceivable life situation, meeting problems requiring solutions, asking questions needing answers. Because the impact of a rapidly changing environment is producing new problems and new questions, new solutions and new answers must be sought. There are changing beliefs, philosophies, and values, changing life styles, changing family patterns, new living situations and working patterns, bringing new eating habits and food forms. These changes are particularly reflected in the food environment. The technology involved in food production from mechanized agribusiness to large food industries is consistently producing a new food environment. There are new products, new food channels. Thus, it is in this context of *change* that a variety of ways to meet needs must be found.

FOOD FACTS AND FALLACIES

■ **How may scientific nutrition concepts be applied to questions concerning food practices?**

Scientifically sound concepts are the result of persistent research and testing. They represent organized tested knowledge. The scientific or problem-solving method, here as in all other branches of modern living, involves four steps:

1. Recognizing that a problem exists, identifying the problem, and determining some desirable goals in relation to it
2. Gathering all possible pertinent data, background knowledge, and principles; and on the basis of this information forming a hypothesis (an educated guess) about the solution to the problem
3. Testing this hypothesis under controlled conditions, which entails isolating the pertinent variables and studying one variable at a time; usually a large number of cases must be observed in detail before valid results accrue
4. Evaluating these test results, and, if the hypothesis seems to be borne out, applying the results to a much larger population, while continuing to observe critically for errors that may become apparent only with time and broad application over a wide range of circumstances

Whenever one is confronted with questionable food information, it is highly legitimate to ask, "What is your evidence?" The scientist maintains an open attitude to new information at all times.

■ **Are the qualities of vitamins and minerals as they occur naturally in foods different from those that are produced synthetically?**

No. Vitamins and minerals produced in a laboratory or added to food do not differ from those that occur naturally in foods. *A vitamin is a vitamin,* no matter what its origin. Its basic molecular structure is identical. Minerals, whether they occur naturally in foods or are added, are the same.

■ **Does cooking food in aluminum cookware harm the food?**

Aluminum is a trace element in the human body and is widespread in nature. There is no evidence to indicate that these trace amounts are harmful or that the amounts that may be ingested in food that has been cooked in an aluminum utensil significantly increases the total amount in the body. Extensive use of aluminum cookware even in quantity cookery in governmental and industrial food service installations, has produced none of the harmful effects claimed by some promoters of this myth. It has no scientific basis in fact.

■ **What is the difference between "organic" and "natural" foods?**

The word "natural" is a generalized term covering all foods that are sold without artificial colorings, preservatives, or any kind of synthetic additives. In other words, nothing has been added after the crop has been harvested. However, while the food was being grown pesticides could have been applied. The term "organic," as used by the followers of the natural food movement, has a more specialized meaning. It refers to a method of agriculture in which no chemical fertilizers have been used. Instead, food has been fertilized with compost, manure, seaweed, or any kind of vegetation that can be incorporated into the soil. Pesticides, herbicides, fungicides, fumigants, or hormones must not have been used. Weeds and insects are controlled through nonsynthetic methods.

■ **Is any food *per se* required for human nutrition?**

No. It is the nutrients in foods, not specific foods as such, that have specific functions in the body. Each of these nutrients may be found in a number of different foods. People require specific nutrients, never specific foods, despite much advertising to the contrary. There is no one food that everybody needs. Many cultures and population groups throughout the world, for centuries, have lived and grown on a variety of food combinations, demonstrating that a variety of foods meet human needs. It is the combination of foods that provides the profile of essential nutrients that maintains health, not any one food or specific food combination alone.

■ **Is pasteurized milk a "dead milk"? Should it be replaced by raw milk?**

No. The process of pasteurization may destroy a small amount of vitamin C, but the quantity of vitamin C in cow's milk is so small that it makes no significant contribution to the human diet and its destruction by pasteurization is therefore not important. However, control of microorganisms by pasteurization and the prevention of the spread of disease by this means far outweighs any imagined dietary loss.

■ **Do citrus fruits, such as oranges and lemons, make the body acid, or produce "acid stomach"?**

Hydrochloric acid secreted by the parietal cells in gastric mucosal glands forms the normally acid medium of the stomach. Citrus fruits have no influence on this secretion. As they undergo metabolism by the body, almost all fruits form an alkaline—not acid—residue.

■ **Does gelatin in large amounts build strong fingernails?**

No. Gelatin is an incomplete protein, which alone builds nothing. Nail formation is influenced by many other factors, such as general body nutrition, disease, environment, and local nail care.

ECOLOGY OF NUTRITION

■ **What is meant by the term "ecology of nutrition"?**

The word "ecology" comes from a Greek word *oikos* meaning "house." There is a vast complex of interrelated forces "housed" in a biologic system, which produces health or disease, good or bad states of nutrition. Some of these revolve around man's internal environment—his state of health and the manner in which he is able to handle foodstuffs and nutrients. Others revolve around man's external environment. These are sometimes far more complex and difficult to sort out and deal with. They include factors that influence and determine the available food supply, such as agricultural development, climate, geography, food production, processing, protection, preservation, distribution, marketing, and the politics that control agencies, industries, and consumers. It is from the resulting food supply that personal food choices are made by individual consumers. Many forces influence these food choices— economics; transportation; psychologic, social, and cultural factors; knowledge; and physical needs. In this context, malnutrition may be defined as the result of imbalance in the ecologic nutritional system.

Contaminated food and water in man's environment may be the transmitters of disease. Many advances have been made in hygiene, sanitation, and preventive medicine in man's struggle to protect himself from the pathogenic organisms that are constantly present in his environment. But all of these problems are by no means solved. Even scientific advances create new difficulties. Everyone is cognizant of air pollution and radioactivity, which are by-products of technical achievements. The study of man's relation to his environment —human ecology—has arisen out of his growing awareness of these pressing needs.

■ **How may food be protected from pathogenic parasites?**

Several pathogenic parasites are a serious concern in conjunction with food:

1. *Trichina worm.* The trichina worm, *trichinella spiralis,* is transmitted through unsanitary garbage eaten by hogs. The larvae become embedded in the pork muscle. If man eats such infested meat the organism grows and multiplies in his intestinal tract, then moves into muscle tissue and causes fever and intense pain. In some fatal cases of trichinosis, millions of encysted larvae have been found in the muscle tissue at the time of autopsy. Two control measures are imperative to prevent trichinosis:

a. Underdone pork should never be eaten; it should be cooked thoroughly until the meat is all white and no pink color remains.

b. Hog food sources must be controlled. Garbage must be cooked before it is fed to hogs. Laws in all states now ban the feeding of uncooked garbage to swine.

2. *Tapeworms.* The beef tapeworm,

Taenia saginata, and the pork tapeworm, *Taenia solium,* are transmitted by the fecal-oral route, usually in the form of mature eggs and segments of the worm. These cysts are eaten by cattle in sewage-polluted pastures or by hogs in polluted garbage. The larvae develop in the animal's intestine, then encyst in the muscle. If man eats the infected meat raw or rare, the adult tapeworm matures in his intestine and continues its reproduction cycle. Important controls are prevention of sewage pollution of pastures, sanitary hog-raising operations, and the avoidance of rare beef and underdone pork.

3. *Amebae.* The most widely known pathogenic species of amebae inhabiting man's intestinal tract is that which causes amebic dysentery—*Entamoeba histolytica* (Gr. *ent,* inside; *histo,* tissue; *lytic,* dissolving). The name indicates its mode of attack. The organisms are ingested as cysts in contaminated food or water. In the intestine the cysts grow into adult forms that produce tissue-destroying enzymes that enable the organism to burrow into the intestinal lining and cause ulcers. Occasionally such embedding may be deep enough to produce intestinal rupture and death. The amoeba may also enter the intestinal lymph vessel and blood vessels and travel to liver, lungs, brain, and other organs, where they may localize and form large, destructive abscesses. Since transmission is entirely by the human fecal-oral route, control centers around strict sanitary measures and personal hygiene. Man is the reservoir, the carrier, and the passer. Fecal contamination of food and water is caused by soiled, unwashed hands and by flies. Carriers who are food handlers contaminate food and utensils, and leaking sewers may pollute water supplies.

■ **What is the difference between bacterial food infections and bacterial food poisonings?**

Food infections result from the ingestion in food of large amounts of viable bacteria that multiply inside the host (man) and cause infectious disease. Each specific disease is caused by a specific organism. Because incubation and multiplication of the bacteria take time, symptoms of food infection develop relatively slowly, usually 12 to 24 hours or more after the infected food has been eaten.

Food poisoning is caused by the ingestion of bacterial toxins that have been produced in the food by the growth of specific kinds of bacteria before the food is eaten. The powerful toxin is then ingested directly and symptoms of the food poisoning develop rapidly, usually within 1 to 6 hours after the food is eaten.

■ **What community problems may result from food-borne bacterial infections?**

A number of different types of diseases may cause community problems as the result of bacterial infections:

1. Salmonellosis. The typhoid and paratyphoid bacilli, which infect man, belong collectively to the genus *Salmonella*. They produce various infections (salmonellosis) of the intestinal tract. Some, such as the typhoid bacillus, also invade the blood and cause general infection. The types of salmonella that are chiefly responsible for human disease are S. *typhi* and S. *paratyphi*. They are largely restricted to man and they spread either directly or indirectly from person to person.

Salmonellae are rod-shaped bacteria that resist cold and survive for long periods in soil, ice, water, milk, and foods. Since they do not form spores, they are easily killed by being boiled for 5 minutes or by pasteurization. Drying and direct sunlight also kill them. The organisms grow easily in simple common foods, such as milk, custards, egg dishes, salad dressings, and sandwich fillings. Seafoods from polluted waters may also be a source of infection.

Immunization practices and regulations controlling the sanitation of community water and food supplies have reduced the incidence of typhoid fever to rare outbreaks. However, paratyphoid organisms continue to frequently infect food. One carrier may infect a large number of persons at one meal by preparing a dish ahead

of time and leaving it in a warm room for several hours, which would incubate the bacilli. The resultant cases of gastroenteritis may vary in intensity from mild diarrhea to severe attacks.

2. Shigellosis. Bacillary dysentery (shigellosis) is caused by rod-shaped bacteria of the genus *Shigella*. Shigellosis is usually confined to the large intestine and may vary from mild transient intestinal disturbance (as is most common in adults) to fatal dysentery (as occurs more often in young children).

The *Shigella* organisms grow easily in foods, especially in milk, which is a common vehicle of transmission to infants and children. The boiling of food and water or the pasteurization of milk kills the organisms but the food or milk may easily be reinfected subsequently through unsanitary handling by the carrier. The several species that may cause shigellosis are spread in much the same way as are those that produce salmonellosis—by feces, fingers, flies, milk, food, and by articles handled by unsanitary carriers.

3. Cholera. Chiefly an Asiatic disease, cholera is caused by *Vibrio comma* (also called *Vibrio cholerae*), an organism that resembles *Salmonella* in many respects. It also is a nonspored bacillus that may be easily killed by boiling, pasteurization, and disinfectants. Transmission is from person to person in the same manner as that of Salmonellae. Attacks of cholera are usually more severe, however. Diarrhea, prostration, and emaciation often proceed rapidly to death, unless treatment is given in time.

4. Brucellosis. Milk from infected cows or goats may transmit the coccobacilli that cause brucellosis (undulant fever). The disease in man is characterized by intermittent fever that recurs daily over a period that may vary from days to years, with general malaise, aching, and stiffness of the back and joints. In mild forms it may be regarded as "intestinal flu." *Brucella* organisms may be transmitted in the milk of goats or cows, or through cuts or scratches on the skin of persons who work with infected animals. Thus butchers, slaughter-house workers, stock raisers, and veterinarians are particularly exposed. The disease is prevented by using only pasteurized milk and other dairy products and by avoiding contact with infected animals.

5. *Leptospirosis.* The genus *Leptospira* is so named because it is the smallest and most delicately formed of the spirochetes (spiral-shaped bacteria). The organisms are transmitted to man mainly in polluted water—by drinking it or by swimming or wading in it and acquiring the organism through cuts or scratches in the skin. The disease in man is characterized by high fever and intense, hemorrhagic jaundice and hepatitis. Careful storage of foods in the home, general cleanliness in housekeeping, and constant control of rats, are necessary for the prevention of leptospirosis.

6. *Tularemia.* The bacterial genus *Pasteurella*, named for Pasteur, includes one species that occasionally causes food-borne disease in man. The organism is *P. tularensis,* named for Tulare county in California where it was first observed. The disease is commonly called tularemia. It is popularly known as rabbit fever because it is frequently transmitted to rabbit hunters, trappers, and handlers (market men and housewives) from wild rabbits that have been infected by ticks, fleas, lice, or other insects that carry the microorganism. It is characterized by focal ulcers at the site of infection, recurrent fever, prostration, myalgia, and headache. Restrictions against the sale of wild rabbits have sharply reduced the incidence of tularemia. Caution should be exercised in eating rabbits of wild or unknown origin.

7. *Escherichia coli infections.* Several *Escherichia coli* species inhabit the human gastrointestinal tract in enormous numbers. Ordinarily *E. coli* cause their host no difficulty, but certain strains produce enteritis, especially in infants. Babies' formulas prepared under unsanitary conditions are the usual route of infection.

8. *Clostridium perfringens food infection. Clostridium perfringens,* the bacterium that causes gas gangrene when it infects deep wounds, is also capable, in certain circumstances, of inducing gastrointestinal illness. Rarely is the illness fatal, and then only in elderly, debilitated patients. Its symptoms are usually mild—diarrhea, acute abdominal cramping, nausea, and headache. Most patients recover in 24 hours, or at most, within a few days. The organism multiplies in cooked meat and meat dishes held for extended periods at warming temperatures or at room temperature. A number of outbreaks of clostridia infection from food eaten in restaurants, college dining rooms, and school cafeterias have been reported. In each case, cooked meat was improperly handled in preparation and refrigeration. Control rests principally upon careful preparation and adequate cooking of meats, prompt service, and immediate refrigeration at sufficiently low temperatures.

■ **What common problems may result from bacterial food poisonings?**

Two basic community problems may be caused by bacterial toxins:

1. *Staphylococcal food poisoning.* Of all the bacterial food poisonings observed in the United States, staphylococcal food poisoning is by far the most common. Powerful preformed toxins in the contaminated food produce illness within 1 to 6 hours after ingestion. The manifestations appear suddenly. There is severe, cramping, abdominal pain, with nausea, vomiting, and diarrhea, usually accompanied by sweating, headache, and fever. There may be prostration and shock. Recovery is fairly rapid, however, and the symptoms subside within 24 hours. The amount of toxin ingested and the susceptibility of the individual eating it determine the degree of severity. The source of contamination is usually a locus of staphylococcal infection on the hand of a worker preparing the food. Often it is only a minor infection, considered harmless or even unnoticed by the food handler. Custard or cream-filled bakery goods are particularly effective culture beds for staphylococcal infection and

are common carriers of the toxins formed during their growth. Other foods that often support the development of staphlococcae are processed meats, ham, tongue, cheese, ice cream, potato salad, sauces, chicken and ham salads, and combination dishes, such as spaghetti encasserole. The toxin causes no change from the normal appearance, odor, and taste of the food, so the victim is not warned.

A careful food history is necessary to determine the source of the poisoning. If possible, portions of the food are obtained for bacterial examination. Few bacteria may be found, since heating kills these organisms but does not destroy the toxin they produce. Prevention of staphylococcal food poisoning rests on enforcement of three practices: (1) strict observance by food handlers of the rules of hygiene; (2) careful and immediate refrigeration of all perishable foods, and (3) reheating foods only immediately before serving—not allowing them to stand for long periods at room temperature. Education of food handlers is vital to the prevention of food poisoning incidence in the community.

2. Botulism. Serious, often fatal, food poisoning results from ingestion in food of the toxin produced by the bacteria *Clostridium botulinum.* Depending on the dose of toxin taken and individual response, the illness may vary from mild discomfort to death within 24 hours. Mortality rates are high. Nausea, vomiting, weakness, and dizziness are initial complaints. Progressively the toxin irritates motor nerve cells and blocks transmission of neural impulses at the nerve terminals (myoneural junction); gradual paralysis follows. Sudden respiratory paralysis with airway obstruction is the major cause of death.

C. botulinum spores are widespread in soil throughout the world. These spores may be carried on harvested food to the canning process. Like all Clostridia, this species is anaerobic (develops in the absence of air), or nearly so. The relatively anaerobic environment in the can and the canning temperatures (above 80° F.) pro-

vide good conditions for toxin production. The development of high standards in the commercial canning industry has eliminated this source of botulism, but a few cases still result each year from the eating of carelessly home-canned foods. Since boiling for 10 minutes destroys the toxin (not the spore), all home-canned food, no matter how well preserved it is considered to be, should be boiled at least 10 minutes before eating.

■ **What does the term "ptomaine poisoning" mean?**

The term "ptomaine poisoning" is a misnomer. It is used by laymen to mean food poisoning. There is no such thing as "ptomaine poisoning" in man. The word "ptomaine" comes from the Greek word *ptoma* meaning "dead body." Ptoamines are members of a large class of basic nitrogenous substances, some of them highly poisonous, which are produced during putrefacation of animal or plant protein. They are easily detectable by the deteriorated appearance of the material almost to a liquid state and by the powerful, obnoxious odor they produce. Food in such a condition is hardly human fare! The word ptomaine is therefore erroneously used when it is applied to other common food infections or poisonings, such as salmonellosis or staphylococcal intoxication.

■ **Are viral infections transmitted by food?**

Yes, although illnesses produced by viral contamination of food are few in comparison with those produced by bacterial contamination of food. Common upper respiratory infections may be transmitted through foods. Persons infected with such viruses may, with soiled hands, handle unwrapped food in stores or cafeterias, or they may sneeze or cough over them. Also, acute viral hepatitis, an inflammatory disease of the liver, is caused by either of two strains of virus: Virus A causes infectious hepatitis (IH); Virus B causes serum hepatitis (SH). Virus B has been found only in blood, and is transmitted only by parenteral inoculation (intravenous transfusion of infected blood or injection with a contaminated needle). Virus A, however, is usually transmitted by the fecal-oral route common to food and water-borne diseases. Explosive epidemics have occurred in towns, schools, and other communities after fecal contamination of water, milk, or food. Shellfish contaminated by living in polluted water have been a source of several outbreaks. Control of community water, milk, and food supplies, and stringent personal hygiene and sanitary practices by food handlers, are essential to the prevention of infectious hepatitis.

■ **What are mycotoxins?**

Toxins that are produced by molds (fungi) are called mycotoxins (Gr. *myco,* fungus; L. *toxicum,* poison). Aflatoxins are examples of these poisonous materials. Aflatoxins were first found in peanut meal fed to poultry and subsequently extracted and found to be produced by strains of *Aspergillus flavus,* a common storage mold. Apparently the toxins are produced immediately after crop harvesting and early in the storage period. Rapid drying, improved storage conditions, and possible use of fungicides would be important control measures.

■ **Are there naturally-occurring poisons in plant food sources?**

Yes. Certain plants contain poisonous substances that occasionally cause human illness or death. Most of these toxic substances are poisonous alkaloids, such as strychnine, atropine, scopolamine, and solanine. Some plants produce toxic substances at one point in their growth cycle and not at others. Some examples of these plants that are poisonous as food include:

Cottonseed. A toxic pigment, *gossypol,* contained in cottonseed, has created problems in preparing protein-rich food supplements for use in combating protein malnutrition throughout the world. Procedures for removing the toxin from cottonseed meal during processing have been devised, and efforts are being made to develop strains of the plant that do not contain gossypol.

Soybeans. A trypsin inhibitor in raw soybeans is responsible for a toxic substance contained in them. Fortunately, this substance is destroyed by heat and is therefore easily inactivated by cooking.

Cycad nuts. Plants of the genus *Cycas,* common in tropical and subtropical areas, are intermediate in appearance between ferns and palms. Many species have a thick, unbranched, columnar trunk bearing a crown of large, leathery, pinnate leaves. The nuts are sometimes eaten in times of extreme need, as during famine; they were investigated in Guam as a possible cause of a disease of the nervous system, amyotrophic lateral sclerosis (ALS), observed in persons who had eaten them. In 1960 they were found to contain the active toxin, *cycasin,* which was isolated and chemically identified. The toxin is now removed from the nuts by a washing process before they are eaten.

Potatoes. The green part of sprouting white potatoes contains sufficient amount of the toxic substance solanine to cause gastroenteritis, jaundice, and prostration. Solanine is a poisonous, narcotic alkaloid. Usually it is removed with the peel before the potato is cooked.

Mushrooms. Certain species of mushroom belong to the poisonous genus, *Amanita.* Wild mushrooms should be strictly avoided as food. A number of edible species of mushrooms are grown commercially.

Rhubarb leaves. The large amount of oxalic acid contained in rhubarb leaves causes illness. These leaves should not be used as leafy greens for cooking and eating. Edible leafy greens are spinach, chard, mustard, turnip, and a few others.

Fava Beans. Favism is the name given to a severe form of hemolytic anemia produced by the ingestion (or by the inhalation of pollen) of fava beans (*Vicia fava*) in persons sensitive to them. This sensitivity is caused by a gentically controlled deficiency of the enzyme glucose-6-phosphate dehydrogenase in the shunt pathway (see hexose monophosphate shunt, p. 11) for glucose oxidation normally found in the red blood cell. This genetic trait was first observed in certain members of the Mediterranean (Sicilian and Sardinian) and African populations, and has more recently been noted in about 10% of Negroes in the United States. The same genetic trait provides some protection against falciparum malaria. It is a good example of an evolutionary genetic adaptation of a population group to a disease process. Susceptible individuals also react to antimalaria drugs such as primaquine, and to the analgesic phenacetin in the same way that they react to fava beans.

Wild plants. Hemlock, wild parsnip, monkshood, foxglove, and deadly nightshade are a few of the many wild plants known to be poisonous. Occasionally they are mistaken for harmless plants that they resemble and are inadvertently eaten.

■ **Are there naturally occurring poisons in animal food sources?**

Yes. A few animal sources provide sources of poison and need careful consideration. One example is the *puffer fish,* so named because it is capable of inflating its body with water or air until it forms a globe. It has a gland containing a powerful neurotoxin, *tetraodontoxin,* which causes death soon after ingestion. Nonetheless, the puffer fish is considered a delicacy in the Orient, and chefs take pride in their ability to remove the gland with great care before cooking the fish. Despite this care, a number of persons each year die of tetraodontoxin poisoning.

Also, during certain summer months clams and mussels in waters along the Pacific Coast from Alaska to California feed on marine organisms, plankton, which infect the fish and produce a toxic alkaloid similar to strychnine. At this season the eating of these fish can be fatal. At different seasons in various locations, herring apparently become poisonous as human food. Just what accounts for these seasonal changes is not known. Other observations have been made of seasonal poisonings from barracuda.

■ **Is there danger of radioactivity in foods?**

Many communities are concerned with the extent of food contamination by radioactive fallout from nuclear weapons testing. The peacetime uses of atomic energy, as well, release small amounts of radioactive materials into the environment. The benefits that are gained from the use of atomic energy in contrast to its biologic cost has been a scientific and philosophical study.

Vegetation may be contaminated directly or through the soil, and animals, especially cattle, can become contaminated both directly and through their forage and water. Man, in turn, ingests radioactivity in milk (strontium^{90}) and meat and their products. However, present montoring systems reveal that present radiation levels are far below those permissible in the human life span.

■ **Why are chemical additives used in food processing?**

In modern food processing, additives are used for a variety of purposes:

1. *Addition of specific nutrients.* Certain foods have proved to be good carriers for factors essential to sound nutrition. To other foods nutrients have been added to replace those lost in processing. Examples include the addition of iodine to salt, ascorbic acid to many fruit juices, vitamin D to milk, vitamin A to margarine, and the B vitamins and iron to cereal products. As the result of enrichment, controlled in many instances by enrichment laws, deficiency diseases, such as goiter and pellagra, have largely been eliminated from the American population. The enrichment of bread and corn meal has been an important factor in the almost total disappearance of pellagra in the southern United States. The addition of vitamin D has made rickets rare in this country.

2. *Production of uniform sensory properties.* Some food additives enhance sensory properties, such as color, flavor, aroma, texture, and general appearance. In their natural state samples of a given food may vary widely in color and flavor according to the season or locality in which they are harvested or according to the species. Nat-

ural and synthetic flavoring agents, colorings, preservatives, and texturing materials add appeal and characteristic uniformity to common food products. An interesting example of color control is the addition of bleaching agents to processed flour. Small quantities of natural pigments in freshly milled wheat flour give it a yellowish color, which many persons find less attractive than pure white. Such flour also lacks the qualities necessary to make the elastic and staple dough necessary for making bread of the texture that is preferred by many people. Bleaching and maturing agents are added to counteract these characteristics.

3. *Standardization of functional properties.* A number of additivies enhance and standardize the functional properties of foods. In this class are emulsifiers, stabilizers, moisture retainers, thickeners, binders, dough conditioners, anticaking agents, jelling agents, and others.

4. *Preservation of food.* Many agents are added to food to help maintain it at its best quality, long past the peak of harvest time or the time of processing. Salt and certain curing agents preserve meat and make possible a variety of meat products. Antioxidants prevent discoloration of fruits and rancidity of fats. Antimycotic agents, such as mold inhibitors, and bacterial control agents such as "rope" inhibitors, preserve bread and other baked products. Sequestrants set apart in an inactive form trace substances in foods, which would otherwise interfere with its processing. For example, in fats sequestrants combine with trace minerals, such as iron and copper, and prevent their catalytic action, which would hasten oxidation—the cause of rancidity in fats. Sequestrants also inactivate certain minerals in the water that is used in making soft drinks, thus preventing turbidity caused by the minerals settling out during processing.

5. *Control of acidity or alkalinity.* The acidity or alkalinity of foods often affects their flavor, texture, and the cooked product. Various acids, alkalis, buffers, and neutralizing agents are used to achieve the desired balance or flavor. For example, acids contribute flavor to candy and help prevent a grainy texture. The flavor of many soft drinks is modified by the addition of acid. Acids and alkalis constitute leavening agents such as baking powder. In making butter, alkali is added to sour cream so that it will churn properly and yield a satisfactory flavor.

■ **Why are chemicals used in agriculture?**

The chemicals used in American agriculture serve a variety of purposes. Today's farmer uses chemicals to control a wide variety of destructive insects, to kill weeds, to control plant diseases, to stop fruit from dropping prematurely, to make leaves drop so that harvesting will be easier, to make seeds sprout, to keep seeds from rotting before they sprout, and many other purposes related to increased yield and marketing qualities.

■ **Is there danger of pesticide residue in food?**

The use of agricultural chemicals brings hazard as well as gain. Recognition of the necessity for control has led to laws governing the use of pesticides, setting tolerance limits on the amount of pesticide residues permitted on crops. The FDA directs a pesticide control program in two phases: (1) initial approval of a chemical for use, and (2) enforcement through continued surveillance. Laws governing the use of pesticides are enforced in three ways— through public education, through constant sampling of field produce, and through market basket studies.

■ **How is milk protected from contamination during processing?**

Because milk is particularly susceptible to contamination by harmful microorganisms, special laws govern its production and marketing. Rigidly enforced government ordinances regulate its handling from farm to consumer. Disease in milk-producing cows is eradicated by veterinary programs under government control. Personnel and equipment involved in the care and milking of the animals and in handling of the milk are required to pass rigid health and sanitation inspections.

Cows are usually milked by machines that pipe the milk to storage tanks without exposure to contaminating dust and insects. In these refrigerated tanks the milk is cooled quickly to about 38° F. and held at that temperature throughout a brief storage period and while it is being transported in refrigerated tank trucks to the dairy.

At the processing plant the milk is subjected to a vacuum treatment to remove objectionable flavors and next it is pasteurized by any of several legal heat treatments. For example, the milk can be held at 145° F. for 30 minutes or at 161° F. for 15 seconds. Pasteurization destroys disease-producing organisms that might be present in the milk and also kills bacteria that could grow during storage and refrigeration. It renders milk and milk products not only safe for consumption but also less likely to spoil during storage and marketing.

Homogenization is usually associated with pasteurization. By this treatment the fat globules are reduced in size and evenly disbursed so that the cream does not separate from the milk. Vitamin D is also added to compensate for the lack of this vitamin in the milk. The standard supplement is 400 I.U. per quart. Finally, the milk is packaged and kept refrigerated until it is delivered to the consumer.

■ **How is meat production controlled?**

Under the meat inspection act of 1906 and the Poultry Products Inspection Act of 1957, the Consumer and Marketing Service of the U. S. Department of Agriculture closely controls the commercial marketing of meat and poultry. Inspectors monitor meat production and marketing. The circular purple stamp mark placed on meat and poultry indicates that it has passed government inspection. Inspectors are concerned with sanitation of the processing plant, inspection of animals at the stockyard before slaughter, immediate examination of the carcass and internal organs, and inspection during meat processing, curing, canning, and smoking. They also regulate disposal of condemned material, the marketing and labeling of products, and inspection of imported meat.

■ **In addition to traditional food preservation by drying and canning, what newer methods are being used?**

Freezing destroys many microorganisms and inhibits the growth of others. Because frozen foods are not sterile, however, they must be handled as perishables from the time they are processed until they are eaten. Rapid, sanitary food preparation, followed immediately by quick freezing, controls bacterial growth and prevents damage to the cell walls, which would break down the texture. Quick freezing is made possible by the use of liquid nitrogen (−320° F.) or fluidized-bed freezers. After the initial quick freezing the food is stored at a low temperature and used before expiration of the recommended storage time. Most frozen food should be held at a 0° F. or lower; −10° F. is better.

In *freeze-drying*, piece-form foods, such as fruits and seafoods, are kept frozen while they dry in a vacuum. This retains the original size and shape of the food but greatly reduces its weight. For example, a freeze-dried strawberry is the same size as the fresh strawberry but weighs only one-sixteenth as much. This lightness is an advantage in handling and transportation. At the present time, foods processed by this technique are less excellent in taste, and meet with less acceptance than do quick-frozen or canned foods.

In *dehydrofreezing*, fruits and vegetables are first dehydrated to about 50% of their original weight and volume, but not until their quality is impaired, then frozen. The quality of dehydrofrozen foods is usually equal to that of foods processed by the standard quick-freezing method. They have the advantages of lighter weight and less bulk, and therefore they cost less to package, freeze, store, and ship. Foods that have been satisfactorily dehydrofrozen include potatoes, carrots, peas, apples, apricots, berries, and cherries. They are used chiefly in commercially prepared combinations, as vegetables in soup or fruits in pies.

Antibiotics have also been used in food preservation. Chlortetracycline and oxytetracycline are used in the preservation of raw poultry. Since about 10% of the population of the United States, however, is sensitive to various drugs, the addition of antibiotics to foods must be carefully controlled. Only small amounts may be employed and residues in tissues are destroyed by cooking. Used under specified conditions, these antibiotics significantly increase retention of quality in fresh poultry and fish during storage.

Ionizing radiation offers a method of food preservation that has been developed only in the past two decades. It was first approved for use on canned bacon and bulk wheat. Gamma radiation was used to kill insect life in bulk wheat, and the electron beam was used to sterilize bacon. Irradiation under approved processes *does not* cause the food to become radioactive or to retain radioactivity that may have lingered in it from previous exposure.

■ **How does the FDA try to control food safety and quality?**

The FDA is a law enforcement agency charged by Congress to ensure, among other things, that the food supply is safe, pure, and wholesome. It seeks to carry out its responsibility through scientific research and public education as well as by surveillance and enforcement. Section 401 of the Federal Food, Drug, and Cosmetic Act is designed "to promote honesty and fair dealing in the interest of Consumers." It directs the Secretary of Health, Education, and Welfare to establish, for any food he deems necessary, regulations governing the definition and standard of identity, reasonable standards of quality, and standards of fill-of-container. The food label must indicate these standards, and must tell what is in the package. It must not be false or *misleading* in any particular.

■ **What is the food additives amendment?**

The Food Additives Amendment to the Federal Food, Drug, and Cosmetic Act of 1938 was passed on September 6, 1958. This amendment, which took effect on March 6, 1960, completely altered the government's method of regulating the use of additives in food. The law provided for the first time that no additive could be used in food unless the Food and Drug Administration, after a careful review of the test data, agreed that the compound was safe at the intended levels of use. An exception was made for all additives that, because of years of widespread use, were "generally recognized as safe" (GRAS) by experts in the field. This approach was a compromise between giving blanket approval to all additives then in use or banning all untested food additives until several years of laboratory safety studies could be conducted.

The result, therefore, is the present GRAS list. It includes several thousand food additives, including salt, sugar, baking powder, spices, flavorings, vitamins, minerals, preservatives, emulsifiers, and non-nutritive sweeteners. All of them are considered harmless as commonly used in foods. Some of them are restricted to uses in certain foods and at certain levels, but most are limited only to their "intended use," and to "good manufacturing practice."

Problems, however, exist with the GRAS list. First, there is an uncertainty as to how many GRAS items there are, and no single compilation of them exists. Quoted statements concerning the number range from approximately 600 to several thousand. FDA officials themselves are uncertain about how many GRAS items there are. Also, in the decade since the GRAS list was formulated, two developments have had direct bearing on the soundness of the original GRAS concept: (1) we have become much more sophisticated about toxicity testing and we have recognized the inadequacy of relying on a lack of reported human adverse effect as the sole measure of safety; and (2) we have also seen the demands of modern technology increase the uses of certain GRAS items well beyond the exposure patterns considered in the original development of the GRAS list. As a result, the government has directed the FDA to re-evaluate all items on the GRAS list for safety. This is an almost impossible task, however, with the present inadequate allocation of funds and personnel to accomplish the task.

■ **What is the "Delaney Clause"?**

The Delaney Clause is an attachment to the Food Additives Amendment. It states that "no additive shall be deemed safe if it is found to induce cancer when ingested by man or animal, or if it is found after tests which are appropriate for the evaluation of the safety food additives, to induce cancer in man or animal." The clause was attached to the amendment just before its final passage. It was under this clause, for example, that cyclamates were banned in 1969. Food additives in general are facing increasing public scrutiny.

11 Food habits

Why do people eat what they eat? For many reasons. Food has many meanings, and a person's food habits are intimately tied up with his whole way of life.

Food habits, like other forms of human behavior, are the result of many personal, cultural, social, and psychologic influences. Everyone is culture bound and ethnocentric, so that he views his own way as the best or right way. The habits of another who differs from him are looked on as foreign or wrong or superstitious or stupid. If people are honest enough to recognize their own biases, many of the misconceptions that prevent understanding other people can be cleared away. Such misconceptions hinder sensitive, constructive care. In the last analysis, it is the cultural and sociopsychologic factors in the individual patient that will prove most influential in determining his nutritional behavior. In each one of us these factors are interwoven into a behavioral complex.

CULTURAL INFLUENCES

■ **What is the concept of culture and how does it influence habit patterns?**

Culture is that complex whole that includes knowledge, belief, art, law, morals, custom, or any other capabilities and habits acquired by man as a member of society. Thus, culture involves the broad aspects of social living, such as language, religion, politics, technology, and so on. However, perhaps even more significantly, culture also involves all the little habits of everyday living, such as preparing and serving food, caring for children, feeding them, and lulling them to sleep. Often the most significant thing that can be known about a culture is what it takes for granted in daily life.

These many facets of a man's culture are *learned.* Gradually, as the child grows up within a given society, the slow process of conscious and unconscious learning of values, attitudes, habits, and practices takes place through the conscious and unconscious influence of parents, teachers, and other enculturating agents of his society. Whatever is invented, transmitted, and perpetuated—his socially acquired knowledge and habits—man learns as part of his culture. These become internalized and deeply entrenched.

■ **What function does culture serve?**

The culture of a people develops over a long period and functions in two main ways: (1) it enables a people to *adapt to its environment,* and (2) it helps *to interpret to them* common (and sometimes terrifying) life experiences. The environment may be harsh and hostile and the way of life developed by this people is what has enabled them to survive. Also, their life experiences such as birth, death, illness, disease, sex, and the phenomena of nature may cause fear or need understanding. Certain rituals, taboos, totems, habits, and practices develop to explain, placate, or protect or to establish human and environmental relationships. A certain poisonous plant, for example, may have become taboo as a food because the tribal ancestors observed that it caused death. Difficulties ensue sometimes when outsiders attempt to change habits of a people without understanding these adaptation and interpretations and thus upset this balance of nature and do more harm than good. This has been the case when some health workers have tried to impose Western culture and habits on peoples in other parts of the world without prior study and appreciation of established customs. Such programs have failed for this very reason.

■ **How does culture influence food habits?**

Food habits are among the oldest and most entrenched aspects of any culture. They exert deep influence on behavior of the people. By and large, food habits are based on food availability, economics, or symbolism. Included among these influential factors are the geography of the land, the agriculture practiced by the people, their economy and market practices, and their history and traditions. Within these patterns, culture determines many things about food:

1. *Cultural determination of what is food.* Items considered to be food in one culture may be regarded with disgust or may actually cause illness in persons of another culture. For example, in America milk is valued as a basic food; in many cultures it is rejected with revulsion as an animal mucous discharge. The use of the staple item bread is another example. Many a diet-obsessed American rejects bread, but in a Greek home bread is the main food. It is *the* meal, and all other foods are considered accompaniments to the bread and are eaten between bites of bread. The religious aspects of a culture also control determination of what food may be used or what is rejected. Pork is unacceptable as food for a Moslem or an orthodox Jew; any meat is unacceptable for the Seventh Day Adventist; the strict Hindu or Buddhist eats no meat, and even the liberal Hindu may not eat beef.

2. *Appetite for specific food.* Culture also influences what foods are acceptable at what time of day. Foods used for one meal may be rejected for another meal. For example, the main breakfast food in a Greek home may be bread and cheese; in Europe, a sweet roll; in America, ham and eggs. Inhabitants of different regions within a country also vary in their choices.

3. *How and where food is eaten.* In a highly urban industrialized society such as America, in which value is placed on action, speed, and productivity, lunch for the business man may be a quick snack that he eats while standing at a lunch counter. Even the form is geared for quick eating—fruit in juice form and meat in a sandwich. However, to the Spanish or Latin American merchant, such a lunch is unthinkable. His less tensely paced culture allows him to close his shop for 2 hours in the middle of the day while he enjoys a leisurely meal and siesta at home with his family.

4. *Appropriate occasion for specific foods.* The force of dietary patterning is seen in the Thanksgiving turkey, the Easter ham, and until recently (and still for strict observers) the Friday fish. Times of religious observance, such as Lent, call for specific food patterns. Food becomes an integral part of transmitting and teaching many aspects of one's particular culture.

■ **In cultures and subcultures using vegetarian diets, how can an adequate quantity and quality of protein be obtained?**

Vegetarian diets may be of four different types:

1. The diet may simply reject meat, but allow milk and eggs—a lacto-ovo-vegetarian diet. In this case complete protein is still available in the milk and egg and supplementary sources in plant proteins. Many cultures of the world exist on such vegetarian diets.

2. It may accept milk but reject egg, and is thus called a lacto-vegetarian diet. The milk still provides a complete source of protein.

3. It may be a strict vegetarian regime, such as the "Vegands" in Great Britain and other countries. In these cases only plant proteins are allowed. Sufficient protein may be achieved through a carefully planned combination of plant sources so that a profile of the essential amino acids necessary for tissue building is provided.

4. Fruitarians are those who follow a still-stricter regime that allows only fruits, seeds, nuts. Such persons have great difficulty in securing sufficient protein.

The real need is not for mere quantity of protein but for *quality* of protein, that is, the obtaining of the eight essential amino acids in sufficient quantity to meet the body's requirements. These eight essential amino acids can be obtained from plant sources through varied combinations of grains, legumes, nuts, and seeds, which compliment one another and cover the lack of a particular amino acid. It must be remembered that no one food, meat or milk for example, is required for human nutrition. It is the essential nutrients in a variety of foods that are required for human nutrition, and these essential nutrients may be obtained in a variety of ways and in a variety of sources and combinations. Value judgments, however, are placed on certain foods in certain cultures. Meat is an example of such a judgment. It is evident that such value judgments are not based on nutritional requirements but are based instead on habit patterns developed within a cultural setting. Meat is the top of the food chain and as such is considered by many as a less efficient means of feeding large populations. Moreover, because of its position in the food chain it tends to be one of the more expensive food items. Hence, its greater use is confined to affluent cultures.

■ **What is food symbolism?**

Symbolism is the act of attaching meaning to a thing—word or object or event—that does not reside in the thing itself, per se, but is attached to it by those who use the symbol. Within every culture there are certain foods that are deeply imbued with symbolic meaning beyond the nature of the foods themselves. These symbols are related to a number of aspects of cultural life:

1. *Major life experiences.* Foods often surrounds events that characterize major life experiences in a culture. Birth of a child is observed in many cultures by a meal that symbolizes a general celebration of the beginning of life. Soon after birth, surrounding a baptism or dedication ceremony, special meals and special foods are used. Stages of development in a young person's life often involve foods. For example, at a coming-of-age ceremony such as the Bar Mitzvah for Jewish boys at the age of 13, honey cakes and wine, canapes, strudle, knishes, and piroggen are generally served. Weddings are surrounded with symbolic foods. Pregnancy is attended by many food symbols, taboos, and practices. Certain foods may be avoided in the belief that they will mark the infant, or certain foods may be denied the pregnant woman in the belief that she will contaminate the food supply. Death also involves food use symbolizing the general fact that each individual life has its end. In some cultures food may be buried with the body to sustain the departed on his journey to the hereafter.

2. *Religion.* Food symbolism plays a large role in most religions of the world. From early times ceremonies and religious rites surrounded acts pertaining to fertility in the harvest season. Food gathering, preparing, and serving followed specific customs and commemorated special events of religious significance. Many of these customs remain. For example, among the Jewish people a number of special feast or fast days commemorate significant events in their history and are a means of teaching cherished beliefs and traditions from one generation to the next. A prime example of the Jewish culture is part of the Passover observance. It is the Seder meal, which is a highly symbolic family meal on the evening before the Passover. At this meal each food signifies a specific aspect of the historical deliverance of the Jewish people from bondage in Egypt.

3. *Politics.* Food use has had political significance in man's history as well. In India the fasts of Ghandi wielded tremendous political power. In America the Boston Tea Party was concerned with important interrelationships between food, eco-

nomics, and a budding nations' political views. Tea was considered to be an almost essential commodity by the American colonists, and the English taxes on tea stimulated the politics of American independence.

4. Social organizations. Foods carry symbolic meanings also, according to the significance given them by various social classes. Some foods are high-status foods; for example, steak and out-of-season foods. Others are low-status foods, such as parts of animals not customarily eaten by the majority of people.

■ **What are the Jewish dietary laws?**

Adherence to Jewish dietary food laws varies among the three basic groups within Judaism: Orthodox—strict observance; Conservative—nominal observance; Reform—less ceremonial emphasis and minimal observance of the general dietary laws. This body of laws is called the rules of kashruth, and food selected and prepared accordingly is called kosher food. Both words come from the Hebrew word *kāsher,* meaning "right" or "fit." The basis of these laws is primarily self-purification and a means of service to God, although they probably also had some hygienic or ethical foundation in their inception. Most of these rules relate to ordinances given to the ancient Hebrews as recorded in the Old Testament books of the law (Leviticus and Deuteronomy) and to the Jewish traditions accumulated through the ensuing centuries. These were collected and interpreted in the Talmud, a body of laws set down in the fourth to sixth centuries B.C.

Since the original Hebrew religion was centered in practices of animal sacrifice, and the blood had special ritual significance, the present day dietary laws apply specifically to the selection, slaughter, preparation and service of meat, to the combining of meat and milk, to fish, and to eggs.

1. The only meat allowed is the meat of cloven hoofed quadrupeds that chew a cud (cattle, sheep, goat, deer), and only the forequarters may be used. The hind quarter may be eaten only if the Sinew of Jacob (hip sinew of the thigh) is removed (Leviticus 11:1-8, Deuteronomy 14:3-8, Genesis 32:33).

2. Chicken, turkey, goose, pheasant, and duck may be eaten (Leviticus 11:13-19).

3. Ritual slaughter follows rigid rules based on minimal pain to the animal and maximal blood drainage. This process of preparing kosher meat involves several steps. The meat is soaked in water in a special vessel. It is then rinsed and thoroughly salted with coarse salt. It is placed on a perforated board tilted to permit blood to flow off, and the meat is left to stand for an hour. After it has drained thoroughly it is washed three times before being used in cooking.

4. No blood may be eaten as food in any form, since blood is considered synonymous with life (Genesis 9:4, Leviticus 3:17 and 17:10-14, Deuteronomy 12:23-27).

5. No combining of meat and milk is allowed. This prohibition is based on the oft-repeated Old Testament command, "Thou shalt not seethe a kid in its mother's milk." (Exodus 23:19, 34-26; Deuteronomy 14:21). Milk or milk food (cheese, ice cream) may be eaten just before a meal, but not for 6 hours after eating a meal that contains meat. In the Orthodox Jewish home it is customary to maintain two sets of dishes, one for serving meat meals and the other for serving dairy meals.

6. Only those fish with fins and scales are allowed; no shellfish or eels may be eaten (Leviticus 11:9-12, Deuteronomy 14:9-10). Fish of the type permitted may be eaten with either dairy or meat meals.

7. No egg that contains a blood spot may be eaten. Eggs may be taken with either dairy or meat meals.

8. There are no special restrictions on fruits, vegetables, or cereals.

SOCIAL INFLUENCES

■ **What is the concept of social class within a culture?**

The structure of a society is largely formed by groupings according to such factors as economic status, education, residence, occupation, or family. Within a given society many smaller groups exist whose values and habits vary. These subgroups within a larger culture are called subcultures. They may be established on the basis of region, religion, age, sex, social class, occupational group, or politics. Even within these subgroups there may be still smaller groups with distinguishing attitudes, values, and habits—the community juvenile gang, the college fraternity, the industrial executives, army officers, the families in a given neighborhood, or a commune. A person may be a member of several subcultural groups, each of which influences his values, attitudes and habits.

Social class, especially, influences value systems. Social classes may be considered as comprising those persons who have similar community status, responsibilities, and privileges. In America social classes are less distinct and rigid than in some countries, but they do exist and they do influence behavior.

■ **What relation does social class structure and value systems have to food habits?**

The American value system, by and large, is based on four general premises: *equality, sociality, success,* and *change.* All of these values influence attitudes toward health care and food habits. The placement of a high value on equality leads health workers to establish standards of quality health care for all people. The high respect accorded to sociality builds peer group pressures and status seeking within social groups. Foods may be accepted because they are high-status foods or rejected because they are low-prestige foods. The esteem in which success is held often leads persons to measure life in terms of competitive superlatives: they want to set the best table, to provide the most abundant supply of food for the family, and to have the biggest eater and therefore the fattest of any baby in the neighborhood. The value that is placed on change leads families or individuals to seek constant variety in their diets, to be geared for action, to seek quick cooking "convenience foods." In response to such market demands food technologists are producing an increasing array of food products each year.

■ **What role does food play in the socialization process?**

The food habits of people in any setting are highly socialized. These habits perform significant social functions, some of which may not always be evident to the persons who have such habits. These social functions include the following relationships·

1. *Social relationships.* Food is a symbol of sociability, warmth, friendliness, and social acceptance. The breaking of bread together binds a group.

2. *Persons involved in social relationships.* People tend to accept food more readily from those persons viewed as friends or allies. People most enjoy eating with those persons to whom they feel close. New foods from persons who seem congenial are more acceptable. Advice about food is accepted from persons who are considered to be authorities and with whom is felt a warm relationship. People tend to distrust food given to them by strangers and outsiders. Emotional feelings about people are transferred to their food—the more alien the authority figure the more he is considered to be unconcerned and it is more likely that his food suggestions will be considered as outlandish or even harmful.

3. *Mother-child relationships.* The maternal role is highly evident in food behavior. Food is symbolic of motherliness, of nurturing. In the family the early feeding process is the vehicle of much conscious and unconscious learning between mother and child. The mother teaches what is acceptable as food, when to eat, how much to eat and why it is eaten. Many mothers are unaware that they impart their own likes and dislikes to their children. A mother's self-esteem is deeply involved in feeding her family. Depending on her education she decides who is an authority to advise her about child feeding. If she is relatively unsophisticated has little education she is likely to view her own mother

and her neighbors as her best guides. If she has somewhat more education she perhaps accepts more readily the advertising of business concerns as the greatest authority. Mothers with middle class or better education place most faith in a professional medical authority.

4. *Food in family relationships.* Eating together as a family group builds closeness and family solidarity. Food habits that are most closely associated with family sentiments are the most tenacious throughout life. The role of each family member is most clearly illustrated to the child as the family eats together. Certain meals have more family significance than others. Dinner is more family-centered than other meals and its pattern tends to be more complex. Its foods are often more symbolic. Strong religious factors associated with food also tend to have their origin and reinforcement within the family meal circle. Increasingly, however, families are eating together less and less as family patterns are changing.

■ **How are social problems related to food habits?**

Among the many effects of rapid social change, with the uprooting and displacing of persons and families, are changes in the food habits of millions of persons.

1. *Poverty.* In many large urban centers, growing numbers of persons who are members of minority groups live in slums where they are unassimilated and often disregarded, alienated, and rejected by the mainstream of a sophisticated, affluent society. Where family income and community sources of food are limited, food choices are often poor at best. These persons tend to live a marginal existence and inadequate housing is attended by problems related to cooking, refrigeration, storage, and sanitation. Malnutrition, broken spirits, and hostility often result.

2. *Family disintegration.* Abject poverty for some workers and affluence for others has resulted from industrialization and changing urban-suburban living patterns. These newly emerging patterns contribute to changes in family patterns and values.

Children who are left to shift for themselves often incur erratic eating habits and tend to fill their stomach with a diet that is nutritionally inadequate. The increased number of teenage marriages, often between young people with limited means of support and little knowledge of food preparation or of child feeding, may lead to poor food choices or poor eating habits.

3. *Alcoholism.* Alcoholism is frequently associated with poor nutrition. Both the alcoholic and his family may be adversely affected. Money spent for alcohol is often diverted from the family budget for food and inadequate funds remain for feeding the family. The alcoholic who does not deprive others of food nonetheless frequently damages his own health by obtaining in alcohol the mere calories requisite for direct energy expenditure. He neglects to eat a proper diet that would supply the many nutrients his body needs, and malnutrition results.

PSYCHOLOGIC INFLUENCES

■ **What role do motivation and perception play in helping to shape food habits?**

Individual behavior patterns including those related to eating are the result of many interrelated psychosocial influences and factors. Factors that are particularly pertinent to the shaping of food habits are motivation and perception.

1. *Motivation.* A motive is the purpose an individual has for acting, something that prompts him to behave in a certain way. Motivation is bound up with personal goals and needs. People of different cultures are not motivated by the same needs and goals. Even primary biologic drives, such as hunger and sex, are modified in their interpretation, expression, and fulfillment by many cultural, social, and personal influences. The kinds of food sought, prized, or accepted by one individual at one time and place may be violently rejected by another individual living in different circumstances. For the person existing in a state of basic hunger or semistarvation, basic physiologic needs are uppermost—needs for food and water. When these needs are

met, higher needs can then be satisfied, such as physical comfort and security, love and affection, self-esteem and recognition, and finally, self-fulfillment and creative growth. All of these levels of need overlap and vary with time and circumstances, but they represent basic human needs that motivate behavior. They are present in one form or another at all times.

2. *Perception.* Perception is the process of adding meaning to what is taken in through the senses. It is perception that enables people to create a relatively stable environment out of an otherwise chaotic assortment of sensory impressions. Perception also limits understanding. Each person must selectively take in only a few, a relatively small number, of the multitude of messages coming in at all times. The number of messages admitted to consciousness is controlled by the amount of information that the brain can resolve at one time. Each phenomenon that the outer world offers is perceived by the individual through social and personal lenses. In every experience of a person's life, what he perceives is a blend of three factors: (1) the external reality, (2) the message of the stimulus that is conveyed by his nervous system to the integrative centers in the brain where thinking and evaluation go on, and (3) the interpretation that each person puts on each datum of experience. A host of subjective elements, such as hunger, thirst, hate, fear, self-interest, values, and temperament, influence response to the phenomena that are presented by the outer world. Those responses are called behavior.

■ **How does psychologic meaning become attached to food?**

Emotional responses to food stem from many sources. The practices and relationships that surrounded one's early infant feeding experiences, for example, build lasting emotional responses. Also, cultural and family conditioning, religious and economic factors, all mold the adult's food behavior. Food feeds the psyche, therefore, as well as the body.

■ **In American culture, what psychologic meaning may be attached to milk?**

Of all commonly used foods, milk is perhaps imbued with more psychologic meaning than any other. These psychologic meanings are frequently appealed to in advertising. To many persons milk symbolizes security and comfort or strength and vitality. This is especially likely to be true if the individual's early relationships with the mother figure were satisfactory, since she was the first feeding partner in supplying the early first food of life—milk. At the same time milk may mean dependence and helplessness, particularly in periods of stress when an individual regresses to prior periods of greater security. For example, ulcer patients on prolonged treatment of milk every few hours may find in such routine a socially accepted form of symbolic regression. In fact, the ulcer itself may in part stem from an inner dependent-independent conflict and a fear of success.

■ **Are sex-related attitudes reflected in foods?**

Yes, quite often. Certain foods, such as meat and bread, carry masculine meanings. They connote the paternal role of hunter, provider, and accepter. These notions about meat have been traced by anthropologists to the beliefs of primitive tribes. Meat was (and still is in many cultures) considered the only food that would make a warrior strong and courageous. A plethora of traditions about the magic power of meat and blood is known to anthropologists. Warriors are forbidden to eat any food but meat. Initiation ceremonies involve meat or blood of sacrificial animals. Some of this ancient tradition has been handed down to modern times in every culture. In some cultures it has been modified by the wish of the group to eradicate ferocity and therefore meat eating is forbidden. In America the tradition that strong men eat meat has been fostered until modern times by frontier history. The survival of the pioneers depended on their physical energy, strength, and aggression. Meat has been the center of the meal, both in terms of menu planning and money expended. In modern industrial America it remains the main concern of the wife that she have a strong husband and active children. Although she may know that eggs are nutritionally equal to meat (*actually better* in ideal amino acid combination), eggs never quite make the grade as a meat substitute. They are offered only as a last resort.

Vegetables and fruits, on the other hand, carry feminine meanings and attitudes, They connote the maternal role of the one who feeds and gives. They are associated with fertility and harvest. This symbolism often has a fascinating anthropologic history. When early human beings first settled down after a purely nomadic and hunting existence to an agricultural life it was the women who tilled the fields while men continued to hunt and fight. The supremacy of the male is bound up with his belief in "feminine weakness" represented by "mere" fruits and vegetables. The less educated (and the less psychologically developed) a man is, the more likely he is to scorn fruits and vegetables on emotional grounds, although he is usually totally unaware of the reason for his preference and attributes it simply to the taste of the food itself.

Fruits are most feminine in meaning. They symbolize love, beauty, sexuality, esteem, luxury. The reproductive notion is basic in the word "fruition" as bearing of fruit. Vegetables carry ideas related to even more primitive and earthy aspects of femininity—vegetate, vegetation. Fruits and vegetables are seasonal, ripe, bright-colored, and pleasantly shaped.

■ **How do food attitudes relate to age?**

Certain foods are considered appropriate at certain ages and not at others. Milk and strained foods, sometimes necessary components of a therapeutic diet for an adult, are considered infant foods and may be rejected, particularly by the person who is uncertain that he has genuinely attained adult status. Such a person may be of any chronologic age.

In the latency period the child's food horizons widen. As he leaves home for school he encounters new foods and is given greater freedom of choice. He also compares his family's food to that of his peers and begins to learn the social status of foods. Certain foods, such as peanut butter, become labeled as children's foods and are promoted as such by advertisers.

During adolescence the tenacious struggle for selfhood ensues. The teenager periodically adopts food fads, exhibits intense likes and dislikes, and displays enormous appetite. His obsession with his body image is basically a sexual problem. It may take the form of muscle-building food for boys and figure-controlling diets for girls.

Adulthood brings certain ideas for food privilege. Foods such as olives, shrimp, gourmet dishes, may be considered adult. Drinks such as coffee, tea, and alcohol are reserved in most groups for adults.

■ **How may food be used to condition behavior?**

Sweets are often used to bribe children; they are given as rewards for good behavior and are withheld for bad behavior. This pattern may carry over into adulthood. Sometimes unusual foods, special ways of preparation, or rare delicacies become symbolic rewards and punishment. In some therapy aimed at controlling obesity, the principle of behavior conditioning is applied. Foods that are problems for the obese person (often sweets, for example) may be associated with unpleasant situations or mixed with unpleasant tastes in order to recondition the person's response to such foods.

■ **How does illness relate to food behavior?**

Illness is a period of psychologic repercussion. Some degree of regression usually is evident. The patient may become demanding, picky, and finicky about his food. Often such behavior is but a way of transferring his anxiety concerning his illness to more acceptable items in his environment. Poor appetite may compound the feeding problem. The patient, even more than the well person, needs to be involved in the selection of his food. The same person who, while well, cares little about the style of food service may, as a patient, find that his appetite is surprisingly dependent on esthetic appeal in preparation and service. The patient with heart disease who complains, "How long do I have to stay on this diet with no salt?" may really be asking, "How ill am I and how soon will I get well?"

12 Nutrition education

■ **How can food habits be changed?**

Perhaps the better question to ask first is, "Should food habits be changed, and if so, what is the wisest way to go about it?" What principles must guide health education work with individuals, families, and communities? How can these principles be applied in practical ways so that people can be reached and helped to meet their health needs through improved food habits? What methods, approaches, and materials may be most effective?

In the search for answers, there are four aspects of nutrition education and applied community nutrition that should be considered: (1) the relationship of cultural forces to changes in food habits, (2) the teaching-learning process itself, (3) the role of health teaching in the practice of the health professions, and (4) community nutrition education. The health workers themselves must be imbued, first, with the concept of *change* if their efforts are to succeed. Life is always a dynamic process. Learning, which is manifested in terms of changed behavior, is in essence based on the principle of change.

CULTURAL FORCES AND FOOD HABIT CHANGE

■ **What principles of approach are wise guides in dealing with health practices within any cultural belief system?**

Wise and experienced health workers in different cultures, sensitized to the needs of the particular culture in which they are working, have formulated these principles of approach:

1. First, make an extensive study of the cultural practices related to health.

2. Carry out an *unprejudiced* analysis of these practices, in the light of the scientific principles known at this point and in consideration of local conditions.

3. Encourage those traditional practices that are beneficial. Do not interfere with those that are harmless. Seek to overcome the harmful practices by means of persuasion and demonstration. Where it is important to health to introduce a food or a treatment that is unacceptable on cultural grounds, devise ways of neutralizing it or of presenting the essential food or aspect of the treatment in a culturally acceptable form.

Three important facts are evident in this approach. First, people will accept new knowledge about health and nutrition only to the extent that the new knowledge can be integrated into existing patterns of custom and belief and philosophy. Second, cross-cultural exchanges are always mutually beneficial. Health workers are no exception. All peoples can learn from one another and thus enrich their own culture. This applies to subcultures within our own culture as well as to foreign cultures. Third, interest in individuals of other cultures and appreciation of the personal and social functions that their belief system and philosophy performs, builds rapport between health workers and the families they seek to serve. Unless such rapport exists among all persons all efforts to educate are wasted.

■ **What is the "channel theory" of food procurement and use?**

The concept of food channels was introduced by Kurt Lewin as a result of his studies concerning food habits and ways of changing them. He concluded that food reaches the family table from its point of origin through a series of channels, from production point to consumer. A channel is comprised of many steps in the complex process of food delivery. It may refer to as simple a step as delivery of a head of lettuce from the kitchen garden to the family table. It may refer to home canning or home cooking, although this channel of home preservation is less used now. The channel may also be one of the many routes through which a food is bought, a market, a way-side stand, a home delivery service. Also, a channel may be the preparation of food for sale by baking, by freezing, or by cooking and serving in a restaurant. It may be the holding of quantities of food at storage points as in refrigeration plants, freezers, and warehouses. Some innovative current food channels have been called "food conspiracies" because they seek to circumvent established food marketing practices of giant food chains by procuring food in quantity directly from the farmer or producer. In any event, the changing social scene is also causing changes in food channels to include a variety of avenues through which food is obtained.

■ **Who are the "gatekeepers" of these food channels?**

Lewin's studies led him to a further conclusion that these channels are controlled at various points by "gatekeepers" and that the flow of food through these channels depends on the ideas about food and the values of these "gatekeepers." Each gatekeeper—farmer, producer, wholesale food dealer, storekeeper, housewife, or other consumer who controls one of the channels through which food is delivered from the field to the table—is more or less consciously influenced by tradition, childhood memories related to specific foods, taste preference, religious or other taboos, political philosophy, beliefs or knowledge about the value or danger of specific items. Some of these psychologic forces operate

through the culture as a whole, but others are highly individual matters. Important among psychologic forces are resistance and conflict.

Nonpsychologic forces also influence these gatekeepers of food channels. They are responsive to such objective pressures as the inability to raise certain foods in certain soils or under certain weather conditions, available means of transportation, the chance to buy a certain food, and available money. Lewin found in his studies that the most significant gatekeeper in the food channel system is the individual housewife—the mother in the home. She was the most significant person who determined what food was to be served and in what condition it was to be delivered to the plate. She selected, from among the many reasons that were presented to her for choosing this or that item, that set of reasons which for her were decisive. In any event, the *personal values of the main gatekeeper,* whoever he may be, are in the last analysis the key to the food habits of a family. However, in the changing patterns emerging in families and communities, this main gatekeeper role is changing also. As families eat less and less together, in a variety of settings using a variety of food forms, increasingly they are making individual choices and serving as their own individual gatekeepers.

■ **What are the most effective means by which health workers can reach and persuade people to improve their food habits?**

Many methods have been used and are being used to bring about desired changes in the food habits of the American people. Approaches range from individual depth therapy as with a disturbed child to propaganda campaigns carried on through the mass media—radio, television, newspapers, magazines, billboards, and other advertising devices. Methods that retain the impact of personal face-to-face meeting while conserving the time of the health worker are most effective. Two types of group techniques that are midway between individual instruction and mass methods are the lecture-request and the discussion-decision sessions. The latter method is superior—those group situations in which the group participates in decisions concerning food habit changes bring a much more long-lasting result. In most settings a blend of both individual and group methods is used.

■ **What are the basic principles of successful nutrition education?**

Experience both in other cultures and in America teach important principles with which health workers can improve their work in nutrition and in health education in general.

1. *Knowledge of people.* Habits are never developed in a vacuum. All people in every culture have *some* knowledge of nutrition. No one comes to a health worker as an "empty slate." He bears the knowledge from his life experiences up to that point.

2. *Understanding reasons for habits.* All beliefs and practices, no matter how strange they may appear, serve psychologic and social functions. Habits need to be evaluated objectively and the overall pattern or system into which the customs and beliefs fit needs to be determined.

3. *Identification of any customs that need to be changed.* Many practices, even though they differ from the health worker's, are beneficial and should be encouraged. Some are harmless and need not be disturbed. Others are harmful. To overcome the harmful ones successfully, a sympathetic approach is necessary to integrate good nutritional practices. Hostility and rejection should never be used. Techniques of persuasion will have to be developed and points must be proved by demonstration and concern.

4. *Meeting individual needs.* A flexible attitude that is sensitive to the needs of individuals in specific situations at specific times allows health workers to be effective. Health workers can most successfully free others if they themselves are free to adjust, adapt, and tailor. There is always more

than one way to do anything. *Health workers must work with open systems.*

5. *Self-knowledge.* Each person has, perhaps without realizing it, a culturally determined system of values. Success is unlikely for the person who attempts to impose his system on the behavior of others. It is quite possible that genuine introspection on the part of the health worker may lead to some major reorientation in certain areas of his own philosophy.

6. *Involvement of key people.* Knowledge of leadership patterns in the community will help develop ways to enlist the cooperation and guidance of key individuals and families.

7. *Main gatekeeper of the food channels.* If the wife and mother in the home is the main gatekeeper who ultimately determines the food habits of her family, it is important that she be reached.

8. *Involvement of people.* Group discussions help to motivate people to action by creating awareness of need. Group decisions, because they reflect the finding of solutions by the persons themselves, usually represent a sense of identification with that solution. This sense of identification is most helpful in producing long-term results. In any event, the person involved must be a part of decisions concerning his plan of care if the plan is to be effective. His personal needs and goals must be the basis of his care.

9. *Communication skills.* The health worker needs to seek a common meeting ground, to perceive the situation as his hearer sees it, to think in the hearer's idioms, and to understand the meanings that words and actions have for the hearers. His assessment of individual needs will enable the health counsellor to adapt his educational methods to the amount of structure required by the learner and the mode of instruction preferred.

10. *Evaluation of results.* Efforts to change behavior must be evaluated. One must always ask, "What happened? Was the teaching realistic? Was it necessary? Did it work? Did it meet the need?" Ques-

tions such as these help the health worker to appraise immediate results and to anticipate long-range effects. They are necessary to maintain perspective and direction.

THE TEACHING-LEARNING PROCESS

■ **What is learning? How does it take place?**

Learning is a very personal thing. It is the continuing process of interaction between the person and his environment, which leads him to change behavior. Several characteristics are basic:

1. *Individual.* Learning is personal and individual. It is something that occurs inside an individual and is activated by the learner himself. It is not poured into people; it emerges from people. It cannot be imposed. Thus, personal involvement is necessary. Learning is relevant to one's needs and problems, and what is relevant and meaningful is decided by the learner and must be discovered by him. One of the richest resources is the learner himself, for learning is an emotional as well as an intellectual process.

2. *Developmental.* Learning is a process that is developmental or evolutionary in character. New learning is built on prior associations—ideas and concepts are constructed as new ideas are put with old. Thus, some necessary components of learning include free and open communication, confrontation with issues and situations, acceptance of self and others, variety of ideas, respect, self-revelation, shared evaluation, active involvement, and freedom from threat. These components build the kind of thought processes that allow new learning to develop and grow.

3. *Interactive.* Learning takes place as the result of a continuous process of interaction with one's environment, the problems it presents, the stimuli and confrontations that it brings. Learning carries from experiences that are cooperative and interdependent, in a nonthreatening atmosphere, which stimulates inquiry, and offers opportunity to apply knowledge to meet personal needs.

■ **What aspects of human personality are involved in learning?**

The teaching-learning process involves three fundamental aspects of human personality, each of which must be taken into consideration in planning a teaching-learning experience.

1. *Cognition.* Cognition is the thought process itself, by which information is grasped. It is shaped by the terms in which the mind thinks about a given body of facts. The thought process usually starts with a diffuse sensation. This is followed by a more focused perception that leads to the construction of a concept and to identification of specific principles involved. The total process of cognition provides the background knowledge that is the basis for reasoning and analysis. The learner senses the contribution of cognition to the learning process as "I know how to do it." This is the mental aspect of learning.

2. *Emotion.* In each individual specific feelings and responses are associated with given items of knowledge and with given situations. These emotions reflect the desires raised and the needs aroused. Emotions provide impetus; they create the tensions that spur a person to act. When he feels unfulfillment, lack, or need he wants to do something about it. If the teacher understands the learner's emotions he can direct this impetus in ways that will forward the learning process. The learner senses the contribution of emotion to the learning process as "I want to do it."

3. *Will.* The will to act arises from the conviction that the knowledge discovered can fill the felt need and relieve the sense of tension. The will focuses our determination to act on the knowledge received, to change an attitude, a value, a thought, a pattern of behavior. The learner senses the contribution of the will to the learning process as "I will do it."

■ **What processes are involved in the overall teaching-learning process?**

Involved in the teaching-learning process are identifiable processes, a variety of operations associated with knowledge and human activity. These are processes through which knowledge is created or learned and processes for using and communicating knowledge. They are an integral part of the content of any subject matter or learning. Essentially, there are three groups of processes involved, each of which overlap and interact in a spontaneous manner, a logical and psychologic balance of development of an idea or concept.

1. *Search.* The first processes are those that are involved with the taking in of information concerning a given problem at hand. This is the initial data intake. It involves processes such as observing, listening, reading, note-taking, listing, charting, identifying, questioning.

2. *Research.* The second stage of thinking is an analytical one. It is a process in which one analyzes the information taken in, researching the material to determine what sorts of relationships exist. Processes at this point include classifying, comparing, contrasting, coding, interpreting, verifying, modifying.

3. *Working plan.* Finally, the third area of activities are those related to the development of a working plan to solve the problem at hand. These are the activities in which the knowledge is applied to meet the needs presented. These processes include solving, constructing, performing, creating, achieving, reconstructing, deciding, testing, and retesting. The interdependent nature of these processes in a dynamic teaching-learning process is shown in the diagram in Fig. 12-1. It is through this kind of basic questioning and inquiry, of looking behind labels to see the process at work—the why and the how—that learning takes place.

■ **What does the term "concept" mean, and how does it relate to learning?**

Concepts are means of thinking and communicating by responding to things and events as a class. They help to provide a framework, a frame of reference, around

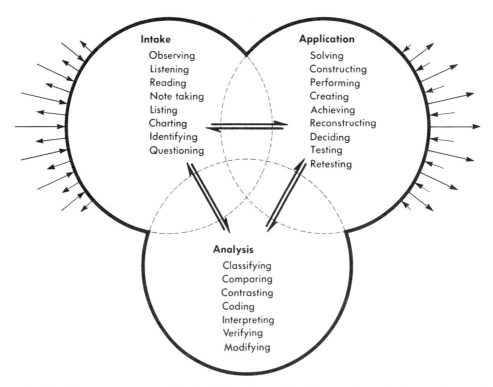

Fig. 12-1. The interactive processes involved in learning—taking in information, analyzing the data, and applying the results of this analysis in decision and action.

which to relate the parts of an idea in order to construct knowledge. Concepts avoid fuzzy abstractions by using concrete references. Concept learning has value, therefore, because it leads to problem solving through the variety of linking relationships possible among the observations or events or parts, and hence to the discovery of new principles forming new knowledge (new to the learner).

For example, a useful conceptual framework for determining human needs and hence for planning relevant patient education and care may be built around four basic factors: (1) the growth and development continuum, (2) the health-disease spectrum, (3) the stress-coping balance, and (4) a basic human needs hierarchy.

COMMUNITY NUTRITIONAL EDUCATION

■ **Why is the concept of the community health center a significant development in health care?**

It is significant because it signals the moving together of the two traditional health systems—the private or curative system and the public or preventive system. Such coordination will prevent much costly and inefficient overlapping and fragmentation, and fresh vision in program planning and development will give needed vitality and human dignity to pressing community health needs. Although the concept of the community health center is not fully formed, it is developing as a result of social pressures and correlated trends in American medicine. Reports indicate that the curative system (largely the professional practitioners and the hospitals) is doing more outreach into the community in home-care programs and extended-care facilities in chronic disease, in health care financing, and in area-wide hospital planning. At the same time the preventive system (largely the public health departments and other government agencies and programs) is organizing its services for the delivery of general health care, care of the chronically ill, rehabilitation work, and overall community planning, especially centered in

families of high risk low income population groups and in broad community health screening programs.

■ **What methods of health education are proving effective in such a setting?**

The community health center provides varied opportunities for health education and care through its facilities and personnel.

1. *The health team.* In the community health center usually a more informal health team approach prevails in the delivery of health care. Specialists in various areas of health care work together with the patient to explore needs and provide services for family-centered health care. There is more involvement of the patient in the planning of his care.

2. *Methods of teaching.* In such a community facility there is opportunity for individual counseling, small discussion groups, classes, use of libraries and exhibits, and various health teaching devices. In small groups patients and their families discuss common problems, and find solutions and support. Also, there is opportunity for acquiring various teaching tools and materials and for expanding and using various innovative approaches involving educational technology. Health education materials, books, pamphlets, leaflets, models, pictures, charts may be organized in a health library under the care of a qualified librarian to provide rich learning resources. An exhibit center for displays of visual and graphic materials related to various aspects of health care is another highly effective means of health education. Self-teaching devices allow for individual learning at a pace suitable to individual needs. With all of these resources available, more attention can be given to planning individual programs of education to suit individual needs.

■ **What community health resources are available to support educational activities?**

1. *Government agencies.* Public health departments conduct many services and educational activities at the local, state,

and national levels. Public health nutritionists are usually available to help in surveying community nutrition needs, in planning nutrition components of community health programs, providing training, consultation, and teaching materials for public health workers and other specialties. Public health nurses are available to work with families through various health services, to help organize and conduct clinics, and to teach community health classes.

2. *Volunteer agencies.* A host of volunteer health agencies, such as the American Heart Association, the American Diabetes Association, and the American Cancer Society, provide educational opportunities and materials through their local chapters. In some large urban areas nutrition committees offer classes taught by local nutritionists, nurses, and physicians. Sometimes these are arranged through cooperation with the local adult evening school. Staff nutritionists provide nutrition consultation services and develop educational materials for use by community physicians and health workers. There are also occasional workshops on specific health problems. Nutritionists and nurses also work with local chapters of the American Diabetes Association in their annual diabetes detection drives and teach classes in the local high schools.

3. *Specific health interest clubs.* Investigation in a local community may disclose organizations formed for the study and dissemination of information related to a specific health problem. They offer support and a sharing of information to persons having common health needs. These groups include the Ileostomy and Colostomy Club, TOPS (Take Off Pounds Sensibly), and Weight Watchers. Community health workers are often invited to speak at meetings of the members.

4. *Schools, churches, civic, and fraternal groups.* A number of lay organizations conduct health-related activities for groups and persons having special needs. One example is the "Meals on Wheels" program conducted in some cities by volunteers who prepare and deliver hot meals to persons in need of such services. These persons are for the most part chronically ill or undergoing rehabilitation, and often are elderly and alone.

5. *Professional groups.* Local professional organizations—medical, nursing, dietetics—provide health education in a number of ways. They sponsor workshops, participate in mass communication through such media as radio and television, and issue staff-written articles for publication in newspapers and magazines. In some communities there is a "Dial-a-Dietitian" program operated by the American Dietetics Association, which offers a telephone answering service through which people may make inquiries about food and nutrition.

6. *Food industry groups.* Food industry groups, such as the National Dairy Council and its affiliated state groups and the National Livestock and Meat Board, provide nutrition education materials and underwrite community nutrition projects.

7. *County interagency Nutrition Council.* In some communities there is an interagency Nutrition Council whose members represent the various nutrition agencies of the county and coordinate the work of all the representative groups. These nutrition councils often collaborate with community-wide health planning groups to coordinate community health activities. They also develop conferences on nutrition and issue teaching materials.

Information concerning nutrition education work in a community may be obtained by writing or telephoning one of the following sources:

1. Agricultural Extension Service, usually located in the state university
2. Home advisers, home economists, and district agricultural extension offices
3. Dietitians in local hospitals
4. Nutrition instructors in high schools, colleges, community colleges, and nursing schools
5. Nutritionists in local health departments or clinics
6. Volunteer health agency office, the

Table 12-1. Clinical signs of nutritional status

	Good	Poor
General appearance	Alert, responsive	Listless, apathetic, cachexic
Hair	Shiny, lustrous; healthy scalp	Stringy, dull, brittle, dry, depigmented
Neck (glands)	No enlargement	Thyroid enlarged
Skin (face and neck)	Smooth, slightly moist; good color, reddish-pink mucous membranes	Greasy, discolored, scaly
Eyes	Bright, clear; no fatigue circles beneath	Dryness, signs of infection, increased vascularity, glassiness, thickened conjunctiva
Lips	Good color, moist	Dry, scaly, swollen; angular lesions (stomatitis)
Tongue	Good pink color, surface papillae present, no lesions	Papillary atrophy, smooth appearance; swollen, red, beefy (glassitis)
Gums	Good pink color; no swelling or bleeding, firm	Marginal redness or swelling, receding, spongy
Teeth	Straight, no crowding, well-shaped jaw, clean, no discoloration	Unfilled caries, absent teeth, worn surfaces, mottled, malposition
Skin (general)	Smooth, slightly moist, good color	Rough, dry, scaly, pale, pigmented, irritated, petechia, bruises
Abdomen	Flat	Swollen
Legs, feet	No tenderness, weakness, or swelling; good color	Edema, tender calf, tingling, weakness
Skeleton	No malformations	Bowlegs, knock-knees, chest deformity at diaphragm, beaded ribs, prominent scapulae
Weight	Normal for height, age, body build	Overweight or underweight
Posture	Erect, arms and legs straight, abdomen in, chest out	Sagging shoulders, sunken chest, humped back
Muscles	Well developed, firm	Flaccid, poor tone; undeveloped, tender
Nervous control	Good attention span for age; does not cry easily, not irritable or restless	Inattentive, irritable
Gastrointestinal function	Good appetite and digestion; normal, regular elimination	Anorexia, indigestion, constipation or diarrhea
General vitality	Endurance, energetic, sleeps well at night; vigorous	Easily fatigued, no energy, falls asleep in school, looks tired, apathetic

local chapter of the American Heart Association, or the American Diabetes Association

NUTRITION ASSESSMENT

■ **What methods are useful in assessing individual nutritional status and needs?**

A number of methods are used in determining individual nutritional needs. These include:

1. *Clinical observation.* Various clinical signs of optimum nutrition may be observed as measures of health. These include such things as general vitality, a sense of well-being, posture, condition of gums and teeth, the skin, the hair, the eyes, and muscle development. Close attention to details can often yield much valuable data concerning nutritional status. Table 12-1 gives a guide for such observations of nutritional status.

2. *Nutrition history.* Using an interviewing schedule such as an activity-associated general day's food pattern, knowledge may be gained of the food habits of an individual. A nutrition history follows three basic steps. First, a general pattern of the day's activity and food intake is obtained, beginning when the person arises in the morning and going through the day until bedtime, so that not only meals but also snacks or informal eating may be accounted for. With respect to each item, questions are asked in terms of general habit—food item, form, frequency, preparation, portion, seasoning. Sometimes pictures or models of portion sizes may be helpful in arriving at a clear picture of the general quantity of food consumed.

Second, the day's pattern should be checked by nutrient groups. Usually this cross-check is made by reflecting back to the patient his original responses concerning the frequency and use of an item and the form in which it is consumed. Weighted phrases such as "only one" or "plenty of," approving or disapproving tones or facial expression, tend to imply judgments and prevent straightforward responses. Throughout such an interview important

clues to food attitudes and values are being communicated.

Third, afterward the food pattern and the cross-check of it are analyzed by some sort of a dietary guide. Calculations of specific nutrients may be made, using reference food tables, or a measure of general nutritional adequacy may be made using a dietary guide.

3. *Twenty-four-hour recall.* The patient is asked to recall every item of nutrient taken during the preceding 24 hours. This is then analyzed in terms of food nutrients or basic nutrient guide.

4. *Food records.* The patient may be asked to keep a food log for a week, more or less, in terms of all items consumed. Notations may also be included as to quantity, method of preparation, setting in which it was eaten, time of day, and so forth. These records may then be analyzed in a similar manner.

5. *Self-administered questionnaires.* Questionnaires may be developed, constructed in a manner that allows patients to respond to questions regarding form and frequency of food use, general marketing habits, food additives, food behavior, attitudes, concerns.

6. *Home visits.* As opportunity permits, visits to the home will yield additional data concerning food use, facilities for storage and preparation, and clues as to food attitudes.

A general dietary guideline by which food habits obtained through one or more of these methods may be analyzed is given in Table 12-2.

■ **What principles of interviewing may serve as guidelines in planning care?**

The interview is a basic tool in the health profession. Therefore, effective interviewing skills are mandatory. Valid health care is person-centered, and interviewing helps to determine valid health needs. The general components of such a goal-directed interview may include the following:

1. *Defined needs and goals.* A clear purpose for the interview is an important

Table 12-2. Daily food guide—the basic four food groups

Food group	Main nutrients	Daily amounts*
Milk		
Milk, cheese, ice cream, or other products made with whole or skimmed milk	Calcium Protein Riboflavin	Children under 9: 2 to 3 cups Children 9 to 12: 3 or more cups Teenagers: 4 or more cups Adults: 2 or more cups Pregnant women: 3 or more cups Nursing mothers: 4 or more cups (1 cup = 8 oz. fluid milk or designated milk equivalent†)
Meats		
Beef, veal, lamb, pork, poultry, fish, eggs	Protein Iron Thiamine	2 or more servings Count as one serving: 2 to 3 oz. of lean, boneless, cooked meat, poultry, or fish
Alternates: dry beans, dry peas, nuts, peanut butter	Niacin Riboflavin	2 eggs 1 cup cooked dry beans or peas 4 tablespoons peanut butter
Vegetables and fruits		4 or more servings Count as 1 serving: ½ cup of vegetable or fruit, or a portion such as 1 medium apple, banana, orange, potato, or ½ a medium grapefruit, melon
	Vitamin A	Include: A dark-green or deep-yellow vegetable or fruit rich in vitamin A, at least every other day
	Vitamin C (ascorbic acid)	A citrus fruit or other fruit or vegetable rich in vitamin C daily
	Smaller amounts of other vitamins and minerals	Other vegetables and fruits including potatoes
Breads and cereals		4 or more servings of whole grain, enriched or restored Count as 1 serving:
	Thiamine Niacin Riboflavin Iron Protein	1 slice of bread 1 ounce (1 cup) ready to eat cereal, flake or puff varieties ½ to ¾ cup cooked cereal ½ to ¾ cup cooked pastes (macaroni, spaghetti, noodles) Crackers: 5 saltines, 2 squares graham crackers, etc.

*Use additional amounts of these foods or added butter, margarine, oils, etc., as desired or needed.
†Milk equivalents: 1 ounce cheddar cheese, 3 servings cottage cheese, 1 cup fluid skimmed milk, 1 cup buttermilk, ¼ cup dry skimmed milk powder, 1 cup ice milk, 1⅔ cups ice cream, ½ cup evaporated milk.

beginning. The interview is based on the needs of the patient, his personal needs and his health needs, in this instance specifically, his nutritional needs. It is important that the nutritionist or other health worker has created a climate conducive to mutual trust and that she has considered the influence of her own behavior and attitudes on the outcome of the interview. The goals, then, that are established for the interview are the patient's goals and the purpose is to determine the best plan of care based on health needs and personal needs.

2. *Actions of the interview.* Various interchangeable and concurrent actions of the interview may be identified. These actions include:

    a. *Observation* should include attention to details of physical appearance, physical signs and symptoms, behavior pattern, and immediate environment if the interview is taking place in the patient's hospital room or home.

    b. *Listening* should be creative, an active process that is sensitive to clues concerning needs. Health workers need to learn to be comfortable as listeners.

    c. *Responses* during the interview may be verbal or nonverbal. Verbal responses include reflection of feelings communicated by the client, or they may be a restatement of the client's response to his words. The questions used should give close attention to words used (avoiding emotion-laden words and bias), and be nonthreatening in nature. Nonverbal responses include the wise use of silence, gesture, posture, movement, facial expression, and touch.

    d. *Interpretation of data* gained during the interview is based on initial goals. It may be that initial goals will need to be redirected in the light of information that comes out.

    e. *Recording of data* in some form is necessary. Usually a minimum amount of recording is best in the presence of the client, listing a few word cues, developing a clear memory for detail with more extensive recording after the patient has left. On some occasions tape recording may be useful, but should never be done without the express permission of the patient.

3. *Terminating the interview.* Terminating the interview will usually relate to

questions such as "Where are we?" and "Where do we go from here?" Plans for follow-up will usually be included. In any event, in most cases leaving an open door for further communication is useful.

4. *Reporting.* Some sort of reporting usually follows the interview, for the benefit of other members of the health team. It may be written charting or it may be oral case conferences. Whatever the form, it usually includes such items as a description of the situation, the identified needs and goals, the care and teaching done, results that followed, and the plan for follow-up care.

5. *Evaluation.* Continuous evaluation proceeds during an interview and in successive ones that may follow. Terminal evaluation is needed when a single interview (if there is to be only one), or a series (if there are several) is completed. Evaluation is always done in the light of initial or revised objectives. It helps to determine how nearly the original goals were met and what changes need to be made in planning care.

A general guide for assessment and care of nutritional needs is given in the outline on the opposite page.

■ **What are some tests for effective individual interviewing and counseling?**

Health teaching involves dynamic interaction between the health worker and the client or patient. It is essential, therefore, that the nutrition counselor periodically reassess his developing comprehension of the dynamics of human behavior, of growth and development, and of learning. There is need to evaluate from time to time his own personal growth and sensitivity in recognizing the needs and perceptions of persons in his care. Key questions to aid in this self-analysis include the following:

1. Do I listen when the patient talks? Am I listening to the choice of words, the repetition of key words, the rise and fall in tone of voice, hesitant or aggressive expressions of words and ideas. Am I listening to overall content, to the main ideas, to topics chosen for discussion? Am I listening for clues to the feelings, needs, and

I. Data intake: assess nutritional needs
    A. The person
        1. Who he is: age, sex, family, occupational role, culture, socioeconomic status, personal characteristics, limitations, strengths
        2. Where he is: physical setting—place of care, its possibilities and limitations; personal setting—mental, psychologic, emotional, and physical, in relation to health or disease, adaptation
        3. His nutritional status: food habits and general nutritional analysis (pp. 300-303 in *Nutrition and Diet Therapy;* also Table 15-1, p. 304), clinical observations and signs (Table 18-1, p. 380)
    B. The disease, if present, or normal physiologic stress (such as pregnany and growth)
        1. The general disease or physiologic process: anatomy and physiology, signs and symptoms, general treatment or management, pathology, course, prognosis
        2. Patient's unique experience with the disease or physiologic stress duration, intensity, medical management, prior diet therapy, adaptation, problems and solutions, knowledge of disease and its care—source, form, attitude, behavior response
II. Hypothesis formulation: identify and define problems and develop plan of care
    A. Explore present needs
        1. Day-to-day nutritional support: maintenance, optimum intake, basic nutritional requirements
        2. Nutritional therapy: treatment by modified diet
        3. Teaching: basic nutrition knowledge, principles of therapeutic modifications
    B. Explore future needs
        1. Continuity of care: home, responsible "significant others," extended-care facility
        2. Plan for medical management: health team conferences, nursing team conferences
        3. Plan for nutritional care: diet modifications, practical food management (family situation, living alone, degree of disability, and so forth), follow-up diet counseling and nutrition education, community resources
III. Hypothesis testing: carry out plan of care
    A. Physical, psychosocial responses: diet and its meaning
    B. Teaching plan: materials needed, content, sequence, methods, approaches, plan for evaluation
    C. Records of action for study
IV. Evaluation: check results
    A. Follow-up care: planned with patient and family and the health team
    B. Reinforcement: to strengthen learning
    C. Revision: as needed

goals, which are not openly expressed? Do I notice the fall of the voice that conveys reluctance, doubt, lack of faith in the therapy recommended, indifference, discouragement, revulsion, or hostility?

2. Does the patient understand what I am saying? Are the words and phrases that I use related to his experience so that he may identify with them and build upon them?

3. Do I respect the necessity for cultural harmony? Does my teaching or counseling conflict in any way with the patient's cultural values and conditioning. Since I know that such conflict will result in lack of confidence and probably in rejection or confusion, do I have the imagination to find ways to integrate my knowledge with this patient's conditioning?

4. Am I comfortable with silences that allow the patient to think through a thought raised? Do I respect the slow thinker, do I allow the patient time to translate our conversation into his own thinking? Am I patient with the person who has a mind of his own and will not change it until he sees convincing cause? Do I recognize the various qualities of

silence in various types of persons? Do I *value* the silence because of these events in his life experience, knowing that until he has gone through that inner process he cannot reach a meaningful decision?

5. Do I accept, without approval or disapproval, what the patient says? Have I set aside my judgmental tendencies, left behind my infantile wish to praise or blame? Do I see evidence of the maturity and freedom of my own approach in the frankness with which patients are able to discuss with me their cravings, their aversions, or their boredom?

6. Do I keep the conversation patient-centered? Do I allow him to set the direction of discussion about himself?

7. Do I reflect, without interpretation, key words and phrases expressed by the patient? This technique is useful to the nutrition educator insofar as it helps him to understand precisely what the patient is telling him. The counselor who calmly restates, without interpretation, those statements that he suspects of masking an emotion-loaded situation, is sometimes able to help the patient face the truth by dispelling fear or anger.

8. Am I genuinely interested? Do I show my interest? Do I indicate my concern by looking directly at him, by my facial expression, nod of head, tone of voice?

9. Has my teaching been practical? Will my suggestions prove workable for this patient in his special life situation? Does he have the resources to carry out such a plan?

10. Has my teaching been important? Does this teaching really matter to the patient's health? Is he making the changes agreed upon? Will they really make a difference in the outcome?

11. If other persons are present and I must discuss the patient with them, do I keep all communication directed to and through him?

12. At the end of the interview, do I leave the door open for further reflection and exploration as needed?

FOOD NEEDS AND COSTS

■ **What are some "nutritional bargains" in food buying?**

Nutritional counseling frequently centers on problems related to wise food buying habits in relation to family food needs and the costs involved. The objective in wise food buying for the family is to maintain optimum nutritional value for money spent on food. Table 12-3 indicates some food choices in less-expensive items that may serve as a guide in counseling situations.

■ **What are some economy buying suggestions in each of the food groups?**

1. *Meats, fish, poultry, eggs.* Meat is usually the most costly food item in the family budget. Thus, considerable study should be given to its selection. The lower grades provide good quality with less fat and they cost less. They have just as much food value as the higher cost cuts. Organ meats are nutritious bargains that can be used frequently. Poultry should be bought as the whole bird, not by pieces. Fish is usually a good buy. Shellfish is more costly, and fresh fish in season is less expensive. Eggs are sold according to grade and size, neither of which are related to food value, so the least expensive available is the best buy.

2. *Milk and cheese.* Fluid skimmed milk, buttermilk, and canned evaporated milk cost less than fresh, whole, fluid milk. Nonfat dry milk is the best bargain of all forms. It is more expensive to have milk delivered, so it is best bought at the store. If cheese is used often, buy it in bulk. Avoid presliced forms, since this adds to the cost. Spread cheeses and imported cheeses are more expensive. Cottage cheese is usually a good buy. It should be bought only as used, however, to avoid waste from spoilage.

3. *Vegetables and fruits.* Vegetables and fruits are the main sources of vitamins A and C, two nutrients found by community surveys to be most often lacking in the average American diet. Buy fresh fruits and vegetables in season. Avoid

Table 12-3. Bargains in the basic four food groups*

Food group	Usually less expensive, more food value for the money	Usually more expensive, less food value for the money
Milk products	Concentrated, fluid and dry nonfat milk, buttermilk, evaporated	Fluid whole milk, chocolate drink, condensed milk, sweet or sour cream
	Mild cheddar, Swiss, cottage cheese	Sharp cheddar, Roquefort or blue, grated or sliced cheese, cream cheese, yogurt
	Ice milk, imitation ice milk, imitation ice cream	Ice cream, sherbet
Meats		
Meat	Good and standard grades	Prime and choice grades
	Less tender cuts	Tender cuts
	Home-cooked meats	Canned meats, sliced luncheon meats
	Pork or beef liver, heart, kidney, tongue	Calf liver
Poultry	Stewing chickens, whole broiler-fryers, large turkeys	Poultry parts, specialty products, canned poultry, small turkeys
Fish	Rock cod, butterfish, other fresh fish in season, frozen fillets, steaks, and sticks	Salmon, crab, lobster, prawns, shrimp, oysters
Eggs	Grade A	Grade AA
Beans, peas, and lentils	Dried beans, peas, lentils	Canned baked beans, soups
Nuts	Peanut butter, walnuts, other nuts in shell	Pecans, cashews, shelled nuts, prepared nuts
Vegetables, fruits	Local vegetables and fruits season	Out-of-season vegetables and fruits, unusual vegetables and fruits, those in short supply
Vitamin A rich	Carrots, collards, sweet potatoes, green leafy vegetables, spinach, pumpkin, winter squash, broccoli, and in season canteloup, apricots, persimmons	Tomatoes, Brussels sprouts, asparagus, peaches, watermelon, papaya, banana, tangerine
Vitamin C rich	Oranges, grapefruit and their juice, cabbage, greens, green pepper, canteloup, strawberries, tomatoes, broccoli in season	Tangerines, apples, bananas, peaches, pears
Others	Medium-sized potatoes, nonbaking types	Baking potatoes, new potatoes, canned or frozen potatoes, potato chips
	Romaine, leaf lettuce	Iceberg lettuce, frozen specialty packs of vegetables
Breads, cereals	Whole wheat and enriched flour	Stone-ground, unenriched, and cake flour
	Whole grain and enriched breads	French, Vienna, other specialty breads, hard rolls
	Homemade rolls and coffee cake	Ready-made rolls and coffee cakes, frozen or partially baked products
	Whole grain or restored uncooked cereals	Ready-to-eat cereals, puffed, sugar-coated
	Graham crackers, whole grain wafers	Zwiebach, specialty crackers and wafers
	Enriched uncooked macaroni, spaghetti, noodles	Unenriched, canned, or frozen macaroni, spaghetti, noodles
	Brown rice, converted rice	Quick-cooking, seasoned, or canned rice

*Cook, F., and Groppe, C.: Balance food values and cents, Berkeley, California, 1967, University of California Agricultural Extension Service, Pub. HXT-42, pp. 6-7.

fancy grades. Purchase less well-formed fruits and vegetables or those with small surface defects that do not affect the eating quality or food value. Lower grade canned products contain the same food value but usually are less expensive because they contain imperfect pieces. If the family size warrants, buy fruits and vegetables in large cans or in quantity. Dehydrated foods vary in price; dried beans and peas and lentils are usually excellent buys and provide good amounts of protein. Avoid specialty dried foods, however, such as potatoes, which are usually more expensive than the fresh product. Frozen fruits and vegetables are usually more expensive than canned or fresh; however, watch for specials in large family-size packages.

4. *Breads and cereals.* Cereals in general are bargains in nutrition. Milled cereals are commonly enriched. Whole grain or enriched cereal products should be purchased to ensure the content of B-complex vitamins and calcium and iron. Grains usually bought in bulk are cheaper; however, adequate storage is needed to avoid spoilage. Usually ready-to-eat cereals cost twice as much per serving as cereals cooked at home, and they do not provide as much nourishment. Try unusual forms of grain when available. For example, bulgur is cooked and dried wheat with the outer brand removed and the remaining kernels cooked to the desired size. It has a toastlike color, is rich in wheat flavor, is equal in food value to whole wheat, and is far less expensive. Avoid processed or specialty preparations of rice and other grains, since this "convenience" process increases the cost. To avoid costly waste of breads and cereals, pack them in a cool, dry place and close packages tightly after each use.

■ **Are there any food plans available to provide guidelines for families on different income levels?**

Yes. To aid the health worker in counseling with families or in working with community groups, several family food plans have been prepared by the U. S. De-

partment of Agriculture through its Consumer and Food Economics Research Division. Five basic plans on different cost levels, with additional variations, are available: (1) liberal plan, (2) moderate plan, (3) low-cost plan, (4) special low-cost plan for use in the southeastern states, and (5) the economy plan. Table 12-4 shows a plan for reducing the cost still further (about 25%).

■ **What government programs exist to help low-income families obtain food?**

Two Federal food assistance programs are administered by the Consumer and Marketing Service of the U. S. Department of Agriculture. These are the donated food program or Surplus Food program and the Food Stamp program. The U. S. Department of Agriculture makes these foods available through its subsidy program to farmers of price support and surplus removal operations, so its primary purpose is financial aid to the farmer, not nutritional support for the poor. These foods include items such as flour, rice, rolled wheat and oats, bulgur, cornmeal, nonfat dry milk, dried beans, canned chopped meat, peanut butter, shortening, margarine, and raisins. Although these foods make an important contribution to persons in extreme circumstances, they often lack the variety needed for nutritional balance or personal need. Human beings need other foods also— fruits, vegetables, meat—and the dignity of a *person-centered approach.*

The Food Stamp program is a more recently developed one, and is supplementing and supplanting the food-donation or food-surplus program in some areas. Families participating in the program exchange their small amount of food money for stamps that are worth more than the money given in exchange. On the average, $10.00 is given in food stamps in exchange for every $6.00 of money invested, although this exchange value has recently been improved somewhat. These food stamps can be spent like money at local food stores for any domestic food.

Problems exist with both of these pro-

Table 12-4. Market basket for lower cost family food plan*

Food group	Food items included
Milk, cheese	Only nonfat dry milk, cheese
Meat, fish, poultry	Stewing beef, ground beef, salt pork, sausage, chicken, fish
Beans, peas, nuts	Dried beans, peanut butter
Flour, cereals, baked goods	Large proportion of flour and cornmeal; only cereals for cooking (no ready-to-eat cereals); rice and macaroni products; bread, crackers, and some sweet crackers
Citrus fruits, tomatoes	Canned orange juice, some fresh oranges, canned tomatoes
Potatoes	Only fresh potatoes (no processed)
Dark green and deep yellow vegetables	Sweet potatoes and carrots
Other vegetables and fruits	Cabbage, onions, bananas, apples; canned apples, corn, fruit juice; dried prunes
Fats, oils	Margarine, lard, and salad dressings
Sugars, sweets	Sugar, syrup, jelly
Accessories	A few seasonings; no soft drinks

*Peterkin, B. B.: Low-cost food plan—choices influence cost, Family Econ. Rev. March, 1967, p. 7-9.

grams and they are not reaching a large segment of the population in need. Some simple teaching materials have been developed to accompany their use to help families plan and prepare more nourishing meals. The core of these materials is a series of 21 illustrated pamphlets "Food for Thrifty Families." The leaflets present a wide range of choices in low-cost foods and easily followed recipes, most of which are adapted for top-of-stove cooking. Program aides, working closely with low-income families, have made effective use of these materials. Copies may be obtained from the Consumer and Marketing Service, U. S. Department of Agriculture.

13 Nutritional deficiency diseases

The primary world health problem today is *malnutrition.* Observation and experience have brought deepened awareness of two important interrelated facts: (1) food alone is not the answer, and (2) a high standard of living does not necessarily solve the problem. Even in the midst of plenty, malnutrition exists.

Important questions need to be asked. First, what is the problem? What is malnutrition? What is its extent and significance in world health today? Second, what is its ecology? Why does malnutrition exist? What complex web of factors combine and contort to cause malnutrition?

As each of these is reviewed, related factors for specific deficiency diseases should be considered. These include the nature of the disease and its clinical manifestation, the cause of the disease, in what inner and outer environment does this disease occur, and what methods of control are most effective in prevention and treatment of the disease? In each case the problems presented are of major public health significance and the answers are by no means simple.

THE ECOLOGY OF MALNUTRITION

■ What is the extent of malnutrition?

Human misery and waste of human life from malnutrition occur in both world hemispheres. Although these effects are far more profound and widespread in less developed areas of the world, they are nonetheless present in more developed nations also. The recent National Nutrition Survey in the United States brought to light more malnutrition than we have been willing to admit. The presence of such ab-

ject need in the midst of affluence and wealth is a reflection on national priorities and value systems. Because of the increasing complexity of society, many persons have only begun to glimpse the magnitude of future needs.

The problem is further compounded by the fact that population growth rates often are highest in those countries that can least afford to maintain an increased population. For example, the population of Latin America is the most rapidly growing in the world. Its rate of growth (up to 3.8% a year) is about 1½ times that of the world rate (2% a year). The rapidity of this expansion will lead the Latin American countries to double their population within a generation. In North America the rate of growth is only 1.4% a year.

Infant and child mortality and morbidity provide an index to the extent of general malnutrition. In Latin America, for example, in the 1 to 4 year age group, the death rate is 20 to 30 times as high as in the United States and Canada. In some areas the rate is even 50% higher. If the rates of infant and child mortality in Latin America were as low as those in the United States and Canada, 250,000 fewer children in this age group would die each year. Still more disturbing examples could be cited for other regions of the world, such as parts of Africa, India, the Orient, and the Middle East. The problem is urgent, and it is becoming more so.

■ What is the difference between primary and secondary malnutrition?

Malnutrition at its fundamental biologic level is an inadequate supply of nutrients to the cell. Nutritional deficiency diseases may be classified as primary or secondary, according to the availability of the nutrient:

1. *Primary deficiency disease.* A primary deficiency disease is a disease that results directly from dietary lack of a specific essential nutrient. For example, scurvy results if the diet is deficient in vitamin C. Beriberi results if the diet is deficient in thiamine.

2. *Secondary deficiency disease.* A secondary deficiency disease is a disease that results from the inability of the body to use a specific nutrient properly, regardless of the quantity that is available for use in the diet. Such inability may result from either of two general types of failure: (1) failure to absorb the nutrient from the alimentary tract into the blood, or (2) failure to metabolize the nutrient normally after it has been absorbed. For example, the malabsorption syndrome is characterized by failure of absorption of fat through the intestinal walls so that fat is lost in the stool. Phenylketonuria is the inability of the body to metabolize the essential amino acid, phenylalanine, so that phenylalanine is lost in the urine, and abnormal metabolites accumulate in the blood.

■ **What factors cause malnutrition?**

Many factors work together to produce malnutrition; it is often complicated by the presence of other diseases. A synergism is, in fact, known to exist between malnutrition and infection. Each compounds the other, and together they cause more serious illness than either would bring alone. For example, a common infectious disease of childhood, such as measles, which would otherwise be mild, may cause death in a severely malnourished child. Infectious diarrhea is a common complication of kwashiorkor and may be the irreversible factor that causes death.

Some of the many related causes of malnutrition can be classed under the three factors that are classically cited by the epidemiologist as the triad of variables that influences disease:

1. *Agent.* Food quantity, imbalance be-

tween community supply and need, food quality, food timing

2. *Host.* Presence of other disease, increased dietary needs, congenital defects, and personal factors, such as ignorance, carelessness, emotional problem, and anorexia

3. *Environment.* Sanitation, culture, social factors, and psychologic factors, economic and political structure, and agriculture

■ **What forms does protein-calorie malnutrition take?**

Millions of children throughout the world are exposed to various degrees of protein-calorie malnutrition. It is a health problem of major proportions, which causes a high rate of morbidity and death in children. Its long-range effects in those who survive are still incompletely understood. In protein-calorie malnutrition a broad clinical spectrum exists between *kwashiorkor,* on the one hand, and *marasmus* on the other. There are many continuous overlapping conditions in between, where features of both are found. Although considerable variability is seen, distinctions usually are based on the nature of the dietary deficiency. In kwashiorkor calories may be sufficient but protein is lacking; in marasmus both calories and protein are deficient.

■ **What is kwashiorkor?**

Kwashiorkor is a disease associated with protein deficiency. The word comes from the Ghan language and was first used in Ghana where early observations and work with children was done. The word may have several meanings, all usually associated with the mystique of jealousy between siblings and with physical sickness. It means literally, "the sickness the older child gets when the next baby is born." Originally a related meaning of "redness" (derived from the characteristic color of the skin in this disease, which results from depigmentation) was attached to the word.

The name is appropriate, for kwashiorkor is the syndrome that develops in a child who, after being weaned from the breast at the age of about 1 year, on the birth of the next sibling, is given a diet consisting largely of starchy gruels or sugar water. Such a sequence of events is typical of many cultures in the underdeveloped parts of the world. Before he was weaned the infant received in the breast milk both protein and calories adequate for growth. The sharply curtailed diet, based on such starchy foods as tubers (manioc, cassava) or grains (maize), may supply adequate calories as carbohydrate but its protein content is qualitatively and quantitatively inadequate. Various clinical pictures are determined by local food patterns involving different degrees of calorie and vitamin deficiency.

Classical symptoms involve retardation of growth and development, with peevish mental apathy, edema, muscular wasting, depigmentation of hair and skin, characteristic scaly changes in skin texture (a "flaky paint" dermatosis), hypoalbuminemia, reversible fatty infiltration of the liver, atrophy of the acini of the pancreas with reduction of the enzymatic activity of the duodenal juice, diarrhea, and moderate anemia. Frequently associated are infections and severe vitamin A deficiency, resulting in permanent blindness. Serious deterioration of patients with kwashiorkor is caused by the infections and diarrhea.

Specific disturbances in water and electrolyte metabolism follow. Total body water increases and there is marked reduction of total body potassium and retention of sodium. Factors probably responsible for these fluid and electrolyte disturbances are hypoalbuminemia, endocrine dysfunction, and circulatory failure. Death may ensue from cardiac arrest caused by potassium deficiency. The inadequate amount of protein, particularly lacking in essential amino acids for normal growth, is apparent in an abnormality of blood lipid transport compound involving protein, and extreme protein depletion in different organs and tissues. Initial treatment during the first 24 hours is aimed at correction of the water and potassium depletion, especially if the diarrhea has been severe

enough to cause continued loss of potassium. This is followed by a refeeding program using a skimmed milk formula, since the tolerance for fat is poor. Gradually the caloric content of the diet is increased by the addition of mixed foods suitable to the child's age, which also gives sufficient vitamins and minerals as well as protein.

Prevention depends on solution of the socioeconomic factors that underlie the disease. Therefore a two-fold program must include: (1) education concerning improved available sources of dietary protein, such as skimmed milk powder, legumes, and fishmeals, and (2) motivation to provide adequate food and the means of procuring it.

■ **What is marasmus?**

The word marasmus comes from a Greek word *marasmos,* which means "wasting." It is applied to the state of chronic total undernutrition in children, which represents a deficiency of both protein and calories in various degrees of severity, and produces a gradual wasting away of body tissues with general emaciation.

The marasmic child is grossly underweight and appears almost cadaverous—a living skeleton of skin and bones. There is atrophy of both muscle mass and subcutaneous fat, giving a shrunken, wizened, "old man" appearance to the face, in contrast to the fat, rounded cheeks of children with kwashiorkor. Edema is minimal or absent, diarrhea is common and may result from infection or from pathogenic microorganisms in the stool, or there may be preexisting nutritional diarrhea complicated by superimposed infection. The growth rate declines progressively; there are both physical stunting and mental and emotional impairment. The infant sleeps restlessly, is fretful, apathetic, and withdrawn. Body temperatures may be subnormal because of the absence of the insulation that is normally provided by subcutaneous fat, and the child must be kept warm. Metabolic activity is minimal. The heart is weak and urine is scanty. Prostration is common.

Such profound deprivation—food, general physical care, and emotional care—may be found in three basic circumstances. (1) The parents may be poor, and they are often ignorant of food values so they do not seek proper food. (2) The parents may have severe mental or emotional problems. This is especially dangerous for the child when the mother is disturbed, for she may reject the child and fail to give it care. (3) There may be other disease, such as tuberculosis, chronic gastroenteritis, dysentery, infectious diarrhea or parasites, and inadequate medical care. All of these conditions thrive in poor socioeconomic settings, and the child is the victim of these circumstances.

Marasmus is most common in infants 6 to 18 months of age. It occurs in slum conditions in any country where socioeconomic deprivation breeds such diseases. Prevention depends on eradicating the underlying causes of the disease and thus on solution of the socioeconomic problems. Treatment follows much the same pattern as that given for kwashiorkor. Since rejection and total deprivation are commonly a part of the etiologic picture, treatment also involves gradually holding the infant as much as the tenderness of his body allows, keeping the child warm, and the provision of much loving care.

VITAMIN DEFICIENCY DISEASES

■ **What is xerophthalmia?**

Xerophthalmia is a disease of the eye in which the cornea and the conjunctiva become dry. It results from extreme deficiency of vitamin A. The dryness is a consequence of metaplasia of the conjunctiva, causing roughness. This usually leads to a loss of secretions and infection usually follows. Early signs are drying, roughness, and wrinkling of the conjunctiva, swelling and redness of the lids, and pain and photophilia. Dry, lusterless patches may be seen on the conjunctiva, and triangular whitish foamy spots (Bitot's spots) occur at the limbus conjunctivae. The cornea loses sensitivity, becomes clouded, and ulcers may form. If the disease is untreated the cornea softens (keratomalacia), and

perforation may occur, resulting in total blindness.

Keratomalacia is still a major cause of blindness in certain underdeveloped countries. For example, in Indonesia many thousands of cases occur each year, and WHO estimates that 5% of all the children in Indonesia have impaired vision or are blind because of vitamin A deficiency.

■ **What is beriberi?**

Beriberi is a disease that usually attacks the neuromuscular system of the body. The two general types of beriberi are infantile and adult. The disease in infants occurs during the first year of life and is characterized by various symptoms: convulsive disorders, respiratory difficulties, and gastrointestinal problems. Terminal symptoms in severe cases include cyanosis, dyspnea, and tachycardia. Sudden death may occur only a few hours after onset.

Adult beriberi, usually seen in young adults with physiologic stress, such as pregnancy and lactation, may be either a dry or wet form according to the presence or absence of edema. The symptoms usually result from involvement of the peripheral nerves and related muscle function. First, there may be a tingling and numbness in the extremities, leg muscle cramps, and later involvement of the muscles of the forearms, the thighs, and the abdominal wall. Paralysis may result. As the heart muscle becomes involved, cardiorespiratory symptoms follow quickly. Vomiting and constipation are usually present.

The disease is caused by a deficiency of thiamine. Thus, it is found in population groups whose diets are based primarily on refined cereal grain, such as the polished rice diet found in the Orient. A person may have subsisted on minimal body thiamine stores until additional physiologic need was presented, and when these increased requirements were not met the disease ensued. In the western world beriberi usually occurs in a milder form and may be associated with other disease. It usually occurs in poverty-stricken areas in conjunction with general states of malnutrition, or among persons with alcoholism, or in pregnant women with a history of poor diet. It also occurs among inmates in some prisons or in hospitals for the chronically ill geriatric patient or for the mentally ill.

■ **What does the term "ariboflavinosis" mean?**

Ariboflavinosis is the term given to a general group of clinical manifestations that characterize the state of riboflavin deficiency. The characteristic findings include seborrheic dermatitis, cheilosis, and eye lesions.

Diets deficient in riboflavin, one of the B-complex vitamins, induce these symptoms. Such diets are lacking in animal protein foods, such as milk, meat, or fish, and the leafy vegetables and legumes—all sources of riboflavin. Riboflavin deficiency frequently develops in association with deficiencies of other B vitamins, such as niacin and thiamine, in situations of poverty, ignorance, chronic alcoholism, or illness, such as prolonged diarrhea.

■ **What is pellagra?**

Pellagra is a disease resulting from niacin deficiency. Its clinical manifestations are of four types. (1) *Gastrointestinal disturbances* include anorexia, general indigestion, weight loss, and diarrhea, which is often severe. (2) *Stomatitis* is a swelling and reddening of the tongue. The entire buccal mucosa becomes involved, with reddening, burning sensation, and tissue erosion. (3) *Dermatitis* is a highly characteristic sign of pellagra. The lesions resemble burned areas and become much more painful upon exposure to sunlight. The dermatitis occurs most often on exposed portions of the skin, but may also be seen in skin folds where the surface is subject to irritation. Infection often occurs as the lesions rupture, and healing leaves darkly pigmented areas. (4) *Neurologic changes* include mental apathy, depression, and anxiety of various degrees. In extreme cases serious disorientation, confusion, and dementia may occur.

The essential amino acid tryptophan is a precursor of niacin. The incidence of pellagra is especially high in populations whose staple food is corn, because corn is low in both tryptophan and niacin. Pellagra may also be a conditioned response complicating other chronic disease involving diarrhea or poor food intake, or in chronic alcoholism with associated malnutrition. In the southern United States, especially in rural areas, pellagra was formerly widespread. However, since wheat flour, cornmeal, and other grains have been enriched and since the general diet has been somewhat improved, pellagra is seen only occasionally in areas of poverty or in association with other diseases affecting food intake or food utilization.

■ **What are the effects of pyridoxine deficiency?**

A deficiency of pyridoxine has been reported to cause convulsions and hypochromic anemia in infants. Adults with multiple vitamin deficiency states characterized by muscle weakness and fatigue have responded to pyridoxine therapy. Additional proof of the effects of pyridoxine deficiency on the nervous system is the fact that an antagonist of pyridoxine, isonicotinic acid hydrazide (isoniazid), which is used in the treatment of pulmonary tuberculosis, causes peripheral neuritis and occasional convulsions. The hypochromic anemia occurring with these neurologic symptoms is thought to be caused by alterations of cellular metabolism of pyridoxine.

■ **In vitamin B_{12} therapy for pernicious anemia, why must the vitamin be given intravenously?**

The defect in pernicious anemia is at the point of absorption of vitamin B_{12}. The anemia is the result of the lack of a material in the gastric secretions, intrinsic factor (IF), which is necessary for the absorption of vitamin B_{12}. Hence injections of vitamin B_{12} rather than oral doses are necessary in order to bypass the absorption defect.

■ **Who are the persons most at risk from a folic acid deficiency anemia?**

The pregnant woman is especially susceptible. The added demands of pregnancy may not be met through an average diet, and supplementation is recommended. A daily supplement of 0.2 to 0.4 mg. of folate during pregnancy should prevent folic acid deficiency in all pregnant women. The infant also is at risk because of the increased physiologic stress of growth, because of infections, or because of ascorbic acid deficiency resulting from a poor diet. Ascorbic acid is closely related to protein and iron in the manufacture of red blood cells.

■ **How does scurvy affect the growing child?**

Since ascorbic acid performs many vital physiologic functions related especially to the formation of connective tissue, collagen, and the integrity of capillary walls, the clinical manifestations of scurvy involve tissue deterioration and changes of hemorrhagic origin. The skin becomes dry, rough, and often has a dingy brown color. Small hemorrhages develop and skin changes usually occur on the arms and legs, the buttocks, and the back. Purpura (hemorrhaging in the skin), which produces a reddish-brown discoloration with the appearance of a bruise, appears first in the lower extremities and then spreads upward. Pinpoint hemorrhages produce small red spots called petechiae, which may coalesce into areas of purpura and finally, if large enough, into even larger areas called ecchymoses. Sometimes the whole extremity may be involved, with extravasated blood.

Deep hemorrhages in the muscle tissue produce brawny areas of induration, resulting from hardening and thickening of the tissue. Clotting in a vein may follow. Hemorrhages in the cavities of the joints also occur, causing local heat, painful swelling, and immobility. The joint pain causes scorbutic infants to lie in a characteristic position, supine, with the knees partially flexed and the thighs externally rotated—the only position of comfort. This position is sometimes called the scorbutic pose.

The gums are spongy, friable, grossly swollen, and bleed easily at the slightest touch. As tissue hemorrhaging continues, thromboses form in the blood vessels and infarcts occur, producing blue-red discoloration. The teeth become loosened and may fall out. Infection is frequent.

Any trauma, even small, produces ulcerated areas. New wounds fail to heal, or if they apparently heal they break open again under the slightest stress. Anemia usually accompanies the disease. It is caused partially by hemorrhagic blood loss, but also by the disrupted metabolic interrelationships of vitamin C with folic acid and with iron. Concurrent deficiencies of other nutrients also contributes to anemia. Infantile scurvy affects the growing bones. The growing ends of long bones are particularly affected. Microscopic fractures, small defects, or cracks occur, associated with bleeding in the subperiosteal space.

Cases of frank scurvy respond quickly and dramatically to therapeutic doses of vitamin C of about 200 mg. or more daily. For example, all bleeding ceases in 24 hours, gums heal in 3 or 4 days, and the leg that has been ecchymotic from hip to heel becomes normal in 3 weeks on such a regimen.

■ **What causes rickets?**

Rickets is a disease directly related to impaired metabolism of calcium and phosphorus. It is manifested in defective bone growth and changes in the body musculature. This impaired mineral metabolism in rickets may have many causes, but by far the commonest cause is a deficiency of vitamin D. Vitamin D may be preformed in food or formed in the body (the skin) through the action of short ultraviolet radiation, such as that in sunlight. Vitamin D is necessary for the absorption of calcium and phosphorus and for their deposit in bone tissue.

■ **Are there vitamin D-resistant forms of rickets?**

Yes. Refractory forms of rickets have been observed, some of which are genetically acquired. A variety of signs appear in different members of the same family. The clinical picture is similar: there are retarded growth and skeletal deformities.

However, these unusual forms may be differentiated by their great resistance to vitamin D therapy. For example, a case has been reported in which the serum vitamin D levels were about 20 times greater than normal, and 1,000,000 units of vitamin D daily were required for healing with the necessary maintenance dose thereafter of 440,000 units daily.

■ **Why is vitamin K given to newborn infants?**

The gastrointestinal tract of the newborn infant is sterile at birth and hence no bacterial synthesis can occur. Bacterial synthesis is the primary source of vitamin K, which is necessary for prothrombin activity in blood and hence for the operation of the blood-clotting mechanism. Without vitamin K there is a fall in prothrombin activity in the blood during the first few days of life, and life-endangering hemorrhages may result. This syndrome has been called hemorrhagic disease of the newborn. The disease can be prevented by giving small doses of water-soluble vitamin K analogues parenterally to newborn infants. The dose, however, must be small, for excess amounts of vitamin K may be toxic, even lethal. The Council on Drugs of the American Medical Association has recommended single doses of the water-soluble analogues equivalent to 1 mg. of synthetic vitamin K for prophylaxis and treatment.

MINERAL DEFICIENCY DISEASES

■ **What causes tetany?**

Any condition that lowers the blood calcium or decreases the availability of the calcium that is present in the blood, or produces alkalosis, may cause tetany. Ionized calcium-phosphate, carbon dioxide, and the acidity of the blood serum exist together in a relationship that must be constant. The control of tetany depends on control of the causative circumstances or conditions. Calcium or ammonium chloride may be given orally if vomiting has subsided. The orally administered dose usually does not take adequate effect in less than 24 hours. Thus for immediate con-

trol, an injection of magnesium sulphate (10% solution, 1 ml./kg. body weight) may be given intramuscularly. Any respiratory depressant effects may be counteracted by parenteral injection of a soluble calcium salt, such as calcium lactate or calcium gluconate. The latter may also be given intramuscularly.

■ **What is the difference between osteomalacia and osteoporosis?**

Both osteomalacia and osteoporosis are diseases of impaired calcium and phosphorus metabolism, with resulting changes in bone formation. They may be distinguished according to cause and result:

1. *Osteomalacia* is the adult form of rickets. It is caused by a deficiency of vitamin D, calcium, or phosphorus in the diet, or by a deficiency of the vitamin D that is produced by exposure to sunlight. Deficiency is more likely to occur during periods of increased physiologic need, such as in pregnancy and lactation, or by factors that hinder the proper metabolism of vitamin D, calcium, and phosphorus. Such hindering factors may be: (1) a defect in renal tubular reabsorption, resulting in imbalances in serum calcium and phosphorus; (2) a malabsorption syndrome, such as sprue or steatorrhea, which makes calcium unavailable to the body and allows it to be lost in the feces, or (3) resistance to vitamin D. The resulting osteomalacia results from a softening of the bones caused by their demineralization, accompanied by general weakness and aching.

2. *Osteoporosis* is a metabolic disorder that usually occurs in persons older than 50 years, especially women after the menopause. It is believed to be caused by age-related decline in secretions of anabolic hormones by the sex glands and pituitary glands. No doubt other factors also contribute, such as lack of stimulating exercise and malnutrition, especially protein malnutrition. The result is a decrease in bone-forming activity (ossification) with a consequent reduction in the amount of bone, although the composition of the bone

remains normal. Hypercalcinuria may occur, especially when prolonged immobilization is a factor, and renal calculi frequently develop. Manifestations include weakness, anorexia, hip and back pain, muscle tenderness and cramping, stooped posture, decreased height caused by shrinkage of the spine, and a tendency of the bones to fracture easily.

■ **In what stress situations may negative iron balance occur and cause anemia?**

Since iron performs important physiologic functions in oxygen transport and cellular respiration, the body guards its small supply, using it over and over again. However, in conditions of physiologic stress, such as growth, menstruation, pregnancy, or hemorrhage, often compounded by poor diet and impaired absorption, a negative iron balance may develop. Anemia is the result.

■ **Why is treatment ineffective in long-standing goiter?**

Goiter is a diffuse enlargement of the thyroid gland, caused by a deficiency of iodine. It may be prevented by sufficient supply of iodine in the diet. The most practical means of ensuring adequate intake is the iodization of table salt. A content of 1 part iodine to 10,000 to 20,000 parts of salt is recommended. Prevention is more effective, however, than treatment, for in long-standing goiter treatment has little effect. The chronic fibrosis that occurs is not reversible.

METHODS OF COMBATING MALNUTRITION

■ **Why is medical care alone an incomplete solution to the problem of malnutrition?**

A direct attack involving case findings, clinical diagnosis, and treatment is of primary concern. All the resources of the medical team are needed for this aspect of the approach. But treating malnutrition and then sending the patient back into the environment that produced it does not solve the problem, because it does not get at the root of the problem.

■ **What is meant by "nutritional rehabilitation" in treating malnutrition?**

Nutritional rehabilitation must follow initial medical treatment. In this program practical help is given to mothers during the recuperation of malnourished children, not only by giving them badly needed food but also by teaching the mothers the rudiments of nutrition and proper food preparation. Gradual restoration of the growth process and its continued support through feeding and habit change is necessary.

■ **What is the role of health education in helping to solve the problems of malnutrition?**

Health education must be a continuous and on-going activity to support medical care and nutritional rehabilitation. This education must begin with the health personnel. Education must also reach the patients themselves, their parents and families, and the public. It must constantly develop in order to accommodate the constant changes in people and the circumstances of their lives in food products and in scientific knowledge. It must be person centered and practical. Often the most significant care in such situations is personal teaching, nutritional rehabilitation, and supportive encouragement.

Ultimately, however, the success of any efforts to combat malnutrition in a community must rest on a developed sense of responsibility in the people involved. The responsibility for providing sound relevant health care rests with members of the health professions. The responsibility for helping to provide a safe and adequate food supply, to explore food enrichment laws, agricultural methods, marketing practices, consolidation of control programs, supporting research, education, and technical developments, rests with the persons who form and administer the economic and political structure of the country. Responsibility for meeting health needs in daily life at the local level rests with community leaders. Responsibility for meeting person and family health needs, for maintaining interest in good nutrition, for making certain that information is correct and clearly understood, and for carrying out the discipline that is required for the development of sound food habits rests with individuals and with the heads of families.

■ **How are various world health groups attempting to combat malnutrition?**

World health groups, such as the World Health Organization, the Food and Agriculture Organization, UNICEF, and others, are actively and earnestly engaged in the mammoth task of combating malnutrition.

Many other national and local groups in the United States and other countries are working toward the same goal. Many food supplements, such as the protein substance "Incaparina," which was developed by the Institute of Nutrition for Central America and Panama (INCAP) in Guatemala City, are being studied and used to add nutrients to inadequate regional diets. Research and education programs are helping to provide knowledge and tools.

14 Nutrition and the life cycle

Nutrition undergirds the quality of life throughout the human life cycle. It supports the right to be well-born. It ensures optimum growth and development. It maintains productive adulthood. It cushions and enriches old age. Through all the successive stages of man, food and feeding behaviors are intimately related with the whole of life—man's psychosocial needs as well as his physical requirements. Aging is a *total life* process, attended from birth to death by constant and dynamic change. Throughout, however, aging remains uniquely *individual*.

NUTRITION DURING PREGNANCY AND LACTATION

■ **What changing concepts are occurring in maternal nutrition?**

Maternal nutrition, through ups and downs of the past 3 decades, has suffered from much ignorance and neglect. That the dictum of a German obstetrician issued early in this century, and repeated after World War I's strict food rationing, that "semi-starvation of the mother is really a blessing in disguise," could have become so entrenched in American obstetrical practice seems incredible. Overwhelming evidence to the contrary, however, is gradually causing the pendulum to swing back. The harm accruing from protein-poor, salt-free, calorie-restricted diets, accompanied by diuretics, has been recognized and changes in clinical and community practice are increasingly evident. These changes reflect the effect of a recent report of the National Research Council. The council re-

port reaffirmed the fact that optimum maternal nutrition is critically important to both mother and fetus. The statement indicated that routine restriction of calories and salt, along with the use of diuretics, is unsound and potentially dangerous. Instead, an optimum diet, meeting increased nutrient requirements, should be actively promoted and supplemented daily with iron and folic acid, and where needed, also with iodine. That pregnancy requires emphasis on sound nutrition is evident.

■ **What is the role of protein in pregnancy?**

The increased demands for protein during pregnancy are highly significant. Large amounts of nitrogen are used by the mother and child. It has been shown that during the last half of gestation, for example, the amount of nitrogen stored by the embryo rises from 0.9 to 55.9 gm. More protein is essential to meet the demands imposed by: (1) the rapid growth of the fetus; (2) enlargement of maternal tissue in the uterus, mammary glands, and placenta; (3) the increase in maternal circulating blood volume, with attendant need for increased synthesis of hemoglobin and plasma protein, both of which are vital to the support of the pregnancy; and (4) the formation of amniotic fluid and storage reserves for labor, delivery, and lactation.

Milk, egg, cheese, and meat are complete protein foods of high biologic value. Protein-rich foods also contribute other nutrients, such as calcium, iron, and B vitamins. Additional supplementary protein is contributed by whole grains, legumes, and other vegetables. The amounts of these

Table 14-1. Daily food plan for pregnancy and lactation

Food	Nonpregnant woman or during first half of pregnancy	Second half of pregnancy	Lactation
Milk, cheese, ice cream, skimmed or buttermilk (food made with milk can supply part of requirement)	2 cups	3 to 4 cups	4 to 5 cups
Meat (lean meat, fish, poultry, cheese, occasional dried beans or peas)	1 serving (3 to 4 ounces)	2 servings (6 to 8 oz.); include liver frequently	2½ servings (8 oz.)
Eggs	1	1 to 2	1 to 2
Vegetable* (dark green or deep yellow)	1 serving	1 serving	1 to 2 servings
Vitamin C-rich food* Good source—citrus fruit, berries, cantaloupe Fair source—tomatoes, cabbage, greens, potatoes in skin	1 good source or 2 fair sources	1 good source and 1 fair source or 2 good sources	1 good source and 1 fair source or 2 good sources
Other vegetables and fruits	1 serving	2 servings	2 servings
Bread† and cereals (enriched or whole grain)	3 servings	4 to 5 servings	5 servings
Butter or fortified margarine	As desired or needed for calories	As desired or needed for calories	As desired or needed for calories

*Use some raw daily.
†One slice of bread equals one serving.

foods that would supply the quantities of protein needed are indicated in the recommended daily food plan in Table 14-1.

■ **How many calories will meet the energy demands of a normal pregnancy?**

Approximately 2,500 calories will meet most needs. Weight is an indicator of energy balance. Thus, weight gain during pregnancy reflects the overall physiologic consequences of pregnancy. The average weight gain is approximately 25 to 30 pounds, but this varies widely. Young women, fed equally well, tend to gain slightly more than older women; and women having their first child tend to gain more weight than women having had several children. Thin women gain more than fat women. In any event, adequate weight gain is essential. A number of studies have shown that a strong, positive association exists between the total gain in weight of the mother and the birth weight of the child. Also, there is an important positive association between the prepregnancy weight of the mother and the birth weight of the child.

■ **What minerals should be emphasized during pregnancy?**

The same as those indicated for nonpregnant adult women should be used, with special emphasis on two particular minerals:

1. *Calcium.* The calcium needs during pregnancy are about 50% greater than normal adult requirements. The importance of calcium to the mother and fetus is suggested by the size of the increase that is recommended. Calcium is the essential element for the construction and maintenance of bones and teeth. It is also an important

constituent of the blood-clotting mechanism and is used in normal muscle action and other essential metabolic activities. Balance studies indicate that the calcium used by the maternal organism increases from about 4 gm. at the middle of pregnancy to about 30 gm. at term. Fetal studies indicate an increase in the quantity of calcium stored from about 1 gm. at the middle of gestation to about 23 gm. at term. Thus for the rapid mineralization of skeletal tissue, especially during the second half of pregnancy, more calcium is essential.

Dairy products are a primary source of calcium. Increases in milk or equivalent milk foods, such as cheese, ice cream, and skim milk powder in cooking, are recommended. Additional calcium is obtained in whole or enriched cereal grain and in green and leafy vegetables.

2. *Iron.* The increase in maternal circulating blood volume during pregnancy has been estimated to be from 20% to 40%. Iron is essential to the formation of hemoglobin. An adequate supply of this mineral is therefore important to maintain the mother's hemoglobin level in her expanded blood volume. Iron is also needed for fetal development, especially for storage of reserve in the liver. About a 3 to 4 month's supply of iron is stored in the developing fetal liver to supply the infant's need after birth. This is necessary because his first food, milk, lacks iron. Also, adequate maternal iron stores fortify the mother against blood losses at delivery.

Liver contains far more iron than any other food. Appetizing ways of preparing it should be discovered and increased frequency of use should be supported. Other meat, dried beans, dried fruit, green vegetables, eggs, and enriched cereals are additional sources of iron.

■ **What are the increased needs for vitamins?**

Increased amounts of vitamins A, B complex, C, and D are recommended during pregnancy:

Vitamin A. 1,000 extra I.U. is recommended for the latter half of pregnancy (about a 20% increase over the usual adult intake). Vitamin A is an essential factor in cell development, maintenance of the integrity of epithelial tissue, tooth formation, normal bone growth, and vision. Liver, egg yolk, butter or fortified margarine, dark green and yellow vegetables, and fruits are good food sources.

B vitamins. There is an especially increased need for B vitamins during pregnancy. These are usually supplied by a well-balanced diet. The B vitamins are important as coenzyme factors in a number of metabolic activities, energy production and function of muscle and nerve tissue. Therefore they play key roles in the increased metabolic activities of pregnancy.

Vitamin C. Special emphasis must be laid on the pregnant women's need for ascorbic acid. A daily increase of 5 to 10 mg. is recommended in addition to the adult recommendation of 55 mg., or nearly a 20% increase. Ascorbic acid is exceedingly important to the growing organism. It is essential to the formation of intercellular cement substance in developing connective tissue and vascular systems. It also increases the absorption of iron that is needed for the increasing quantities of hemoglobin. The expectant mother should be encouraged to eat additional quantities of foods that are common sources of vitamin C, such as citrus fruit, berries, melon, and cabbage.

Vitamin D. The increased need for calcium and phosphorus presented by the developing fetal skeletal tissue necessitates additional vitamin D to promote the absorption and utilization of these minerals. The recommended amount for the latter half of pregnancy is 400 I.U. Frequently supplementary vitamin D may be ordered by the physician. Food sources include fortified milk, butter, liver, egg yolk, and fortified margarine.

■ **If nausea and vomiting occur in early pregnancy, what foods will be tolerated best?**

Small, frequent meals, fairly dry, and consisting chiefly of easily digested energy foods, such as carbohydrate, are most readily tolerated. Liquids are best taken between meals instead of with the food.

■ **If constipation becomes a problem, what foods may help alleviate it?**

This complaint is seldom more than minor. The pressure of the enlarging uterus on the lower portion of the intestine may make elimination somewhat difficult. Increased fluid intake and use of naturally laxative foods, such as whole grains with added bran, dried fruits (especially prunes and figs), other fruits, and juices usually induce regularity. Laxatives should be avoided.

■ **What types of anemia may complicate pregnancy?**

Anemia is common during pregnancy. About 10% of the patients in large prenatal clinics in the United States have hemoglobin concentrations of less than 10 gm./ 100 ml., and a hematocrit reading of below 32. Anemia is far more prevalent among the poor, many of whom live on diets barely adequate for subsistence; but anemia is by no means restricted to the lower economic groups. Several common types are encountered in pregnancy and require nutritional attention:

1. *Iron deficiency anemia.* This is by far the most common cause of anemia in pregnancy. The cost of a single normal pregnancy in iron stores is large—about 700 to 800 mg. Of this amount nearly 300 mg. is used by the fetus. The remainder is utilized in the expansion of maternal red cell volume and hemoglobin mass. This total iron requirement exceeds the available reserves in the average woman. In addition to including iron-rich foods in the diet, supplementation is recommended.

2. *Hemorrhagic anemia.* Anemia caused by blood loss is more likely to occur during puerperium than during gestation. Blood loss may occur earlier, however, as the result of abortion or ruptured tubal pregnancy. Most patients undergoing these physiologic disasters receive blood by transfusion, but iron therapy may be indicated in addition to support the formation of hemoglobin needed for adequate replacement.

3. *Megaloblastic anemia.* The word "megaloblastic" comes from the Greek meaning "large embryo." Megaloblastic anemia is characterized by malformed cells, large nucleated red cells containing basophilic material in its cytoplasm, and little or no hemoglobin. This malformation in red cells is the result of folic acid deficiency. Manifestations include intensification of nausea, vomiting, and anorexia. As the anemia progresses, anorexia is more marked, thus further compounding the nutritional deficiency. The folic acid requirement is greatly increased by pregnancy. Both the trophoblast and the fetus are sensitive to folic acid inhibitors and therefore probably have high metabolic requirements for folic acid and its derivatives. The placenta and the fetus appear to concentrate folic acid efficiently, since the fetus may have an adequate store while the mother is severely deficient in this compound.

Additional nutrients that are essential to the formation of red blood cells are ascorbic acid, vitamin B_{12}, copper, and zinc. Protein, of course, is the essential base for formation and must be in plentiful supply in the form of the eight essential amino acids. The heme portion of the hemoglobin molecule is synthesized from glycine and succinyl-CoA.

■ **What causes toxemia of pregnancy?**

Toxemia is the general term given to an acute hypertensive disorder appearing after about the twentieth week of pregnancy and accompanied by increased edema, proteinuria, and in severe cases, convulsions and coma. It is usually seen in the third trimester toward term. The term "pre-eclampsia" is given to the initial stages of the acute disorder and the term "eclampsia" is defined as being closely related to pre-eclampsia and in most cases is its end result in the convulsive stage.

Toxemia occurs in 6% to 7% of all pregnancies. It accounts for the majority of all maternal deaths (about 1,000 deaths annually in the United States) and for the majority of all deaths of newborn infants (some 30,000 stillbirths and neonatal deaths per year). It is clear in the distribution of cases that toxemia is closely associated with malnutrition and poverty. The states with the lowest per capita income have the highest mortality rates. Most of the mortality from toxemia could be prevented by good prenatal care, which inherently includes attention to sound nutrition.

There is much controversy concerning the cause and treatment of toxemia. However, increasing clinical and laboratory evidence indicates that toxemia is a disease of malnutrition and that the malnutrition affects the liver and its metabolic activities. The characteristic symptoms encountered in toxemia, hypoproteinemia with resulting hypovolemia, closely resemble those symptoms encountered in liver disorders in protein deficiency diseases, such as kwashiorkor. Cases of toxemia have responded to protein therapy, indicating a need for this nutrient. Four nutrient factors seem to be implicated:

1. *Calories.* The concept of calorie restriction to avoid large, total weight gains and to protect against toxemia has been largely refuted by overwhelming evidence. Since its inception in the early 1920s and 1930s, the practice of calorie restriction has found its way into textbooks of obstetrics and has been widely followed by the medical profession, despite the fact that the practice has been subjected to little scientific scrutiny. Reports increasingly indicate that weight gain per se is not a causative factor in toxemia. To the contrary, there is evidence that sufficient weight gain is imperative to support fetal development and to avoid low birth weight babies. In one large group of women studied, who gained in excess of 30 pounds during pregnancy, 91% had no problems at all. Some confusion has resulted from failure to distinguish between weight gained as the result of edema and overall total weight gain caused by accumulation of fat, preparing the body for sustaining the pregnancy and for lactation to follow. Thus, it is clear that

rather than restriction of calories, the diet for pregnant women needs to have an ample amount of calories to meet the energy demands imposed on her and to conserve protein for tissue building functions and the maintenance of optimum levels of plasma proteins.

2. *Salt.* Another practice in the past treatment of toxemia has been that of salt restriction. Because of increased edema during pregnancy, the imposition of salt restriction was made on the rationale that the edema was caused by sodium retention. The increased fluid accumulation in the tissue, however, seems more directly related to the decreased plasma proteins and hence the contraction of the vascular volume resulting from the movement of water from the plasma compartment into the tissue spaces (an imbalance in the capillary fluid shift mechanism, see p. 106). Diuretics have also been commonly prescribed to accomplish the same goal, often in conjunction with salt restriction. However, diuretics only add insult to injury by further reducing an already shrunken plasma volume. Recent studies on pregnant rats have demonstrated the harmful effects of salt depletion. As a result of increased information and awareness, routine salt restriction, as well as the use of diuretics in prenatal care, must be avoided. Rather than restriction of salt, there is the recognition that salt is needed in pregnancy and a normal amount should be used.

3. *Protein.* Protein has a direct relationship to the constant circulation of fluids from the vascular compartment within the blood vessels into the tissue spaces and back to the blood vessels. With the decrease of plasma proteins observed in toxemia and the resulting contraction of the vascular blood volume (hypovolemia), it is clear that protein is an essential nutrient in pregnancy to maintain the integrity of the blood volume in its increased state during pregnancy, as well as the many areas of tissue synthesis required to support and maintain a successful pregnancy. In any event it seems clear that inadequate protein contributes to the complex of malnutrition factors that surround the incidence of toxemia. The diet of the pregnant woman should, therefore, contain optimum quantities of protein of high biologic value to provide resources against toxemia.

4. *Vitamins and minerals.* Part of an adequate diet includes optimum quantities of vitamins and minerals. These are the regulatory agents in the body whose presence is necessary to control tissue synthesis, red blood cell formation, and use of food for energy procurement processes. The pregnant women needs increased amounts of these vital agents. She has a special need for those that contribute to building of skeletal mass in the fetus (calcium, prosphorus, vitamin D), for those that have direct influence on tissue synthesis and energy production (largely B vitamins and ascorbic acid), and especially for those intimately related with the formation of red blood cells. Two particular materials that are related to this function and that pregnancy requires are iron and folic acid. Routine use of an adequate diet plus supplementation of these materials is indicated to ensure adequate red blood cell formation.

NUTRITION FOR GROWTH AND DEVELOPMENT

■ **What is the normal physical growth pattern?**

The normal human life cycle follows four general phases of overall growth:

1. *Infancy.* During the first year of life the infant grows rapidly, with the rate tapering off somewhat in the latter half of the first year. At age 6 months he will probably have doubled his birth weight and at 1 year he may have tripled it. Thus, a baby weighing 7 pounds at birth will weigh approximately 14 pounds at 6 months and about 21 pounds at 1 year of age. This rapid growth rate during the first year of life closely parallels the rapid growth that occurred during the fetal development preceding.

2. *Latent period of childhood.* During

the years between infancy and adolescence, however, the rate of growth slows and becomes erratic. At some periods there are plateaus, at others small spurts of growth. The overall rate, being erratic, affects appetite accordingly. At times a child will have little or no appetite, and at others he will eat voraciously.

3. *Adolescence.* With the onset of puberty the second rapid growth spurt occurs in association with manifold physical changes. Because of hormonal influences, multiple body changes occur including development of long bones, sex characteristics, and fat and muscle mass development.

4. *Adult.* In the final phase of a normal life cycle, growth levels off on the adult plateau and gradually declines during senescence.

■ **What are some ways to measure adequate growth?**

The important consideration in the growth of children, and the wisest counsel that can be given to parents, is that children are individuals; thus physical growth occurs with wide variance. Parents should avoid comparing one child with another and assuming that inadequate growth is taking place when the growth rate does not parallel that of another child. General parameters of growth in children, however, include the following:

1. *Weight and height.* These common general measures of physical growth form a crude index without giving finer details of individual variations. Generally, as the child grows his weight and height are compared to "average" grids of weight and height for his age.

2. *Body measurements.* Body measurements may be helpful indications of growth. These include the recumbent length of the infant as compared to standing height as he grows older, head circumference, measures of chest, abdomen, and leg at the calf, pelvic breadth, skin fold thicknesses, and similar measures.

3. *Clinical signs.* General observation of vitality, a sense of well-being, posture, condition of gums and teeth, skin, hair, eyes, muscle development, and nervous control all contribute measures of state of health and well-being and optimum growth (see Table 12-1, p. 161).

4. *Laboratory data.* Finer measures are obtained by various laboratory tests. These may include studies of blood and urine to determine levels of vitamins and hemoglobin. X-rays of the bones in the hand and wrists may also be taken to indicate degree of ossification, or mineralization of bone.

5. *Nutritional analysis.* A measure of the growth of a child may be based on a nutritional analysis of his general eating habits. This will give some measure of the adequacy of the child's diet to meet his growth needs (see p. 162).

■ **How do the basic nutrients relate to the growth process?**

A review of the nutritional requirements for growth and development reveals their vital relationship to the overall growth process:

1. *Calories.* During childhood the demand for calories is relatively large. For example, 55% of the 5-year-old's calories are involved in the metabolic activities of basal metabolism and food digestion. Physical activity requires 25% of his calories, growth needs 12%, and 8% is represented in fecal loss. Of these calories, carbohydrate is the main energy source. It is also important as a protein-sparer to ensure that protein vital for growth will not be diverted for energy needs. Fat calories are important to ensure certain fatty acids that are essential, especially linoleic acid, although an excess of fat should be avoided.

2. *Protein.* Protein is the *growth element* of the body. The eight essential amino acids that are necessary for formation and maintenance of muscle and nerve tissue and of bone matrix are supplied from protein sources. Protein also serves as an integral part of other body fluids and secretions, such as enzymes, hormones, lymph, and plasma. It is essential to remember that these key amino acids have to be supplied in proper amounts and proportion and timing for tissue protein to be synthesized.

Hence, the necessity for a diet containing a variety of protein food sources is imperative. By and large, the healthy, active, growing child will consume his needed amount of calories and proteins in the variety of food provided him.

3. *Water.* Water is essential to life second only to oxygen. The infant's need for water is even greater than that of the adult, for two reasons: (1) a greater percentage of his total body weight is made up of water, and (2) a larger proportion of his total body water is outside the cell and hence is more easily lost. Generally an infant consumes daily an amount of water equivalent to 10% to 15% of his body weight, as compared with the adult daily consumption of water equivalent to only 2% to 4% of his body weight.

4. *Minerals.* A number of minerals relate to special body function and are essential in growth and development. Two particular minerals involved in growth are calcium and iron. Calcium is the necessary material for bone mineralization, which takes place rapidly during growth. Calcium is also needed for the developing teeth, for muscle contraction, nerve irritability, blood coagulation, and the action of the heart muscle. Iron is necessary for the formation of hemoglobin. Additional food must be added to the milk diet of the infant before fetal stores of iron are depleted to avoid anemia. Several other key vitamins are associated with iron in the formation of hemoglobin and hence are partners in this important function. For example, zinc and copper are two additional minerals associated with iron in growth processes.

5. *Vitamins.* A large number of vitamins are essential for growth and maintenance. Vitamin A is a necessary constituent in the eye for maintenance of the vision cycle. It is also essential for bone and tooth development and in the formation and maturation of epithelial tissue throughout the body. The B-complex vitamins have many functions associated with growth. Thiamine is directly related to energy production and many anabolic activities demanding en-

ergy. Niacin is important in protein metabolism and tissue synthesis. Riboflavin acts as a coenzyme and is particularly involved with increasing size and change in muscle mass and body weight. Several B vitamins are associated with the proper formation of red blood cells and are therefore important during growth. These include cobalamin (B_{12}), pyridoxine (B_6), and folic acid. Vitamin C plays a number of important roles in the growth period, particularly in association with tissue synthesis in the deposition of intercellular cement substance in all tissues. Vitamin D is essential during growth for the absorption and utilization of calcium and phosphorus in bone development. Vitamin K is essential for the formation of prothrombin by the liver, an initial element in the blood-clotting mechanism. Vitamin E has associations with growth in tissue synthesis, muscle metabolism, and red blood cell integrity. Apparently this function is related to the antioxidant role of vitamin E in maintaining the integrity of the cell wall by protecting cell lipids from oxidative breakdown.

AGE GROUP NEEDS
Infant nutrition

■ **How is the premature infant fed?**

The premature infant has an immature digestive apparatus. Fat is poorly tolerated. Therefore the usual milk of choice is skimmed or partially skimmed diluted cow's milk with added carbohydrate as needed. Usually breast milk alone is seldom adequate because it lacks sufficient protein for the rapid growth of the premature infant. However, the mother who desires to breast feed may express her breast milk manually or with a common hand breast pump until the infant is strong enough to nurse at the breast. The breast milk may then supplement the skimmed milk formula at first. Feedings are usually delayed 24 to 36 hours following birth. The comparative inactivity and low heat production of the infant causes relatively large body water content and reduces immediate need for calories. Also his weakness and the danger of aspiration make some feeding delay advisable.

At first the premature infant is usually given sterile 5% to 10% solutions of glucose in water, with small milk feedings added slowly. Usually by the time the infant is a week old he should be receiving about 50 to 60 calories per pound (approximately 2½ ounces of formula per pound per day). There is increased need for supplements of vitamins C and D. Approximately 35 to 50 mg. of ascorbic acid and 500 to 1,000 I.U. of vitamin D are usually given during the second and third weeks, depending on the individual need. Ascorbic acid is needed for the intermediate metabolism of phenylalanine, an amino acid essential to growth. Vitamin D is needed for the rapid mineralization of bones.

Methods of feeding will vary with the infant's strength. The feedings may be given by medicine dropper, by bottle with a soft nipple having larger than usual holes, or by gavage. Care must be taken in all methods to avoid aspiration. This is especially true with the gavage method. The tube used in gavage feeding is a small, soft, plastic one with a rounded tip to avoid tissue trauma and two holes on either side of the tip. The tube is passed through the nose until one inch of the lower end is in the stomach. Proper depth placement in the stomach is guided by markings on the tube made according to the measurement of the individual infant. Correct anatomic placement is tested by placing the free end in water. If bubbles appear in the water, the tube is in the trachea. It should be withdrawn immediately and reinserted. Careful control of the amount of feeding and rate of flow is necessary.

■ **How do food and feeding practices relate to the physical and psychosocial development of the infant?**

Food and feeding practices do not develop in a vacuum. They are intimately related with the early development of the infant, both physically and psychosocially. His physical development demands energy and food supplies it. His first food, however, lacks iron, so that additions in solid foods are needed by the time fetal stores have diminished by the third to the sixth month.

Highly significant is the relationship of food and feeding practices to psychosocial development. The core problem in infancy is the development of *trust vs. distrust.* Feeding is his main means of establishing human relationships. The close mother-infant relationship in the feeding process fills his basic need to build trust. The need for sucking and the development of oral organs (lips and mouth) as sensory organs represent adaptations to ensure an adequate early food intake. As a result, food becomes the infant's general means of exploring his environment. As muscular coordination involving the tongue and the swallowing reflex develop, he will accept solid foods beginning at about the second month. As he grows and his physical and motor maturation develop, he will be able to participate in the feeding process. When these stages of development occur he should be encouraged to explore his new powers. His growing development of trust is evidenced by an increasing capacity to wait for his feedings while they are being prepared.

■ **How is milk produced in the breast?**

The female breast, or mammary glands, are highly specialized secretory organs. The secreting glandular tissue is composed of 15 to 20 lobes, each containing many smaller units called *lobules.* It is in these lobules that the secretory cells, called alveoli or acini, which form milk, or located. They are serviced by a rich capillary system in the connective tissue to supply them with nutrients necessary for milk production. During pregnancy the breast is prepared for this lactation process by enlarging. The alveoli enlarge and multiply, and during the end of the prenatal period they begin to secrete a thin, yellowish fluid called *colostrum.* After delivery the initial breast secretion is colostrum for 2 to 4 days (10 to 40 ml. a day) until the actual milk production begins about the third

day. This colostrum provides initial nutrition for the infant. It contains more protein and minerals than breast milk but less carbohydrate and fat. It is also thought to impart healthful antibodies to the newborn.

Milk is produced under the stimulation of a hormone, *prolactin,* produced by the anterior pituitary gland. After the milk is formed in the mammary lobules by the clusters of secretory cells (the alveoli or acini), it is carried through converging branches of the lactiferous ducts to reservoir spaces under the areola, the pigmented area of the skin surrounding the nipple. These reservoir spaces under the areola are called ampullae. From 15 to 20 excretory lactiferous ducts carry the milk from the ampullae out to the surface of the nipple. Two other pituitary hormones, principally *oxytocin* and to a lesser extent *vasopressin* (ADH), stimulate the ejections of the milk from the alveoli to the ducts, releasing it so the baby can obtain it. This is commonly called the "let down" reflex. It causes a tingling sensation in the breast and the flow of milk. The initial sucking of the baby stimulates this reflex.

■ **How many additional calories are required by the mother for milk production during lactation?**

About 3,000 calories are required in the mother's daily diet to maintain lactation. This represents an additional requirement of 1,000 calories for the overall total lactation process (about 120 calories/100 ml.). This additional caloric requirement represents two factors:

1. *Milk content.* An average daily milk production for lactating women is 850 ml., or 30 ounces. Human milk has a caloric value of about 20 calories per ounce. Thus these 30 ounces of milk have a value of 600 calories.

2. *Milk production.* The metabolic work involved in producing this amount of milk utilizes from 400 to 420 calories. In view of these two amounts, 600 for milk content plus 400 for milk production, 1,000 extra calories will ac-

Table 14-2. Basic twenty-four-hour formula

Age	Ounces of whole milk per pound body weight per day	Sugar*	Water
First 2 weeks	1½ (¾ oz. evap.)	½ oz. (1 tbsp.)†	Add amount necessary
2 weeks to 2 months	1½ to 2 (1 oz. evap.)	¾ to 1 oz. (2 tbsp.)†	to bring total solution
After 2 months	2 (1 oz. evap.)	1 oz. (2 tbsp.)†	to amount required

*May be granulated, corn syrup, or malt-dextrin preparation.
†2 tablespoons granulated sugar or corn syrup = 1 oz.; 4 tablespoons Dextrimaltose = 1 oz.

commodate sufficient milk production to feed the infant.

■ **What additional nutrients are needed to ensure adequate milk production?**

In addition to sufficient calories for milk production, several other considerations are important in the diet of the lactating mother.

1. *Protein.* An increase of 10 gm. of the quantity needed during pregnancy is recommended during lactation, making a total daily protein allowance of about 75 gm. Protein foods of high biologic value should supply this needed protein.

2. *Minerals.* The quantities of calcium and iron required for lactation are the same as those needed during pregnancy. The increased amount required during pregnancy for mineralization of skeletal tissue is now diverted into the mother's milk.

3. *Vitamins.* The increased quantity of vitamin C recommended during pregnancy is the same recommendation for lactation. However, there are increased needs during lactation for vitamin A (2,000 I.U. more) because vitamin A is an important component of milk. There is also increased need for the B-complex vitamins, riboflavin and niacin (about a one third increase over the quantities taken during pregnancy). These vitamins function as coenzyme factors in cell respiration, glucose oxidation, and energy metabolism. Therefore the increased quantities are needed as caloric needs increase.

4. *Fluids.* A practice sometimes neglected because fluids may not be considered a nutrient but which is highly significant to adequate milk production is the increased intake of fluids. Obviously the secretion of milk requires sufficient water intake because its composition is largely water. In addition to water beverages, such as juices, tea, coffee, and milk, all add to the fluid necessary to produce milk.

5. *Rest and relaxation.* In addition to the augmented diet, the mother who breastfeeds her baby requires rest, moderate exercise, and relaxation. Family tensions and anxieties diminish milk secretion. A daily food plan to guide the mother in the selection of a good food source to support lactation is given in Table 14-1, p. 180.

■ **What are the ingredients in an infant formula for bottle feeding?**

The objective in mixing a formula for feeding an infant is to modify cow's milk to make it as nearly like breast milk as possible. A comparison of the ratio of nutrients in the two milks will indicate that the protein content of cow's milk is greater than that of breast milk and hence water dilution is required. The carbohydrate content, however, of breast milk is greater than that of cow's milk, indicating a need for addition of a carbohydrate source in the formula. Thus, the main ingredients are cow's milk, water dilution, and an additional source of carbohydrate, such as corn syrup or Dextrimaltose. A basic 24-hour formula is given in Table 14-2.

A simple evaporated milk formula is usually the most economical. Many special

Table 14-3. Suggested schedule on an approximate four-hour basis

Age	Oz. per feeding	Number of feedings	Time of feedings
First week	2 to 3	6	6, 10, 2, 6, 10, 2
Two to four weeks	3 to 5	6	6, 10, 2, 6, 10, 2
Second to third months	4 to 6	5	6, 10, 2, 6, 10
Fourth and fifth months	5 to 7	5	6, 10, 2, 6, 10
Sixth and seventh months	7 to 8	4	6, 10, 2, 6
Eighth to twelfth months	8*	3	7, 12, 6

*4 oz. milk may be given midafternoon.

Table 14-4. Guideline for addition of solid foods to infant's diet during the first year

When to start	Foods added	Feeding
First month	Vitamins A, D and C in multi-vitamin preparation (according to prescription)	Once daily at a feeding time.
Second to third month	Cereal and strained cooked fruit; Egg yolk (at first, hard boiled and seived, soft boiled or poached later)	10:00 A.M. and 6:00 P.M.
Third to fourth month	Strained cooked vegetable and strained meat	2:00 p.m.
Fifth to seventh month	Zwieback or hard toast	At any feeding
Seventh to ninth month	Meat: beef, lamb, or liver, (broiled or baked and finely chopped) Potato: baked or boiled and mashed or sieved.	10:00 or 6:00 P.M.

Suggested meal plan for age eight months to one year or older

7:00 A.M.	Milk	8 oz.
	Cereal	2 to 3 tbsp.
	Strained fruit	2 to 3 tbsp.
	Zwieback or dry toast	
12:00 NOON	Milk	8 oz.
	Vegetables	2 to 3 tbsp.
	Chopped meat or one whole egg	
	Puddings or cooked fruit	2 to 3 tbsp.
3:00 P.M.	Milk	4 oz.
	Toast, zwieback or crackers	
6:00 P.M.	Milk	8 oz.
	Whole egg or chopped meat	
	Potato, baked or mashed	2 tbsp.
	Pudding or cooked fruit	2 to 3 tbsp.
	Zwieback or toast	

Semisolid foods should be given immediately after breast or bottle feeding. One to two teaspoons should be given at first. If food is accepted and tolerated well, the amount should be increased to one to two tablespoons per feeding.

Note: Banana or cottage cheese may be used as substitution for any meal.

formulas are on the market, but they are more expensive and are usually unnecessary. As the child grows older he will take an increasing amount of formula at each feeding to meet his growth demands. The number of feedings a day will gradually lessen, so that by the time he is a year old he will have reached the general meal pattern of three meals a day. A suggested schedule for feedings is given in Table 14-3.

■ **What is the best schedule for adding solid foods to the infant's diet?**

There is no one set pattern for adding solid foods to the basic milk of an infant's diet during the first year. Individual needs and desires will vary. However, when the infant has developed sufficient muscular coordination involving the tongue and his swallowing reflex has developed, he is ready to eat solid foods beginning at about the second month. These foods may be added in any general order. Usually the first foods given are those that will supply additional iron, plus having a texture sufficiently smooth to be acceptable. Small amounts of cereal and strained cooked fruit are usually given first, followed by gradual additions of egg yolk (followed later by whole egg), strained cooked vegetables and strained meat, toast, chopped meat, potato. By the end of the first year the infant usually is consuming a basic meal pattern of three meals and an interval snack. A general guideline for addition of solid foods to the infant's diet during the first year is given in Table 14-4.

Individual practices will vary widely around this sequence of feeding. By the time a child is approximately 8 or 9 months old he should have obtained a fairly good ability to eat so-called family foods, chopped cooked foods, simply seasoned, without use of a large number of special infant foods.

Nutrition during childhood

■ **What significant physical and psychosocial development occurs during the "toddler years"—ages 1 to 3? How does this relate to food and feeding?**

Two important aspects of growth during the toddler years are important to remember if conflict between the mother and the child is to be avoided in the feeding activities:

1. *Slowed physical growth rate.* After the rapid growth of the first year, the mother may be concerned when she observes the toddler eating less food and at times having little appetite. Beginning with the second year and through the latent years of childhood the rate of gain is less but the pattern of growth changes. Important muscle development takes place as the child begins to walk and to strengthen, for example, the big muscles of the back, the buttocks, and the thighs for erect posture and walking. Bones begin to lengthen, although the overall rate of the skeletal growth slows, and there is more deposit of mineral for strengthening the bones to support the increasing weight. Hence the child, during this period, needs fewer calories (less total quantity of food) but more protein and mineral matter for growth. Hence a variety of food should be offered in *smaller amounts* to provide key nutrients and yet not overwhelm the child.

2. *The struggle for autonomy.* The key psychosocial problem with which the toddler struggles during this period is the conflict between *autonomy vs. shame.* He has an increasing sense of self, of "I," of being a person, distinct and individual, apart from his mother and not just an extension of her. As he begins to walk he has an increasing sense of his independence, a growing curiosity. This curiosity leads him into many areas of conflict and often his constant use of "no" is not perverse negativism as much as it is his struggle with his ego needs in conflict with his mother's efforts to control him. His attention span is fairly short because of his increasing diversion of interest in other things around him. His struggle for autonomy often takes the form of wanting to do things for himself before he is able to do them completely. Therefore, the mother should offer a variety of foods, again in small amounts, and support and encourage some degree of food

choice and self feeding in the child's own ceremonial manner. In this way eating can be a pleasant, positive means of development rather than the basis for conflict. It can help satisfy his growing need for independence and his desire for ritual. The mother needs to maintain a calm, relaxed attitude of sympathetic interest, to understand his struggle, and to give help where needed, but to avoid both overprotection and excessive rigidity.

■ **How much milk should a toddler have?**

Two to three cups of milk are sufficient for the child's needs. Sometimes excess milk intake is a habit carried over from infancy, and it may exclude some solid foods from the diet. As a result the child may be lacking iron and develop a "milk anemia." If the child dislikes milk, milk solids may be used in soups, custards, or puddings, and dry milk can be used in cereals, mashed potatoes, meat loaf, etc. In the variety of foods offered the child there should be an avoidance of emphasis on refined sweets. These may be reserved for special occasions, not used for constant habitual use or bribe mechanisms to get a child to eat.

■ **How does the growth and development pattern of the preschool child—ages 3 to 6—influence his food behavior?**

The preschool child continues to grow in spurts. On occasion he is bounding with energy and his play is hard—running, jumping, testing new physical resources. At other times, as his mental development is growing, he may sit for increasing periods of time engrossed in passive types of activities. He is doing more thinking and is exploring his environment. His core psychosocial problem of development during this period is his struggle between *initiative vs. guilt.* He is beginning to develop a superego—the conscience. As his powers of locomotion increase he has an increasing imagination and curiosity, and this very capacity often leads him into troubled feelings about his changing attitudes, especially toward his parents. This is a period of increasing imitation and of sex identification. In the play there is much grownup role playing in domestic situations. Eating assumes, there-

fore, greater social aspects. The family mealtime is an important means of this socialization and sex identification. The children imitate their parents and others at the table.

Because of his developing social and emotional needs, the preschool child frequently follows food jags that may last for several days. However, this is usually short lived and of no major concern. Again, variety is a keynote in offering food. He usually prefers single foods to combination dishes such as casseroles or stews. With mental development and the learning of language, the child prefers a single food that he can identify and name, because it has retained its characteristic texture, color, and form. He likes foods he can eat with his fingers. Often raw fruit and raw vegetables cut in finger-sized pieces and offered to a child for his own selection helps to meet his needs.

The child should set his own goals in quantity of food. His portions need to be relatively small. Often if he can pour his own milk from a small pitcher into a little glass he consumes a greater amount. The quantity of milk consumed usually declines during the preschool years. The child will consume two to three, rarely four, cups of milk during the day. Smaller children like their milk more lukewarm, not icy cold. Also they prefer it in small glasses that hold about ½ to ¾ of a cup, rather than a large adult size glass. Also, as the child begins to eat increasingly away from home, group eating becomes significant as a means of socialization. He may be involved in nursery or play school situations in which he eats with other children, and here he learns a widening variety of food habits and forms new social relationships.

■ **What physical and psychosocial growth characteristics of the school-age child— ages 6 to 12—are reflected in his eating habits?**

The school-age period has been called the "latent period of growth," because the growth rate slows and body changes occur very gradually. Resources, however, are being laid down for the growth needs to come in the adolescent period. By now the body type is established and growth rates vary widely. Girls usually outdistance boys by the latter part of the period.

The core problem with which the child struggles during these years is the tension between *industry vs. inferiority.* With school there is increasing mental development, ability to work out problems, and competitive activities. He begins moving from a dependence on parental standards to the standards of his peers, in preparation for his own coming maturity. Pressures are generated for self-control of his growing body. There is a temporary disorganization of previous learning and developed personality, a sort of loosening up of the personality pattern for the inevitable changes ahead in adolescence.

The slowed rate of growth during this latent period results in a gradual decline in the food requirement per unit of body weight. This decline continues up into the latter part of the period, just prior to the adolescent period. Likes and dislikes are a product of earlier years. As horizons widen and interests are in many things, there is competition for mealtime and often family conflict ensues. Meals may be hurried or skipped, and the maturing child is left increasingly to himself and prepares food for himself. In some situations meals are makeshift or nonexistent. The school lunch program provides a nourishing noon meal for many children who would not otherwise have one. Midafternoon snacking is common, but it is often sweets of empty calories.

■ **What problems faced by the adolescent —ages 12 to 18—affect his food behavior?**

Two important growth developments occurring during the adolescent period are important to consider:

1. *Rapid growth and body changes.* The rapid growth of the adolescent period requires energy and growth elements. Physical growth differences emerge between the sexes. In the girl there is an increasing amount of subcutaneous fat deposit, par-

ticularly in the abdominal area. The hip breadth increases and the bony pelvis widens in preparation for reproduction. This is often a source of anxiety to many figure-conscious young girls. In the boy physical growth is manifest more in increasing muscle mass and in long-bone growth. His growth spurt is slower than that of the girl but he soon passes her in weight and height and at age 18 weighs about 140 pounds. The development of the sex characteristics that come with puberty also brings many body changes as the result of hormonal influences. The rate at which these changes occur varies widely, and is particularly distinct in growth patterns that emerge between the sexes.

2. *Identity crisis.* The core psychosocial problem with which the adolescent struggles is that of *identity vs. role diffusion.* The profound changes in body image associated with sexual development cause resulting tensions in maturing boys and girls. During this period the identity crisis, largely revolving around sexual development and preparation for an adult role in a complex society, produces many psychologic, emotional, and social tensions. The period of rapid physical growth is relatively short— only 2 or 3 years—but the attendant psychosocial development continues over a longer period. The pressure for peer group acceptance is strong, and fads in dress and food habits are common.

To support the rapid physical growth of this period, caloric needs increase to meet the metabolic demands. Although individual needs vary and girls consume fewer calories than boys, there is an increased appetite characteristic of this period that leads the adolescent to satisfy his hunger with carbohydrate foods and to slight essential protein foods. Protein needs for adolescent growth are large, especially for the developing muscle mass in boys. Minerals particularly needed are calcium and iron. Long-bone growth demands calcium. Menstrual iron losses in the adolescent girl predispose her to simple iron deficiency anemia. Iodine may be another concern in areas where iodized salt use does not ensure sufficient iodine for the increased thyroid activity associated with growth. Vitamins are necessary regulators of these increased metabolic activities. The B vitamins are needed in increased amounts, especially by boys, to meet the extra demands of energy metabolism and muscle tissue development. Intakes of needed vitamin C and vitamin A may be low because of erratic food intake. Peer-group pressure often leads adolescents to greater snacking habits and dependence on only a few foods rather than on a variety of foods.

Most U. S. surveys show the adolescent girl to be the most vulnerable person nutritionally. Two factors combine to help produce this result: (1) because of her physiologic sex differences associated with fat deposits during this period and her comparative lack of physical activity, she gains excess weight easily; and (2) social pressures and personal tensions concerning figure control will sometimes cause her to follow unwise, self-imposed crash diets for weight loss. As a result she may be malnourished at the very time in her life when her body is laying down reserves for coming reproduction. The hazards of such eating habits to her future course during potential pregnancies is clearly indicated.

Nutrition during adulthood

■ What are the stages of psychosocial development during the adult years?

Following the tumultous adolescent years from 13 to 18 the individual emerges into adulthood:

1. *Young adulthood (ages 18 to 40).* In the years of young adulthood the individual, now launched on his own, must resolve the core problem of *intimacy vs. isolation.* If he achieves this goal he is able to build an intimate relationship leading to marriage or self-fulfillment in other personal relationships. But if he fails to do so he becomes increasingly isolated from others. These are the years of career beginnings, of establishing one's own home, of parenthood, of starting young children on their way through the same life stages and early struggles to make their way in the world.

2. *Adulthood—the middle years (ages 40 to 60).* In the middle years of adulthood the core problem that the individual faces is *generativity vs. self-absorption.* The children have now grown and gone to make their own lives in turn. These are the years of the "empty nest," the coming-to-terms with what life has offered, and of finding expression for stored learning in passing on life's teachings. It is a regeneration of one life in the lives of young persons following the same way. To the degree that these inner struggles are not won, there is increasing self-absorption, a turning in upon one's self, and a withering rather than a regenerating.

3. *Senescence—old age (ages 60 to 80+).* In the last stages of life the final core problem is resolved between *integrity vs. despair.* Depending on one's resources at this point, there is either a predominant sense of wholeness and completeness or a sense of distaste, of bitterness, of revulsion, and of wondering what life was all about. If the outcome of life's basic experiences and problems has been positive, the individual arrives at old age a rich person, rich in wisdom of the years. Building on each previous level, his psychosocial growth has reached its positive human resolution.

■ What is the biologic nature of the aging process?

The general biologic process of aging extends over the entire life span and is conditioned by experiences that have gone before. In the latter ages, however, there is a cell loss and reduced cell metabolism. During ages 30 to 90 there is a gradual reduction in the performance capacity of most organ systems. For example, the speed of conducting a nerve impulse diminishes about 15%, the rate of blood flow through the kidneys is reduced 65%, and the resting cardiac output is reduced by 30%. The pulmonary function (the maximum voluntary ventilatory capacity) is reduced 60% and there is a reduced recovery rate following a displacing stimulus. For example, in a glu-cose-tolerance test the blood sugar level takes longer to return to normal and the pulse rate and respiration after exercise take longer to return to normal. There seems to be a gradual overall reduction in the body's reserve capacities, an important cause of which is the gradual reduction of cellular units. For example, nephron units are lost from the kidney as functioning units, or there is a loss of pulmonary func-tional tissue. Some resulting physiologic factors may affect food patterns. For ex-ample, there may be a diminished secre-tion of digestive juices, a decreased motility of the gastrointestinal tract, and a de-creased absorption and utilization of nu-trients.

The gradual diminishing of cells may be in part caused by the gradual breakdown observed in the cell wall as part of the aging process, as a result of the deteriora-tion of the lipids that comprise a large part of its structure. It is in this context that vi-tamin E has been discussed in relation to the aging process. Its antioxidant capaci-ties protect the lipids that construct the cell wall and help, therefore, to maintain its integrity. It should be remembered, how-ever, that aging is a highly individual pro-cess and that persons in the advancing years of life display a wide variation of in-dividual reaction.

■ **What is the role of nutrition in the aging process?**

Nutritional requirements for aging are as follows:

1. Calories. The reduced basal energy requirement caused by losses of function-ing protoplasm and the reduced physical activity combine to create less demand for calories in advancing age. Despite the lowered need for calories, however, there is a continuing need for daily protein intake at the same adult allowance given for age 25—approximately 1 gm./kg. of body weight. This amount provides an allowance for a wide variation in individual needs. The needs for protein are influenced, how-ever, by the biologic value of the protein

(the quantity and ratio of its amino acids) and by an adequate caloric value in the general diet so that protein is not diverted to met energy needs. Approximately one fourth to one half of the protein intake may come from animal sources, with the remain-der coming from plant protein sources. It is estimated that protein should supply from 15% to 20% of the day's total calories. There is usually no need for supplemental amino acid preparations, as some food fad-dists might claim. They are expensive, un-palatable, irritating, impractical, and inef-ficient sources of available nitrogen.

2. Carbohydrates and fats. At least 70% to 75% of the total calories may be provided in the form of carbohydrate or fat to supply energy needs. Otherwise part of the protein will be diverted for this purpose, rather than being used for tissue maintenance. Carbohydrate and fat perform important functions. The optimum amount of carbo-hydrate intake is unknown, but it is usu-ally about 50% of the calories. The fasting blood-sugar level has been found to be es-sentially normal in the aged, so there should be a fairly free choice of carbohy-drate foods according to individual diges-tion or metabolism situations. Fats usually contribute about 20% of the total calories and provide a source of energy and im-portant fat-soluble vitamins and essential fatty acids. The main objective is the avoid-ance of large quantities of fat, with more emphasis on the quality of the fat con-sumed.

3. Vitamins and minerals. The sale of so-called geriatric vitamin preparations, es-pecially of the B complex, implies that the requirement for them increases with age. There may be gradually decreasing tissue stores with normal aging, but there is no difference in requirement from that for nor-mal adults. Individual cases may require increased supply, but a well-selected mixed diet should supply all the essential vitamins in normally needed quantities. Increased therapeutic needs in illness should be eval-uated on an individual basis. There is no need for increased minerals in normal aging. The same adult allowances are sufficient on a continuing basis and are supplied by a well-balanced diet. Two essential minerals that may be lacking, however, in poor diets are iron and calcium. Encouragement may need to be given to some individuals to ensure adequate dietary sources among their many food choices.

■ **What clinical problems may aging persons encounter?**

Various clinical problems may develop during the aging process, which require supportive nutritional therapy:

1. *Chronic disease.* Chronic illness, such as heart disease, often creates additional problems for aging persons. Food needs may be modified by the presence of disease. This may include fat modification or sodium restriction and create problems in procuring and preparing food.

2. *Malnutrition.* Habits set in younger years are accentuated in age. Surveys usually show average adequate caloric intake but frequent evidence of inadequate nutrient intake. For example, there may be fewer animal proteins, more use of grain and other starch, fewer vegetables and fruits, and more sweets and desserts. Also, older persons are frequent prey to claims of food faddists concerning restorative food products, tonics, and regulators.

Numerous factors may contribute to developing malnutrition in an elderly person. Poor teeth or poorly fitting dentures may make chewing difficult. Poor appetite and limited financial means for adequate dental care may discourage efforts to seek improvement in the situation. Also, buccal mucosal changes in the mouth and decrease or change of quality in salivary secretions may cause difficulty in eating. Numerous gastrointestinal complaints may be present, from vague indigestion to specific disease, such as peptic ulcer, or diverticulitis. These may effectively reduce the food intake and curtail the needed nutrients. Financial resources may be limited also, with little money available to purchase needed food. There may be a lack of knowledge of the food needed for a well-balanced diet. Furthermore boredom, loneliness, anxiety, insecurity, and apathy compound the problem. Especially if an older person lives alone, the social value of eating is gone. He may lack adequate cooking, refrigeration, or storage facilities and have no means of transportation to obtain food and bring it back to his home. Often a vicious cycle ensues—his funds are low, he hesitates to spend, he goes without, he feels increasing weakness and lethargy, which leads to still less interest and incentive. Finally, he is ill.

3. *Obesity.* In a different sense, obesity may be considered a form of malnutrition. It is a potential health hazard, indicated in a number of degenerative diseases. Many of the same living situations and emotional factors may cause obesity by contributing to compensatory overeating or poor food choices. Also, there is usually decreased physical activity and a maintenance caloric requirement is lessened.

■ **What approaches will help find solutions to these problems?**

Each situation has to be approached in its own individual context. In all cases there is much need for understanding care and realistic support to build improved eating habits.

1. *Food habits should be analyzed carefully.* The nutritionist or the nurse must listen well to learn the patient's attitudes, precise situation, and limiting factors. Nutritional needs can be met with a variety of foods, and suggestions can be adapted to fit his particular needs and personal situation as well as his personal desires. Suggestions should be administered, therefore, on the basis of knowledge of the practical realities of his living situation.

2. *The practitioner should not moralize.* There is no one food per se that anyone should eat. Thus the statement "eat this because it is good for you" should be struck from everyone's vocabulary. It has little possible value for anyone, much less one who is struggling to maintain his personal integrity and self-esteem in a culture that largely rejects and alienates its aged.

3. *Interest should be encouraged in food variety and seasoning.* A bland and unattractive diet is presumed by many to be necessary for all elderly persons. *It is not.* A variety of food and adventures with new foods, tastes, and seasonings often proves to be the needed stimuli for poor appetite and lack of interest in eating. Sometimes smaller amounts of these foods and more frequent meals are helpful.

4. *Individual approach to problems.* Problems such as weight reduction for the older person should have reasonable approaches. Certainly no drastic measures or diets are indicated, and the plan should be only for a slow, gradual loss as it may be needed. Because individual caloric requirements vary widely and individual personalities and problems are unique, personal and realistic planning with the individual patient, followed by supportive guidance and encouragement, usually pays the greatest dividends.

5. *Exploration of resources.* Consultation with social worker or other community assistance agencies may disclose channels through which the socioeconomic problems surrounding income and housing may be alleviated. Also, counseling with the family members or "significant others" in the elderly person's life may help to sensitize them to the needs of the person, which they may not have been as aware of before.

■ **What community resources are available to help meet these needs?**

The local community may have health professions, such as the Medical Society, the nursing organizations, and the Dietetic Association, which sponsor a variety of programs to help meet the needs of the aged in their respective communities. For example, the Dial-a-Dietitian program of the Dietetics Association may provide sound information concerning nutritional needs. Also, the Meals-on-Wheels program in various communities may provide food for home-bound older persons.

A number of government agencies may also provide resources. The impact of recent Federal legislation covering aid for elderly persons for medical care under the Social Secuitry Act can hardly be minimized. This is the so-called Medicare Bill (Title XIX), which has increased the demand for high-quality medical care and its availability to elderly persons. Some elderly persons may not be aware of the resources for health care that are provided for them under this bill.

The Department of Health, Education, and Welfare also conducts activities at a national level to coordinate care for the aged. The Federal Council on Aging conducts conferences and publishes the newsletter, *Aging,* and provides other resource materials for community workers. The Department of Agriculture, through its agricultural extension services, state universities, and county home advisers on the local level, provides much practical aid for elderly persons and community workers. Also, skilled professionals in public health departments work in the community through local and state agencies. They provide health guidance for elderly persons and operate chronic disease programs.

Other volunteer organizations are available as a resource. These include the Heart Association and the Diabetes Association, who conduct activities related to the needs of older persons. Two particular national organizations sponsor local community groups—Senior Citizens of America and American Society for the Aged, Inc. Often these groups provide in their larger urban centers programs to involve elderly people. Often they give them channels of communication that meet social needs as well as provide nutritional support through their activities and educational programs.

III
Clinical nutrition

15 Child health problems

A child's response to illness is conditioned by his prior life experiences and the common patterns of growth and development. Sick or well, all children confront indispensable tasks of physical and psychosocial growth. The stress of illness invariably causes some degree of regression, as coping responses are mobilized. Nutritional care provides basic support for healing processes, both through its physiologic functions in building tissue integrity and through its psychosocial role as a communication vehicle.

Child health problems will find solutions, therefore, within the context of basic needs of ill children: quality medical and physical care, sensitive emotional support, and optimum nutritional therapy. In planning nutritional care, consideration must be given to the general age group needs of the child, any necessary diet modifications, the individual child's food behavior, and his family's attitudes and habits.

GASTROINTESTINAL PROBLEMS

■ **What general gastrointestinal disturbances may surround the early feeding of infants and children?**

Several functional disturbances sometimes cause great concern for young parents:

1. Infantile colic. This name is given to a condition characterized by intermittent periods of loud, continuous crying. It is usually self-limiting, however, ending spontaneously during the first 3 months of life. But to young, tense parents this brief interval of time may seem an eternity. Treatment usually involves careful history tak-

ing, discovering parental attitudes and reviewing feeding practices. The child may be underfed by a zealous young mother and have abdominal discomfort. In other cases the formula may be changed rapidly from day to day by an experimenting mother. Treatment mostly involves explanation and moral support to the parents, with reassurance that their child is growing normally, after review of feeding practices and examination of growth pattern.

2. Simple functional vomiting. Regurgitation or "spitting up" is common in most young infants. Its cause is usually gastric distention from over feeding or from air swallowing during feeding or crying. Related factors may be ineffective burping and leaving the baby in a supine position rather than a prone position after feeding. Also, overactivity and semiacrobatics at the hands of doting fathers and grandparents soon after the infant has been fed may stimulate regurgitation. The temperature of the feeding may be a factor, since feedings that are too hot may induce vomiting. Milk at room temperature is better tolerated, and even cold feedings have evoked no difficulty in a number of infants. Treatment usually revolves around simple attention to causative factors and reassurance to the young mother.

3. Constipation. The old adage, "It is not what he eats, but what eats him!" is correctly applied to constipation in childhood. *Psychogenic* constipation may occur during ages 1 to 2, while the child is being toilet trained at the hands of a compulsive, anal-fixated mother who believes in an arbitrary timetable of elimination. Correction of the problem involves adjustment of the parent-child relationships and a resulting easing of the conflict and tensions. The mother needs to learn two simple physiologic facts—toxins are not absorbed from fecal material and a *daily* stool is not essential to the child's health. Each child has his own individual biologic rhythm. Occasional, simple, *physiologic constipation* is usually transient. It is aided by moderately reducing the milk intake, increasing the carbohydrate intake (for example, increasing the sugar somewhat in the formula), increasing fruits and vegetables, and increasing the water intake.

■ **What treatment is indicated in diarrhea in infants and young children?**

Mild diarrhea is fairly common in infants and children, and usually responds to simple treatment. This consists of reducing the food intake, especially of carbohydrates and fat in the formula, and increasing the water intake, sometimes including oral electrolyte replacements in it.

Prolonged diarrhea is a much more serious problem, especially if it is associated with infection. Because of his relatively high water content and his large area of intestinal mucosa in proportion to body surface area, the infant's fluid and electrolyte reserves may be rapidly depleted. Marked dehydration and acidosis may result. These are medical emergencies calling for immediate parenteral fluid and electrolyte therapy. The loss of potassium can be dangerous, since hypokalemia affects the action of the heart muscle.

Oral feedings may be resumed after initial replacement of fluid and electrolytes. Water, glucose, and balanced salt solutions may be used, followed by milk mixtures, breast milk, or substitutes, such as Probana (a high-protein formula with banana powder), or Nutramigen (a casein hydrolysate free of galactose) as the stool volume decreases. Calories are increased to normal requirements as soon as possible, to provide energy needs and thus allow protein to build tissue. Such agents as pectin and kaolin may thicken the stools but most authorities agree they have little or no therapeutic usefulness in severe infant diarrhea. Pediatricians generally discount the previous practice of completely starving patients with acute diarrhea, a practice that was based on the erroneous belief that avoidance of oral intake put the bowels at rest. Also, an adult remedy, tea, should not be given to the child. The xanthines in tea stimulate and excite children, and in some cases cause diuresis, which in turn only aggravates the fluid imbalance.

■ **What is celiac disease?**

The name *celiac* comes from a Greek word *kolia* meaning "belly" or "abdomen." The term "celiac disease" is given to a number of diseases, all of which result in similar clinical manifestations of intestinal malabsorption: (1) general malnutrition; (2) multiple foul, bulky, foamy, greasy stools; (3) distended abdomen caused by an accumulation of improperly digested and inadequately absorbed material and by abnormal gas accumulations; and (4) secondary vitamin deficiencies.

A number of different clinical entities have been identified as producing these same symptoms. In electron microscopic study of the intestinal mucosa, tissues have consistently shown eroded mucosal surfaces without the number or form of villi normally seen and with sparse microvilli. This erosion effectively reduces the absorbing surface areas by as much as 95%. As the result of these and other studies the various diseases comprising the celiac syndrome have been grouped according to cause.

Impaired digestion of fat. Inadequate absorption of fat may be caused by decreased length of small bowel, as in surgical resection, or by increaesd intestinal motility as a result of diarrhea. Also, obstruction of the intestinal lymphatics as a result of *exudative enteropathy* may cause abnormalities. *Inflammatory disease,* such as intestinal infections or parasitic infestations, regional enteritis, or ulcerative colitis, may also cause lesions. A more-recently discovered cause is that of *gluten-induced celiac disease,* a biochemical dysfunction of the mucosal cells apparently related specifically to *gluten,* a protein in certain grains—wheat, rye, oats, and barley.

The principle causes of the celiac syndrome are cystic fibrosis of the pancreas, gluten-induced celiac disease, idiopathic disease or steatorrhea, such as in tropical sprue, and exudative enteropathy. All of these conditions are characterized by excessive intestinal loss of serum protein, often with abnormalities of the intestinal lymphatics. The two most common of these entities encountered in children are (1) gluten-induced enteropathy (this is the entity that usually bears the name celiac disease), and (2) cystic fibrosis of the pancreas.

■ **How is gluten-induced celiac disease treated?**

Dietary management is the main form of treatment following control of initial fluid and electrolyte problems through medical care. Oral feedings are important as soon as toleration permits to combat the progressive malnutrition that ensues and its deficiency states of anemia, rickets, and an increased bleeding tendency. The diet is better defined as a *low-gluten* rather than a *gluten-free* one, because it is impossible to remove all the gluten completely and

there is evidence that a small amount of gluten is tolerated by most patients. Obvious sources of the grains in question—wheat, rye, oats, and barley—are eliminated. However, specific instructions must be outlined to the child's parents, because these grains are also used as thickeners or fillers in many commercial products. Careful label reading should become a habit. The basic diet principles for management of patients with celiac disease on a low-gluten program are summarized in the list below.

■ **How is cystic fibrosis treated?**

Cystic fibrosis is a generalized hereditary disease of children that involves the exocrine glands and affects, in turn, many tissues and organs.

Clinical manifestations include (1) pancreatic deficiency with greatly diminished digestion of food caused by the absence of pancreatic enzymes; (2) malfunction of mucus-producing glands, with accumulation of thick, viscid secretions and subsequent respiratory difficulty and chronic pulmonary disease; (3) abnormal secretions of the sweat glands containing high electrolyte levels; and (4) possible cirrhosis of the liver arising from biliary obstruction and increased by malnutrition or infection.

Diet principles for patients with celiac disease

1. Calories—high, usually about 20% above normal requirement to compensate for fecal loss
2. Protein—high, usually 6 to 8 gm./kg. body weight
3. Fat—low, but not fat free because of impaired absorption
4. Carbohydrate—simple, easily digested sugars (fruits, vegetables) should provide about one half of the calories
5. Feedings—small, frequent feedings during ill periods; afternoon snack for older children
6. Texture—smooth, soft, avoiding irritating roughage initially, using strained foods longer than usual for age, adding whole foods as tolerated and according to age of child
7. Vitamins—supplements of B vitamins, vitamins A and B in water-miscible forms, and vitamin C
8. Minerals—iron supplements if anemia present

Table 15-1. Principles of dietary management for patients with cystic fibrosis

Principle	Reason
High calorie	Energy demands of growth and compensation for fecal losses; large appetite usually ensures acceptance of increased amounts of food
High protein	Usually tolerated in large amounts; excess above normal growth needs required to compensate for losses
Moderate carbohydrate	Starch less well tolerated, simple sugars easily assimilated
Low to moderate fat, as tolerated	Fat poorly absorbed, but tolerance varies widely
Generous salt	Food generously salted to replace sweat losses; salt supplements in hot weather
Vitamins	Double doses of multivitamins in water-soluble form (vitamin E supplements sometimes used as low blood levels of the vitamin have been observed); vitamin K supplements with prolonged antibiotic therapy
Pancreatic enzymes	Large amounts given by mouth with each meal (may be mixed with cereal or applesauce for infants) to compensate for pancreatic deficiency—powdered pancreas containing steapsin, trypsin, and amylapsin (Pancreatin, or other pancreatic extracts such as Cotazyme or Viokase).

Treatment therefore is based on three factors: (1) control of respiratory infection, (2) relief from the effects of extremely viscid bronchial secretions, and (3) maintenance of nutrition. The multiple stools characteristic of the disease are similar to those seen in celiac disease. However, they also contain more undigested food because only about half of the child's food is absorbed. Thus the child with cystic fibrosis has a much more voracious appetite.

The basic objective of nutritional therapy is to compensate for the large loss of nutrient material resulting from the insufficiency of pancreatic enzymes to digest it. Apparently protein hydrolysates, split fats (emulsified, simple fats), and simple sugars are assimilated readily. There is a wide variation, however, in tolerance for fat; and the amount of fat intake is usually prescribed according to the character of the stools. Large increases of protein seem to be well tolerated and are needed for replacement of losses and for growth. Diet programs for cystic fibrosis are similar to those outlined for celiac disease, with food varying in form according to the age of the child. The diet differs, however, in that gluten sources need not be restricted, and, of course, there is greater emphasis on quantity of food. These principles of dietary management for patients with cystic fibrosis are summarized in Table 15-1.

■ **How may the child with a cleft palate be fed?**

Feeding difficulties in infants and young children may result from abnormalities in the structure of the mouth. When the parts of the upper jaw and the palate separating the mouth and the nasal cavity do not fuse properly during fetal development, the anatomic abnormality creates difficult feeding problems. The premaxillary and maxillary processes normally fuse early in gestation, between the fifth and eighth week of intrauterine life, and fusion of the palate is completed about one month later. If this fusion fails to occur, cleft lip (harelip) or cleft palate results.

Since the infant is unable to suck adequately, early feedings are tiring and lengthy. A softened nipple with enlarged opening, through which the infant can obtain milk by a chewing motion, is helpful. In some instances a medicine dropper or gavage feedings may be used initially. The infant should be held in an upright position and fed very slowly in small amounts to avoid aspiration. There should be frequent rest periods and burping to expel the large amount of air swallowed. If acid foods such as orange juice are irritating, ascorbic acid supplement may be prescribed. As solid foods are added they may be mixed with milk in the bottle and given in thin gruel or thickened form through a large nipple opening.

Surgical repair of the cleft palate is usually carried out over the growth years, depending on the extent of the deformity and the growth of the child. Following surgery special care is essential. The infant or child is usually fed a fluid or semifluid diet, with a medicine dropper or spoon. Great care must be exercised to protect the suture lines and avoid any strain.

FOOD ALLERGIES

- **What are the principle food allergies in children?**

The main food offenders that cause allergic manifestations in children are protein foods—milk, egg, wheat. A wide variety of environmental, emotional, and physical factors influence the child's reaction, however, and a suitable regime is sometimes difficult to find. Children tend to become less allergic to food sources as they grow older and respond more at later ages to inhalent allergens.

Milk. Cow's milk has long been the most common cause of allergic disease in young infants. Current observation indicates that milk allergy occurs in about 1% to 2% of all infants and accounts for some 30% of the cases among allergic infants. The allergy to milk usually causes gastrointestinal difficulties, such as vomiting, diarrhea, and colic. The diagnosis is usually made by clinical symptoms, family history, and trial on a milk-free diet. A substitute formula is used, such as soybean preparation (for example, Sobee or Mull-Soy) or a meat formula. However, pediatricians agree generally that there may be a tendency among some clinicians to overdiagnose milk allergy in

infants and children with general gastrointestinal disturbances, irritability, and skin rash. Thus, a remission of symptoms on a milk-free diet should always be followed by a trial on milk again to determine if it does indeed cause the symptoms to reappear. Only then should the child be labeled as allergic.

Other than gastrointestinal responses, milk allergy may be manifest by skin problems, such as rashes, eczema, and respiratory difficulties, such as wheezing and runny nose. These symptoms tend to be more often caused by food if gastrointestinal problems are also present with them.

Egg, wheat, and other foods. The albumin in egg white is the potential allergen, and hence it is usually added to the infant's diet following earlier use of egg yolk alone. Wheat is also a fairly common food allergen. The prevalence of wheat in the common American diet makes its restriction a problem. Other grains have to be substituted.

- **How is diet therapy for a child with food allergies planned?**

In an allergic child's diet, foods are usually added slowly, common offenders being excluded in early feedings. In some cases a series of diagnostic diets, such as the Rowe Elimination Diets, may be used to identify the offending food. Guidance in the substitution of special food products and in the use of special recipes should be provided for the child's mother by the nutritionist and the nurse.

Common foods that tend to create allergic reactions in general use with infants and children include the following, which should be avoided: egg, fish, wheat, strawberries, tomatoes, pork, bacon, citrus fruit, nuts, peanut butter, chocolate, pineapple, milk or milk products. Careful diet counseling with the parents and the child is an important aspect of treatment. If specific foods have been definitely identified as offenders, elimination of these will be indicated. Evident forms of the food can easily be removed, but many occurrences are in commercial products and other hidden sources, which will make label reading and attention to recipes of prime consideration. As the child grows older the allergic reaction to the given food may wane and it may be gradually readded to the diet.

OBESITY

■ **Is the nature of obesity the same in all children?**

No. The pattern of the growth years and the study of developing obesity during these years points to two types of obesity in children:

1. *Developmental obesity.* At birth fat accounts for about 12% of the infant's body weight. During the middle of the first year there is usually more fat in males than in females. By the time the infant is 1 year old, fat accounts for about 24% of the body weight. As the child continues to grow through the childhood years, this general percent of fat remains essentially constant, relative to the desired weight or height and age. The peak for onset of juvenile obesity occurs during the first 4 years of a child's life and is apparently established by the time the child is 11 years old. About the twelfth year the percent of body fat increases in girls and the development of lean body mass begins to rise sharply in boys.

This developmental form of obesity begins early in life, therefore. The cells become supersaturated with fat and additional cells are recruited from connective tissue for fat deposit. With the increasing weight, additional bone and muscle cells must also increase to help carry the load. As a result these children are usually taller, have an advanced bone age, and have been consistently obese since infancy. Their percentage of lean body mass is high and so also is the fat deposit.

2. *Reactive obesity.* The reactive type of obesity in childhood usually results from intense and oft-repeated episodes of emotional stress. As a result of the stress period the child overeats and his weight often assumes an up-and-down type of weight pattern. His body composition is high in fat,

but not in the lean body mass observed in the developmental type of obesity.

■ **How may food practices during the growth years be altered to counteract childhood obesity?**

Several factors appear reasonable in considering feeding patterns of the early growth years.

1. *Fat content of infant formulas and quantity fed.* With the knowledge regarding the rapid growth of the first year and the normal laying down of fat during that period, questions can be raised concerning the fat content of infant diets and formulas. Some modification may be in order. The attitude of mothers who insist on the emptying of the bottle with every feeding of the formula beyond the infant's obvious desire for food can also be questioned.

2. *Sex differences in early years.* If the sex differences at the early age of 2 or 3 years in calorie expenditure are considered, it should be realized that all toddlers are not going to eat the same amount of food. The basic metabolic rate is higher in the male than in the female during the second and third year of life. Therefore parents should be prepared for very early differences among young boys and young girls.

3. *Overfeeding in the preschool years.* Overfeeding during the years of slow, erratic growth can make a large contribution to the development of continuing obesity. The peak onset of developmental types of obesity is during these early preschool years. Mothers of young children would be well-advised to offer them the enjoyment of a wide variety of food in realistic, smaller portion sizes.

4. *Decreased activity of elementary school years.* Prior to the beginning of the school years the child engages in much strenuous physical play, testing developing strength and motor capacity. Usually this is more independent, spontaneous activity and there is not yet a set schedule for the day. With the continuing experience of school, however, the child becomes more sedentary in his recreational pattern as well as in school activities. This great

change in energy expenditure, in conjunction with a latent slower growth pattern, during ages 7 to 11, calls for guidance from parents concerning food intake habits.

5. *Adolescent sex differences in body composition.* The increasing tendency for fat deposit in the teenage girl in comparison to greater increase in lean body mass in the teenage boy makes weight control a greater problem for the girl. Guidance from parents in a supportive, accepting manner, especially for young girls, is needed. Also young girls need sound counseling concerning food choices.

DENTAL CARIES

Over 99% of the children in the United States at one time or another are affected by dental caries, and there seems to be little pattern to its incidence. Three factors combine to produce tooth decay.

1. *The susceptible host.* Inherent differences in caries susceptibility vary widely among individual children. The interplay between the anatomical shape of the tooth plus the environment that sustains its development during its formative period appear to be causative. Since already formed teeth are stable structures, it is evident that this positive nutritional influence can have effect only during growth and development of the enamel-forming organ and fetal development of the tooth bud. Thus, important nutrients in the diet of the mother during this time are protein and certain vitamins and minerals, especially vitamins A and D, calcium, and phosphorus. There is also some indication that either fluoride ingestion in the drinking water by the mother during her pregnancy and afterward by the child or the topical application of fluoride applied to the young child's teeth will directly influence tooth formation and health.

2. *Oral bacteria.* In humans, streptococci comprise the highest number of bacteria in the dental plaque, the gelatinous coating of the teeth. They seem to have a particular affinity for carbohydrates and act upon them rapidly. It has been shown

in control tests that only 13 minutes after carbohydrate was present as a substrate, streptococci alone lowered the pH of the dental plaque from 6.0 to 5.0. However, the oral flora is complex and bacterial affects can vary from symbiosis between two or more microorganisms. It is their substrate that is mandatory for the metabolism of caries-producing organisms, and this substrate is carbohydrate.

3. *The diet.* As carbohydrate food accumulates in the mouth it provides the necessary media for the normal growth of acidogenic microorganisms that cause tooth decay. Sites of particular susceptibility are irregularities on tooth surfaces where food particles may be retained, or gummy materials that may adhere to the teeth and remain longer in contact with them. Persistent and continuous eating of adhesive carbohydrates, therefore, is a prime factor in tooth decay. The other dietary element involved in dental caries is fluoride. Repeated studies consistently confirm about 60% reduction in the incidence of dental caries in children, both in prenatal and postnatal exposure to fluoridated water.

■ **What dietary measures may help to reduce dental caries?**

Although the problem of dental caries is by no means solved, two nutritional factors seem apparent in its cause and hence in its treatment. First, adhesive carbohydrates (sweets, candy bars, caramels) consumed at frequent intervals *do* increase dental caries. Also, carbohydrates in liquid form are less cariogenic than those in solid form. Second, fluoridated public water supplies decrease the dental caries rate.

GENETIC DISEASES

■ **What concept is involved in genetic disease?**

Some key terms involved in the basic concept of genetic disease include the following:

1. A *chromosome* is a rod-shaped body developed in the cell nucleus. Each human cell contains 46 chromosomes arranged in 23 pairs. One pair forms the sex chromosomes carrying the sex trait, and the remaining 22 pairs control the other various characteristics of the cell and of the individual.

2. *Autosomes* are any of the chromosomes other than the pair that carries the sex characteristics.

3. *Genes* (Gr. *gennan*, to produce) are self-reproducing particles in the cells, located at definite individual points (loci) on the chromosomes. Each gene is a long, double-stranded molecule (helix) of DNA (deoxyribonucleic acid), with a special arrangement of its components—its so-called genetic code. A *mutant gene* (L. *mutare*, to change) is an altered form of a gene that can be transmitted to the offspring. Why genes mutate is not known. Probably temperature, irradiation, or infection are involved. A mutant gene is an abnormal gene that keeps on reproducing itself in successive generations.

4. The genes on the respective pairs of chromosomes are almost identical with each other, so they, too, form pairs or so-called links of genes. A gene trait is *recessive* (does not manifest itself) if it does not match its partner. The recessive gene must be carried by both parents to cause a defect.

5. A *heterozygote* is an individual in whom the members of one or more gene pairs are unlike. Such a person is called a "carrier" of the trait, but he does not manifest its symptoms. Transmission of recessive traits to successive generations follows the pattern established by Mendel. If two carriers marry, the risk for each birth is 25% manifest trait, 50% carriers, 25% normal (neither carrier nor manifesting the trait).

Relationships involved in inheritance of genetic disease are shown in the diagram in Fig. 15-1.

■ **What is phenylketonuria (PKU)?**

Genetic control of metabolism is exercised at two basic levels: (1) control of heredity, and (2) control of cell function. Cell metabolism, which sustains life, is made possible by the presence of a thousand or more protein enzymes that control essentially all of the chemical reactions that take place in cells. Each one of these enzymes is a specific protein, synthesized by a specific DNA pattern in a specific gene. Therefore, when a specific

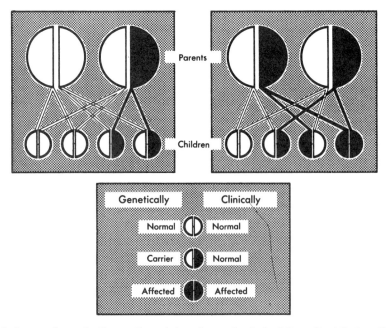

Fig. 15-1. Pattern of genetic disease. Transmission of recessive traits follows Mendel's law. If two carriers marry, one child will be normal, one child will manifest the trait, and two children will be carriers.

gene is abnormal (mutant) the enzyme whose synthesis it controls cannot be made and in turn the metabolic reaction controlled by that enzyme cannot take place. The result is a genetic disease manifesting symptoms relative to those reaction products. Phenylketonuria is one such disease.

The metabolic defect in phenylketonuria is the absence of the liver enzyme *phenylalanine hydroxylase,* which catalyzes the oxidation of the essential amino acid phenylalanine to tyrosine, another amino acid (Fig. 15-2). Since the gene is defective, the enzyme cannot be produced and the reaction at this point does not proceed normally. Phenylalanine then accumulates in the blood and its alternate metabolites, the phenyl acids, are excreted in the urine. One of these acids, phenylpyruvic acid, is a phenylketone, hence the name, phenylketonuria. This acid gives the characteristic green color reaction with ferric chloride (the basis for the "diaper test" of the infant's urine to detect the presence of phenylketonuria).

The most profound effect that may occur in untreated PKU is mental retardation.

The IQ is usually below 50 and most frequently under 20. The damage to the central nervous system probably occurs within the first 2 years. The patient may learn to walk, but few learn to talk. There is increased motor irritability, hyperactivity, convulsive seizures, and bizarre behavior, such as disorientation, failure to respond to strong stimuli, catatoniclike positions, fright reactions, and screaming episodes.

Another clinical symptom involves pigmentation abnormalities. Because tyrosine is used in the production of the pigment material melanin, PKU children usually have blond or light brown hair and blue eyes, the skin is fair and susceptible to eczema. Tyrosine also is involved in the production of epinephrine by the adrenal gland, accounting for the low blood level of epinephrine in the child.

The urine frequently has a strong musty odor from the presence of large amounts of phenylacetic acid. Sometimes this is the first noticeable symptom that leads the mother to seek medical care for the child.

■ **What blood levels of phenylalanine guide the treatment of PKU?**

Normal phenylalanine blood levels

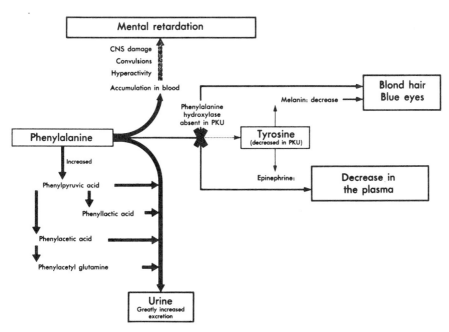

Fig. 15-2. The metabolic error in phenylketonuria. Because of the absence of the enzyme phenylalanine hydroxylase, the essential amino acid phenylalanine cannot be converted to tyrosine.

range from 1 to 3 mg./100 ml. of blood. In the untreated PKU child they may run as high as 60 times this amount. Treatment is designed to maintain the blood levels within acceptable ranges of 2 to 6 mg/100 ml. to prevent symptoms. Treatment is by dietary maintenance. A low-phenylalanine diet is used to reduce the serum phenylalanine and prevent the high levels that cause the clinical symptoms. Since phenylalanine is an essential amino acid necessary for growth, it cannot be totally removed from the diet. Blood levels of phenylalanine, therefore, are constantly checked and the diet is calculated to allow the limited amount of phenylalanine (usually between 10 and 20 mg./kg. body weight). The diet of a normal child contains 100 to 200 mg. of phenylalanine per kilogram of body weight.

■ **How is the diet of the PKU child managed?**

The first food of the infant is milk, and milk has a relatively high phenylalanine content. So the first need for the PKU infant is a milk substitute. The formula is usually made from Lofenalac, a special casine hydrolysate balanced with fats, carbohydrates, vitamins, and minerals. One measure of Lofenalac powder in 2 ounces of water makes a formula of 20 calories per ounce and is usually well accepted by the infant. A small designated measure of milk is usually added to this formula to adjust the needed phenylalanine content.

As the child grows, solid foods are added to the diet as calculated according to their phenylalanine content. These food additions are selected from a list of phenylalanine food exchange groups or equivalents. The diet is prescribed by the physician according to the child's blood phenylalanine test and calculated by the nutritionist in terms of the number of food choices allowed daily from each food group. Then a meal pattern of feedings is made out for the mother to follow. It is not known yet how long such a diet must be continued. One physician has suggested that it may be possible to relax the dietary

controls as early as age 4, but at present it is probably wise to continue the diet at least until the child is 6 to 8 years old.

■ **Is there any public assistance available to help families with PKU children bear the financial burden of continuing care?**

Yes. Funds are available through the Crippled Children's Program. Investigation of these funds should be made through the public health agency in the local community.

■ **Are screening tests on newborns for the presence of PKU usually routine procedures?**

Yes. Surveys indicate that the incidence may be more than originally thought—about 1 in every 10,000 births. Moreover, because the possibility of severe mental retardation from undiagnosed and untreated phenylketonuria is so profound, routine screening is usually done. A number of tests have been developed to detect the disease and mandatory screening laws are being passed in most of the states to ensure that all newborns are tested. Usually the Guthrie test is used. This is a highly specific blood test, sensitive as early as the third day of life. A simple heel puncture is made and the blood is absorbed on specially-treated absorbing paper. Another definitive blood test is the fluorimetric procedure developed by McCaman and Robins. In California both of these tests are approved for use under the regulations that are now part of the State Administrative Code, Title 17.

■ **What is galactosemia?**

Galactosemia is also a genetic disease caused by a missing enzyme. The metabolic defect transmitted by a single autosomal recessive gene is illustrated in Fig. 15-3. The incidence of galactosemia is lower than that of phenylketonuria; it occurs about once in 25,000 to 50,000 births. The missing enzyme is *galactose-l-phosphate uridyl transferase* (G-l-PUT). This is one of three enzymes that control steps in the conversion of galactose to glucose. Milk, the infant's first food, contains a large amount of lactose (milk sugar) that

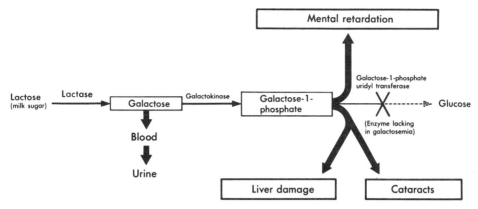

Fig. 15-3. Metabolic error in galactosemia. Because of the absence of the enzyme galactose-1-phosphate uridyl transferase, galactose cannot be converted to glucose.

is acted on by the intestinal digestive enzyme lactase to produce the two monosaccharides glucose and galactose. After galactose is initially combined with phosphate to begin the metabolic conversion to glucose, it cannot proceed further in the galactosemic infant. Galactose-1-phosphate and galactose rapidly accumulate in the blood and in various body tissues. This excessive tissue accumulation of galactose damages vital organs and special tissues. Liver damage brings jaundice, hepatomegaly with cirrhosis, enlargement of the spleen, and ascites. Death usually results from hepatic failure. If the infant survives, the continuing tissue damage and accompanying hypoglycemia in the optic lens and the brain cause cataracts and mental retardation.

■ **How is the diet managed for a galactosemic infant?**

The main indirect source of dietary galactose is the galactose in milk. Therefore *all* forms of milk and lactose must be removed from the diet. In this instance a galactose-free diet is used. The milk substitute usually used for infant feeding is Nutramigen, a complete protein hydrolysate that is free of galactose. Careful attention, however, must be given to avoid lactose from other food sources as solid foods are added to the infant's diet, since lactose is a common food additive in many commercial products. Parents must be edu-

cated concerning these sources and must check labels on all commercial products carefully.

■ **Is there a similar disease of lactose intolerance?**

Yes. This condition is caused by the deficiency of lactase, the digestive enzyme that breaks down the milk sugar, lactose (a disaccharide), into its constituent monosaccharides, galactose and glucose. Thus, although the dietary management would be identical to that used in galactosemia, the cause is different.

JUVENILE DIABETES

■ **How does juvenile diabetes differ from maturity-onset diabetes?**

Juvenile diabetes is different in that it is characterized by a greater degree of insulin deficiency, if not an absolute lack. Hence, it is a more labile form of the disease, responding only to insulin treatment and diet. Maturity-onset diabetes, on the other hand, tends to be a milder form, less labile, and often controlled by diet alone or diet and oral hypoglycemic agents.

■ **What are the principles of dietary management for the juvenile diabetic?**

Two important principles should prevail in the care of the diet for a child with diabetes.

1. *Quantity and nutrient ratio.* The diet during the formative years of any child should provide an optimum nutritional

base essential for growth and development and health. These physiologic needs for growth and the psychosocial development paths that accompany each stage of normal development are important bases to remember in planning the diet for the diabetic child. Thus, the nutrient ratios in a balanced diet for children with diabetes includes adequate quantities of protein, carbohydrates, and fat to meet growth and energy demands.

2. Distribution of the diet. The distribution of the food through the day is imperative to achieve the necessary balance with the insulin dosage for control of the diabetes. Thus, the distribution pattern is based on the absorption rate and activity of the insulin used and on the general family meal pattern. Usually these needs are met with three fairly equal meals at breakfast, lunch, and dinner, with an added snack in midafternoon and evening. A midmorning snack may also be required by a younger child.

Regularity and routine are important factors in building consistent habits on a day-to-day basis. The three balance factors always involved that must be considered are food, insulin, and exercise, with additional consideration during periods of infection.

■ **What should a teaching program for a diabetic and his family include?**

An important base for maintaining the health of a diabetic child is sound education at the onset of the disease, for both the child and his family. This teaching-learning program should include basic needs for routine care:

1. An understanding of diabetes
2. A realistic diet plan to meet normal needs, provide a basis for balance of the diabetes, and fit in with the family food patterns
3. Techniques of insulin administration and minor adjustment
4. Urine testing for sugar and acetone
5. Keeping of reasonable daily records according to need
6. Personal cleanliness in skin care
7. Recognition of the early signs of insulin shock and how to treat it
8. Recognition of early signs of acidosis and the need for immediate medical care
9. Adjustments in illness and infections

Provision should be made for the active involvement of the child and his family in practice sessions and feedback discussions. Some follow-up form of support should be provided for the family on a continuing basis.

16 Adult health problems

The stress of illness or chronic disease in the adult also brings forth physiologic and psychosocial responses to cope with the problems involved. Responses to disease, however, are highly individual. Care is based on identifying and meeting individual needs. The coping mechanisms one patient brings to his disease and its tensions are different from those operating in another. Each person represents the sum of his life experiences. Physical, psychologic, social, economic, and cultural forces have molded him. It is these resources that he draws on in illness and that provide a basis for his ongoing care.

The hospital setting is often a formidable one for a patient and may fail to provide the positive, personal supports he needs. Outpatient clinical care may also proceed on an impersonal basis. In each setting it is imperative that a plan for identifying individual needs, physical and personal, be developed and a plan of care and health education be followed, which is based on these individual needs. To this end a greater involvement of the patient in planning his own care is essential.

The principles of diet therapy, therefore, in clinical problems stem from several basic concepts:

1. *Normal nutrition base.* A therapeutic diet still needs to meet basic individual nutritional requirements and is based thereon.

2. *Disease application.* Modification of the nutritional components must have specific rationale based on the specific indi-vidual disease situation. Dietary changes may include modifications in one or more of the basic nutrients, or in energy value, or in texture or seasoning of food.

3. *Individual adaptation.* A workable plan for a specific person must be based on his food habits and life situation. This can only be achieved through careful planning with the patient. Whatever the problem, such as those discussed here as examples, nutritional care is valid only to the extent that it involves these knowledges, skills, and insights.

OBESITY

■ **How do the basic laws of energy exchange apply to obesity?**

The enigma of the problem of obesity stems generally from two factors, its unsure definition and its multiple causes. The basic physical laws of energy exchange account for obesity—an intake of more energy potential as measured in food calories than output in total energy metabolism, including basal needs and physical activities (see Chapter 5, p. 40). Table 16-1 indicates a general scheme for measuring basal energy needs and additions for different levels of physical activities. However simple this statement of energy balance seems, the maintenance level of calories varies widely with individuals in like circumstances. It is also influenced by their activity level. Obese persons generally consume fewer calories than nonobese ones, but their activity level is usually lower also. Obese, sedentary persons, therefore, simply

Table 16-1. General approximations for daily adult basal and activity energy needs

Basal energy needs (av. 1 cal. per kg. per hr.)		Man (70 kg.) calories 70 × 24 = 1,680	Woman (58 kg.) calories 58 × 24 = 1,392
Activity energy needs			
Very sedentary	+20% basal	1,680 + 336 = 2,016	1,392 + 278 = 1,670
Sedentary	+30% basal	1,680 + 504 = 2,184	1,392 + 418 = 1,810
Moderately active	+40% basal	1,680 + 672 = 2,352	1,392 + 557 = 1,949
Very active	+50% basal	1,680 + 840 = 2,520	1,392 + 696 = 2,088

cannot afford to eat as much as their leaner counterparts, since their maintenance level is comparatively low.

■ **What additional factors may contribute to the problem of obesity and weight control?**

The complexity of "simple" obesity is further increased by multiple causes. Among these factors, in addition to physical energy exchange factors, are the following:

1. *Physiologic factors.* The normal physiology of the growth years contributes to an accumulation of fat tissue deposits. There are critical periods in the development of this obesity during childhood, in early infancy, and in early stages of puberty. For the female a critical period is after age 21 because of lessened activity with no adjustment of caloric intake. Other times are during the first pregnancy and after menopause, because of the hormonal factors that are operating. For the male a critical period is between the ages of 25 and 40, because of decreasing activity with no consequent change in the large food habits formed during adolescence. Both men and women tend to gain weight after the age of 50 because of the lowered basal metabolic rate and decreased exercise, with failure to adjust eating habits and caloric intake accordingly. Other practical factors that influence physical obesity are the overfeeding of infants and children and a lack of dietary adjustment by adults during periods of increased susceptibiilty to weight gain.

2. *Inheritance factors.* There is some evidence that seems to indicate a genetic factor in obesity, but the significance of these results for human obesity is unknown. It is true that obese children are more likely than nonobese children to have obese parents. It is probable, however, that the greater influence is a familial one, in that the home situation molds food habits. Excessive food preparation and consumption is the normal family habit pattern, one that tends to be perpetuated in the adulthood and passed on to successive generations.

3. *Social factors.* Class values place different judgments on the incidence of obesity. For example, in lower social classes obesity tends to be more the norm and is a more accepted state. With upward social mobility, however, there is less and less acceptance of obesity and increased social group pressure to maintain a lighter weight. These values vary between men and women and also among individual members of various social classes.

4. *Psychologic factors.* The relation of emotional factors to obesity is well established. The obese state may well be the individual's protective resolution of deeper emotional problems. In such cases, to remove the obesity without providing an alternative and satisfying resolution for the emotional problems may well create still further problems.

■ **What practical management plans are used with obese patients in general practice?**

By and large, in common practice the general approach to the control of simple

Table 16-2. Calorie adjustment required for weight loss

To lose 1 pound a week—500 fewer calories daily
Basis of estimation

1 lb. body fat	=	454 grams
1 gm. pure fat	=	9 calories
1 gm. body fat	=	7.7 calories (some water in fat cells)
454 gm. × 9 cal. per gm.	=	4,086 calories per lb. fat (pure fat)
454 gm. × 7.7 cal. per gm.	=	3,496 calories per lb. body fat (or 3,500 calories)
500 cal. × 7 days	=	3,500 calories = 1 lb. body fat.

obesity is an attempt to incorporate all of these etiologic factors. It is based on the underlying energy exchange factors and the patient's situational needs. Thus it has three main principles: (1) individual decision and support, (2) individual diet with calorie and situational adaptations, and (3) a planned follow-up program.

The degree of patient motivation is a prime factor. The initial interviews seek to determine individual needs, attitudes toward food, and the meaning food has for the patient. Recognition is given to the emotional factors involved in the reduction program and support is provided by the team of physician, nutritionist, and nurse to meet the patient's particular needs.

A guide for the calorie adjustments required for weight loss is given in Table 16-2. Based on these estimates, careful interviewing follows to determine a realistic plan for outlining an individual program. Follow-up care provides support to carry out the program and allows for individual adjustments as the program proceeds. The follow-up program may include both individual counseling and group discussion sessions. Groups have proved useful in many instances to provide support and enlightenment for the members.

■ **What is the "behavior conditioning" approach to obesity control?**

Based on the recognition that the food behavior pattern of an individual is causing his obesity problem, programs have been initiated, which attempt to intervene in these behavior patterns. A recondition-

ing program ensues in which the undesirable food behavior is cast in an unpleasant context in order to change it to a more desirable behavior. For example, foods that are particularly difficult for the individual to control are reintroduced into the individual's life situation, mixed with unpleasant taste additives or eaten in unpleasant situations.

DIABETES

■ **What is diabetes?**

Diabetes is a metabolic disorder resulting from a lack of insulin, a hormone produced by the beta cells of the islets of Langerhans in the pancreas. Whether this lack is an absolute lack per se or whether the lack is at the level of availability in the blood is not entirely clear. Recent insulin assay tests developed to measure the level of insulin activity in the blood (I.L.A.) have found insulinlike activity levels in early diabetes to be two or three times the normal insulin levels. Investigators have postulated that the insulin is present but it is bound with a protein, hence making it unavailable. The degree of this insulin lack varies widely among individual diabetics. Thus, a spectrum of diabetes exists from severe cases to mild asymptomatic ones.

Diabetes has been found to be a hereditary disease. It is usually defined in terms of the clinical symptoms produced as a result of the lack of insulin. These symptoms appear as the diabetes develops. Initial complaints include increased thirst, urination, and hunger, with accompanying weight loss in the case of the child or obesity as a predisposing factor in the case of the adult. Clinical laboratory data further reveals glycosuria (sugar in the urine), hyperglycemia (elevated blood sugar level), and abnormal glucose tolerance tests. With a glucose load, the blood sugar rises to a higher level and takes a longer period to return to normal. As the disease continues, other symptoms may occur, such as blurred vision or skin irritation or infections. If control is not established, fluid and electrolyte imbalance ensues, bringing acidosis (ketosis), loss of strength, and eventual coma.

■ **What are the normal blood sugar controls?**

Blood sugar enters the system from dietary carbohydrates, protein, and fat, and from liver glycogen. These sources maintain a steady supply of blood glucose. A normal blood sugar level is 70 to 120 mg./ 100 ml.; to prevent a continued rise above 120 mg., several routes of glucose use are necessary:

1. Conversion to glycogen for storage in the liver (glycogenesis)

2. Conversion to fat (lypogenesis) and storage in adipose tissue
3. Conversion to muscle glycogen
4. Cell oxidation for energy

Although its precise role in relation to these routes of handling blood sugar is not entirely clear, insulin has an effect on these control mechanisms. It is believed to function in several ways:

1. It facilitates the transport of glucose through the cell membrane.
2. It enhances the conversion of glucose to glycogen and its storage in the liver.
3. It stimulates the conversion of glucose to fat.
4. It influences glucose oxidation through the main glycolytic pathway by aiding the necessary initial phosphorylation reaction.

The constant balance between these control measures, the input sources of blood glucose and the control outlets for blood glucose, is shown in Fig. 16-1.

■ **What is glucagon?**

Glucagon is another hormone that is secreted by the pancreas in the adjacent

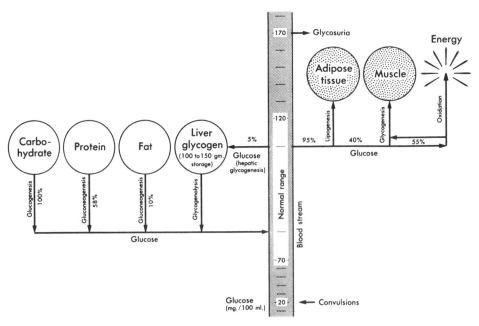

Fig. 16-1. Sources of blood glucose (food and stored glycogen) and normal routes of control.

alpha cells in the islets of Langerhans. This new hormone was given the name "glucagon" because of its stimulating effect on *glycogenolysis,* the conversion of glycogen to glucose. It has an opposite action to insulin and is sometimes used to control more brittle and unstable diabetes. It acts as a counterbalance to excess insulin, that is, as treatment for insulin shock or hypoglycemic reactions. Its molecular structure has been identified and it has been prepared commercially from pancreatic extracts. It is available for injection by a labile diabetic who needs the antidote for insulin.

■ **What happens in uncontrolled diabetes to cause the symptoms of hyperglycemia and ketosis?**

In uncontrolled diabetes glucose cannot be oxidized properly through the main glycolytic pathway in the cell to furnish energy, and therefore it builds up in the blood, causing hyperglycemia. Without cell glucose, fat formation is curtailed, and fat breakdown increases, leading to excess ketone formation and accumulation, the condition of diabetic ketosis. The appearance of one of these ketones—acetone—in the urine indicates the development of ketosis. Tissue protein is also broken down in an effort to secure energy, causing weight loss and nitrogen excretion in the urine.

■ **What are the objectives of nutritional care in diabetes?**

There are three basic objectives in the care of a diabetic patient:

1. *Optimum nutrition.* The patient's basic requirement is adequate nutrition for growth and development and maintenance of an ideal weight. The leaner side of the average weight for height is wise, and any degree of overweight is to be avoided.

2. *Avoidance of symptoms.* An effort is made to keep the patient relatively free of symptoms such as glycosuria and hyperglycemia.

3. *Avoidance of complications.* Complications in tissues such as the eye (retinopathy), in nerve tissue (neuropathy), and in renal tissue (nephropathy) occur in uncontrolled diabetes. An effort is therefore made for more careful control to prevent these complications. Coronary artery disease occurs in diabetics about four times as often as in the general population, and peripheral vascular disease occurs about 40 times as often. It is believed that these chronic manifestations may be reduced or retarded by good care and control.

■ **How is the diet for a person with diabetes planned?**

The fundamental principle of the diet for an individual diabetic patient may be stated simply: *it is always based on the normal nutritional needs of that individual.* His diet is expressed in terms of his total requirement of calories and the ratio of these calories in carbohydrates, proteins, and fats.

1. *Calories.* Calorie specifications are based on *ideal weight,* with allowances for physical activity or added stress, such as growth. If the patient is obese, as many adult diabetics are, the diet prescription would indicate a sufficient reduction in calories to bring about a gradual weight loss. If the patient is a fast-growing, lean, adolescent boy, or a large, lean laborer expanding much energy, the calories would need to be much higher.

2. *Protein.* As a general rule of thumb, the protein in grams is about 5% of the number of total calories. Normal age-group requirements for protein govern the amount indicated for the individual patient, with perhaps the optimum or upper range being the guideline. For the adult man an average of 65 gm. is the recommended daily balance. Thus for the diabetic, 65 to 80 gm. may be used daily.

3. *Carbohydrate.* Carbohydrate should be adequate for need but not excessive. The range is from 100 to 250 gm. As a general rule the carbohydrate in grams is equal to 10% of the number of calories. Refined or "free" sugar should be avoided in *habitual* use.

4. *Fat.* The key word for use of fats is *moderation.* Some physicians advise substitution of vegetable fats for some of the animal fats in the diet to increase the ratio

of unsaturated fatty acids. This is based on the general indication of a relationship between saturated fats and coronary artery disease and the greater risk factor of such disease in diabetes.

A general rule of thumb for outlining the final prescription is the setting of calories and protein according to known standard individual requirements. Then, after the protein calories have been deducted from the total calories, the remaining calories are divided approximately half and half between carbohydrate and fat.

■ **How is the meal pattern planned?**

An important consideration is the distribution of the total diet through the day, since balance is the key concept to diabetes control. This distribution will be influenced by the type of control used—insulin, oral hypoglycemic agent, or diet alone.

1. *Insulin.* The schedule of the day's food intake pattern should be balanced with the type of insulin used and its pattern of absorption and activity peaks.

Short-acting insulin—regular crystalline, semilente. Short-acting insulins cover about a 4-hour period of time, and thus only the one meal following their use. These insulins are usually used in situations where short-term periods of control are indicated, such as in surgery, during labor and delivery, or in periods of illness.

Medium-acting insulin—NPH (neutral protamine Hagerdorn), lente, globin. NPH is the most widely used insulin preparation. Medium-acting insulins usually are given in the morning a half hour before breakfast, reach their peak of activity in 8 to 10 hours (about midafternoon), and last from 20 to 24 hours. The meal distribution may be considered a ⅕, ⅖, ⅖ pattern, with allocations for midafternoon and bedtime snacks. The morning snack is usually more necessary only for the younger child, seldom for the adult.

2. *Oral hypoglycemic drugs.* General indications for the use of these medications

include: (1) maturity onset type of diabetes, (2) no history of ketosis or coma, and (3) the diabetes has been present for less than 10 years. With all of these oral medications a fairly even distribution of the diet is also important. These medications are thought to operate on the basis of the stimulation they provide for limited function of insulin-producing cells in the pancreas. Thus, there is insulin activity going on as the result of their use and distribution of the food to balance with this activity is needed.

3. *Diet alone.* Even if the diabetes requires only diet control, there is still need to consider distribution through the day and a fairly consistent balance of meals. Since there is a limited tolerance for handling glucose, a load of glucose at any one point is to be avoided. There is better overall control with a balance of meals through the course of the day.

■ **How is the diet outlined for the patient in terms of a practical meal-planning guide?**

Using these two factors, the individual patient's diet prescription and the meal distribution pattern needed, an individual meal pattern can be outlined using his personal life situation and food habits as a base for individual adaptation. A careful diet history is an important first step, therefore, in adapting the needed dietary pattern to the individual patient's life situation. If the diet is to be a useful therapeutic tool in the care of his diabetes, it must be realistic and workable for him. A flexible system of food exchange groups is generally used to provide a reference guide for food choices for the patient to use in his own meal planning. This system consists of six groups of foods: milk, vegetables, fruits, bread, meat, and fat, grouped according to approximate like composition. Thus, within any one group, food items can be freely exchanged, since all foods in that group in the portions indicated are of approximately the same food value. Materials for use in instructing the patient concerning the use of this food exchange system may be obtained from the local community's public health nutritionist or hospital dietary staff or the American Diabetes Association.

■ **What should be included in a diabetes education program?**

A diabetes education program should be based on the assessed needs of individual patients. This assessment should include both an educational and a nutritional assessment and an evaluation of the disease status. A checklist such as the following may be used to guide selection of content:

1. The disease—general facts of diabetes, its nature, symptoms, and care
2. The diet—basic knowledge of food values, individual diet plan, and ways of using substitutes; practical guides in marketing and food preparations may be needed
3. Insulin or oral hypoglycemics—details of insulin administration and care of equipment, or use of oral drugs; relation to food intake and exercise
4. Urine testing—methods of testing urine for sugar and acetone, and recording of results
5. Exercise—its value in diabetic control and general health; its relation to balance with insulin and food
6. Skin care and hygiene—for control of infection and maintenance of good circulation
7. Insulin shock—recognition of symptoms and knowledge of action to counteract those symptoms
8. Diabetic acidosis—recognition of symptoms and the need for immediate medical care
9. Personal identification—the necessity for a card or tag identifying diabetic needs, especially if on insulin
10. Educational resources—reading materials and community organizations providing services

Various materials and resources are available for use in a follow-up program. Such a program may involve both individual counseling and group instruction.

The skilled personal diet counseling given a patient with newly diagnosed diabetes is the most valuable means for initiating a stable course. Regulation of the diabetes depends on securing the necessary cooperation of the patient himself. Sound knowledge is the basis of wise action and consistent habits. Therefore, the initial dietary interview and the planning of the diet *with the patient* to meet his individual needs are of primary importance. A number of visual aids and types of equipment are available, including food models, charts, diagrams, pamphlets, programmed instruction material, demonstration equipment and other audio-visual materials. Various references and reading material may be suggested for patient education. A number of community resources may be used, such as the American Diabetes Association and the Public Health Department.

■ **What is Medic Alert?**

Medic Alert is an identification program for persons with health problems, devised through the creative efforts of a California physician. It is a nonprofit service foundation with more than 150,000 American members and affiliated groups in a number of foreign countries. A small stainless steel medallion, worn on a bracelet or necklace, carries the individual's assigned identification serial number, a brief warning of the medical problem, and the telephone number. The telephone number may be called collect, day or night, to reach the central answering service in the foundation's Turlock, California, headquarters, where all member's records are on file and are available to medical personnel. A small membership fee is paid only once. It covers the stainless steel medallion with emblem and a supplemental wallet card. Additional information may be obtained by writing Medic Alert Foundation International, Turlock, California 95380.

GASTROINTESTINAL DISEASE

■ **What factors are involved in diet therapy for various gastrointestinal disorders?**

Diet therapy for any disorder of the gastrointestinal tract will be determined by consideration of four basic factors:

1. The secretory functions that provide the necessary environment and agents for chemical digestion
2. The neuromuscular functions that provide the necessary motility for mechanical digestion and move the food mass along
3. The absorptive functions that enable the end products of digestion (the nutrients) to enter the body's circulation and nourish the cells
4. The psychologic influence, the individual's particular emotional makeup, and his manner of dealing with life's day-to-day problems

■ **What is the cause of peptic ulcer disease?**

The precise cause of peptic ulcer disease is not known. However, two fundamental factors are involved: (1) the amount of gastric acid and pepsin secreted, and (2) the degree of tissue resistance to withstand the digestive action of these secretions. In the development of gastric ulcers, which are less common, although the presence of acid is essential, the degree of tissue sensitivity seems to be the paramount factor. In the patient with the more common duodenal ulcer, excess production of acid and pepsin is the primary factor. In either case, hydrochloric acid in the gastric juice is generally acknowledged to be the essential factor in the development, perpetuation, and recurrence of peptic ulcer. It is understandable that the majority of these mucosal lesions would occur in the duodenal bulb where the gastric contents, emptying into the duodenum through the pyloric valve, are most concentrated in acid. Peptic ulcer usually occurs in men between the ages of 20 and 50 years, a time in life when career and personal strivings may be at a peak. The ulcer-prone individual tends to be anxious and tense, aggressive, and a competitive type of person. The first symptoms of peptic ulcer are usually increased gastric tone and painful hunger contractions when the stomach is empty. Nutritional deficiencies may be present in low plasma protein levels, anemia, and loss of weight. Hemorrhage may be the first sign of the ulcer in some patients. Diagnosis comes from clinical findings, x-ray tests, and visualization by gastroscopy.

■ **What is the basis for treatment of peptic ulcer?**

Three basic factors form the basis for care of peptic ulcer: (1) *drug therapy* and antacids to counteract hypermotility and hypersecretions, (2) *rest*, both physical and mental, aided as needed by sedative therapy, and (3) *diet therapy* to provide maximum restorative powers and prevent further tissue damage.

■ **What two schools of thought govern the dietary management of peptic ulcer?**

Two basic philosophies underline the approaches to care of peptic ulcer:

1. *Traditional conservative dietary management.* In general the traditional management of peptic ulcer has followed a restrictive pattern. The food on such a dietary regimen must be both acid neutralizing and nonirritating. The acid-neutralizing therapy begins with milk and cream feedings every hour or so to neutralize free acid with milk protein, suppress gastric secretion with cream, and generally soothe the ulcer "by coating the stomach." These assumptions have not been supported by research, however. There are gradual additions of soft, bland foods following this initial therapy over a period of time, keeping some food in the stomach at all times to mix with the acid to prevent its corrosive action on the ulcer. These bland foods are usually limited to choices of white toast or crackers, refined cereals, egg, mild cheeses, a few cooked, pureed fruits and vegetables, and later, ground meat. This nonirritating therapy is concerned with eliminating chemical, mechanical, and thermal irritation.

2. *Liberal individual approach.* Accumulating experience and research, however, has begun to challenge the validity of

some of the traditional management practices. A number of studies have refuted the rationale usually given for these practices. In the light of such studies, reasonable principles of diet therapy are derived:

a. *The individual must be treated as such.* A careful and initial history will give information about daily living situations, attitudes, food reactions, and tolerances. On the basis of such a history, a reasonable and adequate dietary program, *which the patient can follow,* may then be worked out.

b. *The activity of the patient's ulcer will influence dietary management.* During acute periods of active ulceration more vigorous therapy may be necessary to control acidity and initiate healing. However, when pain disappears, feeding should be liberalized according to individual tolerance and desire, using a variety of foods. Optimum nutrition and emotional outlook, and hence recovery, are more likely to be supported by such a liberalized individual program. During quiescent periods and for long-term prophylaxis when the patient is asymptomatic, he fares best from judicious choice of a wide range of foods and the establishment of regular, unhurried eating habits.

■ **What basic principles of diet therapy can guide peptic ulcer treatment?**

The following is a summary of the diet therapy principles for peptic ulcer:

1. There must be *optimum total nutrition* to support recovery and maintenance of health, based on individual needs and food tolerances.

2. *Protein* must be adequate for tissue healing needs and for buffering capacity.

3. *Fat* should be used in moderate amounts for suppression of gastric secretion and motility. Where cardiovascular disease is a concern, reduction of saturated fat may be desired and substitutions made of polyunsaturated fat.

4. *Meal intervals and size* should be adequate to maintain individual control of gastric secretions. There should be frequent, small feedings during more active stress periods. Regular meals, moderate in size and sufficient in number for individual need, should be an established habit.

5. *Positive individual needs on a flexible program* rather than negative blanket restrictions on a rigid regimen should be the guide. In any event, picayune dictums and uncompromising prohibitions have no place. Objective research that eliminates prejudiced ideas, and individual counseling that meets personal needs, together form the keystone of wise peptic ulcer therapy.

■ **What general functional disorders of the intestine may be treated with nutritional therapy?**

General functional disorders of the intestine, such as "irritable colon," constipation, or diarrhea, are treated by attention to the underlying cause and symptomatic care. Adjunct therapy with diet may involve fluid intake, modification of the diet's fiber content, and adjustment of specific foods according to individual tolerances.

■ **What is diverticulosis?**

Diverticulosis is a term given to the formation of small tubular sacs branching off from a main canal or cavity in the body. In this case the term is commonly applied to the formation of these small protrusions from the intestinal lumen, usually the colon, producing the condition *diverticulosis.* More often this condition occurs in older people and develops at points of weakened musculature in the bowel wall. The condition is asymptomatic unless the diverticula become inflamed, a state called *diverticulitis.* Fecal residue may accumulate in these small pouches and cause increased irritation. There is pain and tenderness, usually localized in the lower left side of the abdomen, nausea, vomiting, distention, and intestinal spasm, accompanied by fever. If the process continues, intestinal obstruction or perforation may result, in which case surgery would be indicated.

During acute periods, oral feedings may be limited to clear liquids with gradual progression to full liquids. Follow-up diet therapy is based on texture modifications, using at first a residue-free diet if necessary, then maintenance according to individual need on a low-residue diet. Residue is contributed to the diet mainly by four food groups: vegetables, fruits, grains, and milk. Hence, a low-residue diet will involve some modification in each of these groups. The fruits and vegetables will usually be in strained or soft form to remove a maximum amount of cellulose. The grains will be used in refined forms to remove the outer husk and bran layers that contribute the cellulose. Milk is a questionable item, eliminated entirely on a residue-free diet, and limited in use usually in cooked form on a low-residue diet. Milk produces a residue, curd, upon contact with the acid medium of the stomach.

■ **What is sprue?**

The term sprue is given to a general malabsorption syndrome occurring in adulthood. The adult nontropical sprue is similar in nature to childhood celiac disease (see p. 200). In fact, most adults with sprue give a history of having had episodes of celiac disease as a child.

The characteristic diarrhea in sprue consists of multiple foamy, malodorous, bulky, and greasy stools. Poor absorption of fat is evident in the large amounts of fat appearing in the stools as soaps (saponification of fatty acids with calcium salts) and fatty acids. Poor absorption of iron produces a microcytic hypochromic anemia. In other persons a lack of folic acid will produce a macrocytic anemia. Poor absorption of vitamin K may lead to hemorrhagic tendencies. Poor calcium absorption may produce a disturbed serum calcium-to-phosphorus ratio with a resulting tetany-like response. The condition varies widely among individuals, with subsequent differences in severity of symptoms and nature of treatment. Usually the treatment

involves omission of gluten sources. Gluten is a protein found mainly in wheat, with additional amounts in rye and oat (see p. 201). The low-gluten diet will therefore outline sources of wheat, rye, and oat that will need to be eliminated from the diet.

■ **What is the treatment for ulcerative colitis?**

The cause of ulcerative colitis is unknown, and no specific cure has been devised. However, general plans of management are based on efforts to control infections, the inflammatory process, and restore nutrients deficient for tissue healing.

New drug therapy, with more potent antibiotics, has improved the condition in many patients. Ulcerative colitis usually occurs in young adulthood and may have a psychogenic overlay. The common clinical manifestation is a chronic bloody diarrhea that occurs at night as well as during the day. Ulceration of the mucous membrane of the intestine leads to various associated nutritional problems, such as anorexia, nutritional edema, anemia, avitaminosis, protein losses, negative nitrogen balance, dehydration, and electrolyte disturbances. There is weight loss, often general malnutrition, fever, skin lesions, and arthritic joint involvement. Principles of treatment involve three important factors: rest, nutritional therapy, and sulfanamides. There must be physical, gastrointestinal, and emotional rest. There must be vigorous nutritional therapy.

1. *High protein.* Massive losses of protein from the colon tissue result through exudation and bleeding. Also, their loss is associated with impaired intestinal absorption. Only if adequate protein is provided for tissue synthesis can healing take place. The diet should supply from 120 to 150 gm. of protein per day. Protein supplements in between-meal feedings using skimmed milk powder, Sustagen, Geveral, Protenum, or Meritene are helpful to achieve the necessary intake. Tasteful ways of including protein foods of high biologic value (egg, meat, cheese) must be devised. Milk causes some difficulty in many

patients, so it is usually omitted at first, then gradually added in cooked form, such as in cream soups or puddings.

2. *High calorie.* At least 3,000 calories a day are needed to restore nutritional deficits from daily losses in the stools and the consequent weight loss. Also, only if sufficient calories are present to support and protect protein's main catabolic function will the negative nitrogen balance be overcome.

3. *Increased minerals and vitamins.* When anemia is present, iron supplements may be ordered. However, in many patients oral iron preparations are poorly tolerated and blood transfusions are used instead. Extra vitamins associated with the healing process and with the metabolism of the increased calories and protein are especially needed. These are ascorbic acid and the B vitamins, thiamine, riboflavin, and niacin. Usually additional supplements of these vitamins are ordered. Folic acid therapy may also be involved. Potassium therapy may be indicated, because of losses from diarrhea and tissue destruction.

4. *Low residue.* To avoid irritation to the colon, the diet is fairly low in residue. In acute stages it may be almost residue-free (based mainly on lean meat, rice, white bread, pasta, strained cereal, cooked eggs, sugar, butter, and cream). As soon as tolerated, the diet needs to be increased with high-protein feedings. Only heavy roughage need be avoided, since the primary concern is the positive supply of necessary nutrition in as appetizing a manner as possible.

Perhaps no other condition better illustrates the need for a close working relationship between physician, nurse, dietitian, and patient than does chronic ulcerative colitis. The appetite is poor, but the nutritional therapy is imperative.

LIVER AND GALLBLADDER DISEASE

■ **What causes hepatitis? Why is nutritional therapy significant in its treatment?**

The exact organism responsible for hepa-

titis is not clearly defined. It is probably one of a group of related viruses. There are several types of hepatitis, mainly epidemic, or infectious, hepatitis (IH) and homologous serum, or serum hepatitis (SH). However, the resulting clinical syndrome is very much the same. In infectious hepatitis the viral agent is transmitted by the oral-fecal route, a common one in many epidemic diseases. Thus, the usual entry is through contaminated food or water. In serum hepatitis the organism is usually transmitted in infected blood through transfusions or by contaminated instruments—syringes and needles. The viral agents of hepatitis produce diffuse injury to liver cells, especially in parenchymal cells. In milder cases the tissue injury is largely reversible, but with increasing severity more extensive necrosis occurs. Massive necrosis in some cases leads to liver failure and death. Jaundice, the most obvious manifestation, serves as a rough index of the severity of the disease.

After an incubation period of 2 to 6 weeks in infectious hepatitis and 10 to 17 weeks in serum hepatitis, symptoms develop. These include general malaise, lassitude, anorexia, diarrhea, headache, fever, enlarged and tender liver, and enlarged spleen. Convalescence varies from 3 weeks to 3 months, and is a significant period during which time optimum care is essential to avoid relapse.

Nutritional therapy is significant as the keystone of treatment for several reasons:

1. *Optimum nutrition* provides key nutrients for the recovery of the injured liver cells and the overall return of strength. It is the major therapy and the principles of the diet modifications relate to the liver's function in the metabolism of each nutrient.

2. Since the viral agents of hepatitis are unknown, there is no precise correlating drug therapy. Hence, treatment is all the more dependent on nutritional therapy. Two additional factors that support nutritional therapy are bed rest and adequate fluid intake.

The principles of the basic diet to sup-

Table 16-3. High protein, high caloric formula for milkshakes

Ingredients	Amount	Approximate food value	
Milk	1 cup	Protein	40 gm.
Eggs	2	Fat	30 gm.
Skimmed milk powder or	6 to 8 tbsp.	Carbohydrate	70 gm.
Casec	2 tbsp.	Calories	710
Sugar	2 tbsp.		
Ice cream	1 in. slice or 1 scoop		
Cocoa or other flavoring	2 tbsp.		
Vanilla	few drops, as desired		

port healing in hepatitis include the following:

1. *High protein.* Protein is essential for liver cell regeneration. It also provides lipotropic agents, such as methionine and choline, for the conversion of fats to liproproteins and removal from the liver, thus preventing fatty infiltration. The diet should supply from 75 to 100 gm. of protein daily.

2. *High carbohydrate.* Sufficient available glucose must be provided to restore protective glycogen reserves and to meet the energy demands of the disease process. Also, an adequate amount of glucose ensures the use of protein for vital tissue regeneration. The diet should supply from 300 to 400 gm. of carbohydrate daily.

3. *Moderate fat.* An adequate amount of fat in the diet makes the food more palatable, and hence the anorexic patient will be more encouraged to eat. Former regimens limiting the amount of fat on the basis of preventing fat accumulation in the diseased liver are not currently used. However, values of better overall nutrition from improved food intake outweigh these concerns and a moderate amount of easily utilizable fat in the form of whole milk, cream, butter, margarine, vegetable oil, and cooking fat is beneficial. The diet should incorporate from 100 to 150 gm. of such fat daily.

4. *High calorie.* From 2,500 to 3,000 calories are needed daily to furnish energy demands of the tissue regeneration process, to compensate for losses caused by fever

and general debilitation, and to renew strength and recuperative powers.

5. *Meals and feedings.* Positive support is necessary to encourage the feeding process. The patient is anorexic and has little desire to eat at a time when nutritional therapy is the key to recovery. The food may need to be in liquid form at first, using concentrated formulas such as the one in Table 16-3, for frequent feedings. As the patient can better tolerate solid food, every effort should be made to prepare and serve appetizing and attractive food.

■ **Why is protein a key factor in the nutritional therapy for cirrhosis?**

Liver disease may advance to the chronic state of cirrhosis. This term comes from a Greek word, *kirrhos,* meaning "orange." The term was first used because the cirrhotic liver was a firm, fibrous mass with orange-colored nodules projecting from its surface. Some forms of cirrhosis result from biliary obstruction or liver necrosis of undetermined cause, or in some cases from previous viral hepatitis. The most common problem, however, is fatty cirrhosis associated with malnutrition. The malnutrition may develop from other causes, but is usually the result of a long history of alcoholism.

Protein is a key factor in treatment because the underlying malnutrition causes a protein deficiency. This deficiency produces multiple problems: (1) Low plasma protein levels lead to failure of the capillary fluid shift mechanism (see p. 106) when decreased plasma colloidal osmotic pressure causes ascites to develop. (2) Lipotropic agents are not supplied to effect fat conversion to lipoproteins and damaging fat accumulates in the liver tissue. (3) Blood-clotting mechanisms are impaired, since factors such as prothrombin and fibrinogen are not adequately produced. (4) General tissue catabolism and negative nitrogen balance continue the overall degenerative process. Early signs include gastrointestinal disturbances and pain. In time jaundice may appear, increasing weakness, edema, ascites, gastrointestinal bleeding tendencies and iron deficiency or hemorrhagic anemia (a macrocitic anemia from folic acid deficiency) may also be present. As the disease progresses, fibrous scar tissue increasingly impairs blood circulation through the liver and portal hypertension develops. Contributing further to the problem is the ascites, localization of edema fluid within the peritoneal cavity. The impaired portal circulation may lead to esophageal varices, with danger of rupture and fatal massive hemorrhage.

Protein is, therefore, given according to tolerance. The daily protein intake should be 80 to 100 gm. to correct the severe undernutrition, regenerate functional liver tissue, and replenish plasma protein. However, if signs of impending hepatic coma appear, the protein is adjusted to individual tolerance. Sodium is usually restricted to 500 to 1,000 mg. daily to reduce the fluid retention, and if esophageal varices develop it may be necessary to give soft foods to prevent the danger of rupture. Optimum general nutrition should be maintained by a sufficient number of calories, mostly in the form of carbohydrate and vitamins supplied according to individual need deficiency. Moderate fat is used, and alcohol is strictly forbidden.

■ **What is hepatic coma?**

As cirrhotic changes continue in the liver and portal blood circulation diminishes, collateral circulation develops, bypassing the liver. The normal liver, by means of its urea cycle, is by far the most important organ in the body for the removal of ammonia from the blood, converting it to urea for excretion. However, in the diseased liver these normal reactions cannot take place. Ammonia-laden blood approaches the liver, cannot follow the usual portal pathway, and is detoured through the collateral circulation. It reenters the systemic blood flow still carrying its ammonia load, and produces ammonia intoxication. This condition results in coma and is called hepatic coma. Ammonia is formed predominantly in the gastrointestinal tract as a result of enzymatic action on dietary protein. Gastrointestinal bleeding adds still another source, and intestinal bacteria produce more ammonia.

As the condition advances the patient manifests various disorders of consciousness and alterations of motor function. There is apathy, mild confusion, inappropriate behavior, drowsiness, and finally coma. The fundamental principle of therapy is removal of the sources of the excess ammonia. Antibiotics, such as neomycin, as well as purgation by enema and a suitable laxative, may be administered to reduce ammonia-producing bacteria. The diet is the main adjustment of protein. A low protein intake is indicated. Protein is reduced as individually necessary to restrict the exogenous source of nitrogen in amino acids. The unconscious patient will receive no protein, but the usual amounts with impending difficulty range from 15 to 50 gm., depending on whether symptoms are severe or mild. Calories and vitamins are ordered according to need; about 1,500 to 2,000 calories are sufficient to prevent tissue catabolism, which would be still another source of amino acids and available nitrogen. Carbohydrates and fats sufficient for energy needs are essential. Vitamin K is usually given parenterally, along with other vitamins that may be deficient. Fluid is carefully controlled in relation to output.

■ **What is the treatment for cholecystitis?**

Cholecystitis is an inflammation of the gallbladder, usually resulting from a low grade chronic infection. The infectious process produces changes in the gallbladder mucosa, which affect its absorptive powers. Normally the cholesterol in bile, which is insoluble in water, is kept in solution by the hydrotropic action of the other bile ingredients, especially the bile acid. However, when mucosal changes occur in cholecystitis, the change in absorptive powers of the gallbladder affects the solubility ratio of the bile ingredients, excess water may be absorbed or excess bile acid may be absorbed. Under these abnormal conditions cholesterol may precipitate and cause gallstones (almost pure cholesterol) to form, a condition called *cholelithiasis*. Also, a high dietary fat intake over a long period of time predisposes to gallstone formation because of the constant stimulus to produce more cholesterol as a necessary bile ingredient to metabolize the fat. The treatment for cholecystitis, therefore, revolves around modifications in the amount of fat in the diet.

Surgical removal of the gallbladder is usually indicated. In any event, conservative therapy or postsurgical therapy calls for reduction in dietary fat. Fat is the principle cause of contraction of the diseased organ and the subsequent pain, and it should be greatly reduced. Calories should therefore come principally from carbohydrate food, with sufficient protein to meet basic needs. Food tolerances are highly individual, and blanket restriction of so-called "gas-formers" seems unwarranted.

■ **Why is a fat-free or low fat diet still used following gallbladder surgery?**

Even after the affected organ, the gallbladder, has been removed surgically, ingestion of fat will still cause pain as a result of contraction at the site of surgical removal. Hence for some time after surgery it is wise to follow a modified fat regimen.

CARDIOVASCULAR DISEASE

■ **How is the problem of atherosclerosis related to diet?**

The cause of atherosclerosis, a basic pathologic process in coronary heart disease, is unknown. Fatty degeneration and thickening occurs in arterial walls, with plaque formations largely consisting of cholesterol, narrowing of the vessel lumen, developing of blood clots and eventual occlusion of the involved artery. The tissue serviced by that artery is therefore without nutrient supply or oxygen and dies. This dead tissue is called an *infarct*. When the artery is one supplying the cardiac muscle (myocardium), the result is an acute myocardial infarction.

The search for a cause of atheroclerosis has led to a consideration of diet as a highly significant risk factor in the disease process. Attention has focused on lipid metabolism for two reasons: (1) the artery deposits and plaque formations are largely cholesterol and other fatty materials, and (2) an elevated blood cholesterol level (hypercholesteremia) and elevation of other serum lipids is usually present.

■ **What modifications in fat are used in diet therapy?**

Dietary substitution of foods high in polyunsaturated fatty acids for foods high in saturated fatty acid has had the effect of lowering blood cholesterol. However, what the significance of these lowered cholesterol levels is in terms of the disease process is unknown. Hence, principles of diet therapy have centered about controlling both the amount and kind of fat. About half the calories of the average American's diet is contributed by fat. It is suggested that this be moderated to about 35% or lower if weight reduction is needed. About two thirds of the total fat in the American diet, furthermore, is of animal origin and therefore mainly saturated fat. The remaining one third comes from vegetable sources and is mainly unsaturated fat. The fat-controlled diet reduces the animal fat and uses instead more plant fat, bringing the ratio of polyunsaturated fat calories to about half of the total fat calories.

The Council on Foods and Nutrition of the American Medical Association has outlined a series of three fat-controlled diets, each one on three calorie levels, with the ratio of polyunsaturated fatty acids to saturated fatty acids ranging from 1:1, to 1.5:1. These diets may serve as guides:

1. Modified fatty acid content—35% fat, 40% of total calories
2. Moderate fat reduction—fat 25% of total calories
3. Severe fat reduction—fat 10% of total calories

■ **Why may calories and texture also be modified?**

In the acute phase of cardiovascular disease additional dietary modifications in calories may be needed. The basic therapeutic objective is *cardiac rest*. Thus, a brief period of undernutrition during the first few days after the attack may be advisable. The metabolic demands for digestion, absorption, and utilization of food require a generous cardiac output; small intakes of food decrease the level of metabolic activity to one which the weakened heart can accommodate. During the recovery stages the calories may be limited to 800 to 1,200 calories to continue cardiac rest from metabolic loads. If the patient is obese, as is frequent, his calorie level may be continued for a longer period to affect some desired weight loss.

Texture may also be modified in order to reduce the effort involved in eating. Early feedings may be soft in nature or easily digested. Smaller meals, served more frequently, may give needed nutrition without undue strain or pressure.

■ **What is hyperlipoproteinemia?**

Lipoproteins are the major vehicular form of fat in the blood serum. Hence elevation of these materials is called hyperlipoproteinemia. Other terms used for this condition interchangeably are hyperlipidemia and hypertriglyceridemia. In any event the condition is characterized by an elevation of the serum lipids in the blood. The lipoproteins in the blood are produced in two places: (1) in the intestinal wall after initial absorption, and (2) in the liver.

The intestinal wall lipoproteins are called chylomicrons (see p. 20). They have the highest lipid content of all the lipoproteins, containing mostly triglycerides with a very small amount of protein as a carrier substance; hence they have the lowest density of all the lipoproteins. The other major lipoproteins produced in the liver transport fat to the tissues for use in energy production and interchange with other metabolites. These are the pre-beta, beta, and alpha lipoproteins. Thus, the four types of lipoproteins in the blood may be grouped or classified according to their fat content and their density, those with the highest fat content having the lowest density. These four groups are, in order of lipid content:

1. Chylomicrons—lowest density, mostly triglycerides with a small amount of protein
2. Pre-beta lipoproteins—very low density lipoprotein
3. Beta lipoproteins—low density lipoprotein
4. Alpha lipoproteins—the highest density lipoprotein

The causes of hyperlipoproteinemia in general are varied. Sometimes it is secondary to other diseases and hence treatment is directed toward the causative disorder. In other cases it may be primary, in that the cause is not as obvious. It may be caused by some disorder of lipid metabolism, by an abnormal diet or an abnormal response to a normal diet, or by other obscure causes. It is sometimes inheritable. Treatment of primary hyperlipidemia is usually undertaken for several reasons: most commonly it is associated with a high risk of premature atherosclerosis. This is especially important in certain children and young adults. Another reason, less common but sometimes urgent, is to relieve the recurrence of abdominal pain and the risk of acute pancreatitis that may attend severe hyperglyceridemia. Also, annoying and alarming skin lesions called xanthomas may be caused by elevated blood lipids; however, they frequently disappear with proper treatment. In cases of elevated blood lipids, cholesterol is usually elevated also.

■ **What basic types of hyperlipoproteinemia have been identified?**

Five types of abnormal blood lipid patterns have been identified. They are given
below, with the indicated nutritional therapy for each:

Type I. There is a marked increase in
chylomicrons with normal or decreased
beta and pre-beta lipoproteins. This is a
rare, familial type usually found in children. A genetic deficiency of lipoprotein
lipase is the cause. This is the enzyme that
effectively clears chylomicrons from the
blood following intestinal absorption (see
p. 20). Therapy is aimed at keeping the
diet low enough in dietary fat to make the
patient asymptomatic and free of recurrent
bouts of pain. The fat is maintained at
about 25 to 35 gm. a day, an extremely low
level, and the P/S ratio is unimportant.
There is no cholesterol restriction, and carbohydrate is elevated, since it serves as
the major contributor of calories. Often
medium-chain triglycerides (MCT) may
be used as the dietary supplement. These
fats are absorbed directly into the portal
vein and transported to the liver without
requiring chylomicron formation for transport.

Type II. There is an increase in serum
beta lipoproteins. The pre-beta form may
be moderately increased or normal. The
cholesterol is elevated, 300 to 600 mg./100
ml. The triglycerides are normal or moderately elevated. This type is common and
occurs in all ages. A familial form may
occur in early life before age 1, and clinical symptoms are evident in young adult
subjects. Treatment involves lowering the
intake of cholesterol to less than 300 mg./
day, and decreasing the intake of saturated
fats while increasing that of polyunsaturated fats. The familial Type II is usually
not as responsive to diet therapy as is the
nonfamilial Type II.

Type III. This is a relatively uncommon
pattern characterized by the elevation in
the plasma of an abnormal form of beta
lipoprotein. It is characterized by eleva-
tions also in cholesterol and triglycerides
and some elevation in the pre-beta lipoprotein fraction. A characteristic diagnostic
finding consists of orange-yellow streakings
of the palmer creases (palmer xanthosis).
Male patients have an increased incidence
of coronary and peripheral vessel disease,
often before the age of 35. Female patients tend to develop these same manifestations 10 to 15 years later. This type is
usually familial and apparently transmitted
as a recessive trait. The diet therapy initially involves a reduction in weight to an
ideal body weight. Then the maintenance
diet is designed to reduce the cholesterol
and elevate the unsaturated fatty acid content. Thus, it is a diet balanced in fat and
carbohydrate, about 40% of the calories
coming from each.

Type IV. This is a very common lipoprotein pattern, most frequently seen after
the second decade of life and often associated with diabetes and glucose intolerance. It probably represents a form of premature atherosclerosis. The triglycerides
are elevated, sometimes to extremely high
levels. The cholesterol may be normal but
increases usually in relation to the triglyceride increase. About 50% of the patients
with Type IV patterns have abnormal glucose tolerance tests and many have hy-
peruricemia as well. This pattern may be
familial, also. It is usually compounded by
obesity. Diet therapy is primarily aimed,
initially, at weight reduction to an ideal
body weight. When the weight is reduced
the patient usually has lower triglyceride
concentrations. Sometimes weight loss even
returns the triglycerides to normal. An
ideal body weight is an essential part of
treatment. After weight reduction, the
maintenance diet is low in carbohydrate
and cholesterol and high in unsaturated
fatty acids. Alcohol intake is usually restricted, along with carbohydrate, since
these materials tend to increase endogenous triglyceride concentrations.

Type V. This pattern is often seen secondary to acute metabolic disorders, such
as diabetic acidosis, pancreatitis, alcoholism, and nephrosis. There is an elevation in
the chylomicron fraction and in the pre-
beta fraction of lipoproteins. Usually the

triglycerides and the cholesterol fractions are elevated. Patients with familial Type V may have symptoms after age 20 and may have all the features of Type I, that is, enlarged spleen, bouts of abdominal pain, and sometimes pancreatitis. They have varying degrees of intolerance to both dietary and endogenous fat. The diet concentrates on restricting calories and reducing the weight to an ideal level. Sometimes weight reduction alone will return the plasma lipids to normal concentrations. After weight reduction the diet essentially involves low carbohydrate and low fat pattern of intake. The protein content of the diet is usually high to supply energy and tissue needs, since carbohydrate and fat are so restricted.

■ **What is the basic problem in congestive heart failure?**

The basic problem is one of fluid imbalance, the development of tissue fluid, edema, as a result of the weakened myocardium's inability to maintain an adequate cardiac output to sustain a normal blood circulation. The tissue edema brings added problems in breathing and places stress on the laboring heart. There are several causes for this edema:

1. *Imbalance in capillary fluid shift mechanism.* Since the heart fails to pump out the returning blood fast enough, the venous return is retarded and a disproportionate amount of blood accumulates in the vascular system concerned with the right side of the heart. The venous pressure rises, overcoming the balance of pressure necessary to maintain filtration in the normal capillary fluid shift mechanism (see Fig. 8-2, p. 106). Thus, fluid which normally would flow between the interstitial spaces and the blood vessel is held, instead, in the tissue spaces rather than being returned to circulation.

2. *Hormonal mechanisms.* The aldosterone mechanism (Fig. 8-5, p. 112) compounds the edema problem. Since the heart fails to propel the blood circulation forward, the deficient cardiac output effectively reduces the renal blood flow. This decreased renal blood pressure triggers the

release of renin, an enzyme from the renal cortex that combines in the blood with its substrate, angiotensinogen, to produce angiotensin I and II. Angiotensin II acts as a stimulant to the adrenal gland, which in turn produces aldosterone. This hormone causes a reabsorption of sodium in an ion exchange with potassium in the distal tubules of the nephron, and water absorption follows. Ordinarily this is a life-saving homeostatic mechanism designed to protect the body's water supply. However, in congestive heart failure it only adds to the edema problem.

The ADH mechanism (Fig. 8-6, p. 113) also adds to the edema problem. The cardiac stress and the reduced renal flow cause the release of vasopressin (ADH), the antidiuretic hormone from the pituitary gland. This hormone stimulates still more water reabsorption in the distal tubules of the nephrons.

3. *Increased cellular free potassium.* As the reduced blood circulation depresses cellular metabolism, protein catabolism in the cell releases protein-bound potassium, increasing intracellular osmotic pressure from free potassium. As a result sodium ions in the surrounding extracellular fluid increase to prevent hypotonic dehydration (p. 105). This increased extracellular sodium in time adds to more water retention.

■ **How may sodium in the diet be controlled?**

Dietary sodium comes from two sources: salt (NaCl) used as a seasoning in food, and sodium that occurs naturally in foods. Hence, sodium-restricted diets involve control of these two sources. Four basic levels of sodium restriction have been outlined by the American Heart Association and are in general use:

1. *Mild sodium restriction (2 to 3 gm.).* This level may be achieved by light use of salt in cooking but no added salt at the table, and the omission of obviously salty foods where salt is used as a preservative or flavoring agent.

2. *Moderate sodium restriction (1,000 mg.).* This level is attained by the deletion of salt as such in cooking or at the table,

and no use of salty foods. Beginning at this level some control of natural-sodium foods is begun. Higher sodium vegetables are limited and meat and milk are used in moderate portions.

3. *Strict sodium restriction (500 mg.).* In addition to the deletions thus far, meat, milk, and egg are allowed in smaller portions. Milk is limited to two total cups in any form, meat to 5 to 6 ounces total, and no more than one egg. Higher sodium vegetables are deleted.

4. *Severe sodium restriction (250 mg.).* No regular milk may be used. Low-sodium milk is substituted. Meat is limited to 2 to 4 ounces total and eggs are limited to three a week.

■ **Why is sodium restriction usually indicated in the treatment of hypertension?**

Hypertension alone is not a disease. It is a symptom complex that is present in a number of disorders. It is a common clinical problem in cardiovascular disease. Little is known of its cause. However, studies have indicated a link in sensitivity to high salt use. Apparently this relationship may be through the renin-angiotensin mechanism. Improvement of hypertensive patients through use of a low-sodium dietary regimen has been observed clinically. Drug therapy is usually the basic treatment, but adjunct sodium restriction sometimes enhances the effectiveness of the drugs.

RENAL DISEASE

■ **What diet therapy is indicated in acute glomerulonephritis?**

Usually some antecedent streptococcal infection is related to the onset of glomerulonephritis. It has a more or less sudden onset, and after a brief course the majority of patients, especially children, recover completely. In others the disease may progress or become latent only to develop later into chronic glomerulonephritis. There is some dispute, however, as to whether acute and chronic glomerulonephritis are one continuous disease. The inflammatory process involves primarily the glomeruli; as a result of loss of glomerular function, de-

generation of the conjoined tubules follows.

Symptoms include hematuria, proteinuria, and varying degrees of edema, hypertension, and renal insufficiency. There may be oliguria or anuria (acute renal failure) and chronic renal failure.

The diet therapy centers about protein and sodium.

1. *Protein.* Controversy exists concerning the use of a low-protein diet. There seems to be no advantage in restricting protein. In short-term, acute cases in children, nutrition with *adequate protein* is of greater concern unless oliguria and anuria develop. This complication usually lasts no more than 2 or 3 days, however, and is managed by conservative treatment.

2. *Sodium.* Salt also is usually not restricted unless complications of edema, hypertension, or oliguria become dangerous. In such cases, the 500 to 1,000 mg. sodium diet may be used. In most patients, especially children with acute poststreptococcal glomerulonephritis, diet modifications are not crucial. Major treatment centers on bed rest, drugs, and optimum nutrition.

3. *Water.* Intake should be adjusted to output as a rule, including losses in vomiting or diarrhea. During periods of oliguria the intake of water may be 500 to 700 ml./day.

■ **What is the nephrotic syndrome?**

The primary degenerative defect is in the capillary basement membrane of the glomerulus, which permits the escape of large amounts of protein into the filtrate. Tubular changes in epithelium are probably secondary to the high protein concentration in the filtrate, with some protein uptake from the tubule lumen.

The primary symptom, therefore, is massive albuminuria. Other findings include additional protein losses in the urine, including globulins, and specialized binding proteins for thyroid and iron, which sometimes produce signs of hypothyroidism and anemia. Blood levels of plasma proteins drop and serum cholesterol levels rise. As serum protein losses continue, tissue proteins are broken down and general malnutrition ensues, there are fatty tissue changes in the liver, sodium retention, and edema. Severe ascites and pedal edema mask gross tissue wasting.

Treatment is directed toward control of the major symptoms, edema and malnutrition, from the massive protein losses:

1. Protein. Replacement of the prolonged nitrogen deficit is a fundamental and immediate need. The plasma albumin level may have been reduced to 20% or less of its normal value. This is a major factor in the development of nephrotic ascites and edema. Daily protein allowances, therefore, are high, 100 to 150 gm. or more will be needed.

2. Calories. Calorie intakes daily of 50 to 60 calories/kg. body weight are essential to ensure protein use for tissue synthesis. Appetite is poor, however, and much encouragement and support are needed to ensure that the patient actually consumes the diet. Thus the food must be appetizing and in a form most easily tolerated.

3. Sodium. Sodium is usually restricted to help combat the massive edema. Usually the 500 mg. sodium diet is satisfactory to help initiate diuresis. Low-sodium milk may be needed to help maintain the desired high protein intake and yet restrict sodium.

■ **What are the treatment objectives in chronic renal failure?**

Chronic renal failure is characterized by progressive degenerative changes in renal tissue. Few functioning nephrons remain, and these gradually deteriorate. Uremia is the term given the symptom complex of advanced renal insufficiency. Although the name derives from the common findings of elevated blood urea levels, the symptoms result not so much from the urea concentrations per se as from disturbances in acid-base balance and in fluid and electrolyte metabolism and from accumulation of other obscure toxic substances not clearly identified.

Individual patients vary in degree of symptoms and need individual management according to laboratory test data indicating cations of renal function. Usually there is anemia, lassitude, weakness, loss of weight, and hypertension. Sometimes aching and pain in bone or joint are present. Later signs and progressive illness include skin, oral and gastrointestinal bleeding from increased capillary fragility, muscular twitching, uremic convulsions, pericarditis, Cheyne-Stokes respiration (an irregular, cyclic type of breathing), ulceration of the mouth, and fetid breath. Resistance to infection is low.

Treatment aims at correction of the individual nutrient imbalances according to the progression of the illness and the patient's response to the treatment being used. In general, however, overall treatment has several basic objectives:

1. To reduce and minimize protein catabolism
2. To avoid dehydration or overhydration
3. To correct acidosis carefully
4. To correct electrolyte depletions and avoid excesses
5. To control fluid and electrolyte losses from vomiting and diarrhea
6. To maintain nutrition and weight
7. To maintain appetite and morale
8. To control complications, such as hypertension, bone pain, and central nervous system abnormalities

■ **How are these objectives met through diet therapy?**

The general diet must be adapted to meet individual nutrient adjustment needs:

1. Protein. The basic problem involved is to provide sufficient protein to prevent catabolism, yet avoid an excess that would elevate urea levels. Some drastic nonprotein, nonpotassium regimens, such as the Borst diet, composed of butter, sugar, and cornstarch served as soup, pudding, or butterballs, are drastic extremes. With recent advances in the use of hemodialysis, such drastic extremes are not necessary. Moderate protein, adjusted to individual need, will usually range from 30 to 70 gm. and have a high biologic value to supply essential amino acids.

2. *Sodium.* Sodium needs vary also. Both severe restriction and excess are to be avoided. Usually the needed balance is achieved, however, with a sodium intake between 400 and 2,000 mg.

3. *Potassium.* In renal failure the patient's potassium levels may be either depressed or elevated. Thus, individual therapy must be guided by blood potassium determinations. The damaged kidney cannot clear potassium adequately so the daily dietary intake is kept at about 1,500 mg.

4. *Water.* A balance between intake and output must be carefully maintained. Extremes of water intoxication from over loading, or dehydration from too little water, may result. The capacity of the damaged kidney to handle water is limited, and in many cases solids can actually be excreted better with a controlled amount of water. As little as 600 ml. daily may be indicated for some patients, but the usual needs range from 800 to 1,000 ml. daily. Careful records of intake and output are imperative.

5. *Carbohydrate and fat.* With protein controlled, the diet must supply sufficient nonprotein calories to ensure protein use for tissue synthesis and to supply energy. Carbohydrate should always be given with protein to increase utilization of the amino acids. About 300 to 400 gm. of carbohydrate is the average daily need. Sufficient fat is added (usually 75 to 90 gm.) to give the patient 2,000 to 2,500 total calories daily.

■ **What is the modified Giordano-Giovannetti diet?**

This diet is the result of separate work by two Italian physicians, Carmelo Giordano and Sergio Giovannetti. In 1963 Dr. Giordano put his uremia patients on a synthetic diet of carbohydrate (sugar and starch) and fat (margarine or vegetable oil) made into a flavored pudding, served with an additional vegetable and fruit and supplemented with a formula of essential amino acids. All of his patients improved clinically and positive nitrogen balance was achieved. He formulated his approach on the principle of feeding only essential amino acids, which caused the body to use its own excess urea nitrogen to synthesize the nonessential amino acids needed for tissue protein production.

Using the same principle, Dr. Giovannetti subsequently treated chronic uremia patients with a similar diet, adjusted, however, to more nearly meet the tastes of the Italian diet. It was composed of a low-protein basal diet of bread and Italian pastas made with a special low-protein wheat starch, fats, and sugars, selected low-protein vegetables and fruit, supplemented with essential amino acids, and a small amount of egg protein (selected because it has the highest biologic value of the protein foods) (see p. 35). He achieved the same positive effects in reduction of blood urea concentrations and the correction of negative nitrogen balance, and the improvement of clinical symptoms. The diet effectively reduced the production of protein catabolites and prevented wastage of body protein.

In 1965 the same principle formed the basis of a diet used in England for similar patients, adapted in this case to British tastes—milk for tea, a low-protein bread product in wafers instead of Italian pasta. The same improvement in clinical symptoms was observed in this modified diet of 18 to 20 gm. of protein.

Since this regimen was first developed it has been used in a number of United States clinics in a modified form for uremic patients, and similar relief of clinical symptoms has been observed. The modified Giordano-Giovannetti regimen that has emerged in use is based on an intake of 18 to 20 gm. of protein of animal source—6½ ounces of milk and one egg—and vegetable protein, including the minimal requirements of all the essential amino acids. Methionine may be low, in which case this one essential amino acid may be added in the dietary supplement. The daily food plan is summarized in the list on the opposite page.

Practical diet plans and food exchange lists, recipes, and food preparation sugges-

Food plan for the modified Giordano-Giovannetti diet

1 egg

6 ounces milk or one additional egg

Low-protein bread (one loaf) approximately ½ pound, 650 calories and 1.5 gm. protein

Fruit—2 to 4 servings

Vegetables—2 to 4 servings

Fruit and vegetable choices to total 3 to 12 gm. of protein and 1,300 to 1,900 mg. of potassium

Free-food list—use as desired for extra calories. This list includes foods containing little or no protein, such as butter, oil, jelly, honey, condiments such as herbs and spices, beverages such as tea, coffee, Sanka, carbonated beverages, hard candy, sugar, cornstarch, tapioca, and so on.

Nutrient supplements as prescribed. These may contain an amino acid supplement— formula of minimum adult requirements of essential amino acids or only methionine, 0.5 gm. if additional food source is given in milk and eggs, a multivitamin supplement and an iron supplement.

tions have helped to make the diet useful in the home situation. Careful instruction for the patient and his family is essential, with much follow-up help and support to carry out the plan.

■ **What are the principles of treatment for renal calculi?**

The principles of treatment revolve around the cause of the stone formation:

1. Fluid intake. A large fluid intake produces a more dilute urine and helps to prevent concentration of the stone constituents.

2. Urinary pH. An attempt to control the solubility factor is made by changing the urinary pH to an increased acidity or alkalinity, depending on the chemical composition of the stone formed.

3. Binding agents. Materials that bind the stone element and prevent its absorption in the intestine increase fecal excretion. For example, sodium phytate is used to bind calcium, and aluminum gels are used to bind phosphate. Glycine may have a similar effect on oxalates.

4. Stone composition. Dietary constituents of the stone are controlled to reduce the amount of the substance available for precipitation.

■ **What forms of diet therapy are used for renal calculi?**

Diet therapy for renal calculi is directly related to the chemistry of the stone involved:

1. Calcium stones. By far the majority of renal stones, about 96%, are calcium compounds. A low calcium diet of about 400 mg. daily is usually given. This is about half that of an average adult intake of 800 mg. The lower level is achived mainly by removal of milk and dairy products. A still lower test diet of 200 mg. of calcium may be used to rule out hyperparathyroidism as an etiologic factor. Since calcium stones have an alkaline chemistry, an acid ash diet may also be used in conjunction with the low calcium regimen to create a urinary environment less conducive to precipitation of the basic stone elements. A listing of foods according to their ash produced is given in Table 16-4. Cranberry juice seems to have a strong urinary acidifying effect or bacteriostatic value and is frequently used as a dietary adjunct.

2. Uric acid stones. About 4% of the total incidence of renal calculi are uric acid stones. Since uric acid is a metabolic product of purines, dietary control of this

Table 16-4. Acid and alkaline ash food groups

Acid ash	Alkaline ash	Neutral
Meat	Milk	Sugars
Whole grains	Vegetables	Fats
Egg	Fruit (except cran-	Beverages (coffee and tea)
Cheese	berries, prunes,	
Cranberries	and plums)	
Prunes		
Plums		

Table 16-5. Summary of diet therapy principles in renal stone disease

Stone chemistry	Nutrient modification	Diet ash (urinary pH)
Calcium	Low calcium (400 mg.)	Acid ash
phosphate	Low phosphorus (1,000 to 1,200 mg.)	
oxalate	Low oxalate	
Uric acid	Low purine	Alkaline ash
Cystine	Low methionine	Alkaline ash

precursor is indicated. Purines are nucleoproteins found in active tissue, such as glandular meat and other lean meats, meat extractives, and to a lesser extent in food sources, such as whole grains and legumes. A low purine diet thus eliminates or controls these foods. An effort is also made in conjunction with the low-purine diet to produce an alkaline ash, since the stone constituent, uric acid, is an acid material.

3. **Cystine stones.** About 1% of the total stones produced are cystine in composition. Their occurrence is relatively rare, and usually hereditary. Cystine is a nonessential amino acid produced from the essential amino acid methionine. Thus, a diet low in methionine is used for managing cystinuria and cystine-stone disease. It is used in conjunction with high-fluid and alkali therapy.

A summary of the diet therapy princi-ples in renal stone disease is outlined in Table 16-5.

SURGERY

■ **Why is protein an essential element in postoperative nutritional care?**

Adequate protein intake in the postoperative recovery period is of primary therapeutic concern to replace losses and supply increased needs. Negative nitrogen balances of as much as 20 gm./day may occur, which represents an actual loss of tissue protein of over a pound a day. In addition to protein losses from tissue catabolism there is loss of plasma proteins through hemorrhage, wound bleeding, and exudates. Increased metabolic losses result also from extensive tissue destruction and inflammation or from infection and trauma. If any degree of prior malnutrition or chronic infection existed, the patient's protein deficit may become severe and cause serious complications. Thus, the body's protein needs involve the following requirements:

1. *Tissue synthesis in wound healing.* Tissue protein can only be synthesized by essential amino acids brought to the tissue by the circulating blood. These 8 essential amino acids must come either from ingested protein or by intravenous injection. Tissue protein deficiencies are best met by oral feedings. As early as possible an intake of 100 to 200 gm. daily should be attempted, to restore lost protein tissues and synthesize new tissue at the wound site.

2. *Avoidance of shock.* A reduction in blood volume, a loss of plasma protein, and a decrease in circulating red blood cell volume contribute to the potential danger of shock. Where protein deficiencies exist, this danger is enhanced.

3. *Control of edema.* When the serum protein level is low, edema develops as a result of a loss of colloidal osmotic pressure to maintain the normal shift of fluid between the capillaries and the surrounding interstitial tissues (see p. 106). This edema may affect heart and lung action and local edema at the surgical site also delays closure of the wound and hinder the normal healing process.

4. *Bone healing.* In orthopedic surgery, where extensive bone healing is involved, protein is essential for proper callous formation and calcification. A sound protein matrix must be present for the anchoring of mineral matter in the bone.

5. *Resistance to infection.* Amino acids are necessary constituents of the proteins involved in body defense mechanisms—antigens, antibodies, blood cells, hormones, enzymes. Tissue integrity itself is a defense barrier against infection.

6. *Lipid transport.* Proteins are necessary for the transport of lipids in the body and therefore for the protection of the liver, a main site of fat metabolism, from danger by fatty infiltration. Protein provides essential lipotropic agents to form lipoproteins, the transport form of fat in the body.

It is evident, therefore, that multiple clinical problems may easily develop where protein deficiencies exist. There may be poor wound healing and dehiscence, delayed healing of fractures, anemia, failure of gastrointestinal stomas to function, depressed pulmonary and cardiac function, reduced resistance to infection, extensive weight loss, liver damage, and increased mortality risks.

■ **Why is water balance an important concern following surgery?**

Adequate fluid therapy is of paramount importance to ensure the patient against dehydration. During the postoperative period there may be large fluid losses from vomiting, hemorrhage, exudate, diuresis, or fever. Where drainage is involved there is still more fluid loss. Intravenous therapy will supply initial needs, but oral intake should begin as soon as possible and be maintained in sufficient quantity.

■ **What additional nutrients are necessary dietary constituents in the postoperative diet?**

Additional components of the diet give supportive therapy to protein:

1. *Calories.* Carbohydrate must be supplied in adequate quantities to allow protein to do its tissue-building work. Carbohydrate supplies the energy required for increased metabolic demands. Thus, as protein is increased, the total calories must be increased also. A minimum of 2,800 calories per day must be provided before protein can be used for tissue repair and not be converted in part to provide energy. In acute stress, as in extensive radical surgery or burns, where protein needs are as high as 250 gm. daily, 4,000 to 6,000 calories are required. In addition to its protein-sparing action, carbohydrate also helps to avoid liver damage from depletion of glycogen reserves. Fat calories must be adequate but not excessive. Excessive body fat is to be avoided, since fatty tissue heals poorly and is more susceptible to infection, hematoma, and serum collections.

2. *Minerals.* Replacement of mineral deficiencies and insurance of continued adequacy is essential. In tissue catabolism, potassium and phosphorus are lost. Electrolyte imbalances in sodium and chloride result from fluid losses. Iron deficiency anemia may be developed from blood loss or from faulty iron absorption.

3. *Vitamins.* Vitamin C is imperative for wound healing. Its presence is necessary for formation of cementing material in the ground substance of connective tissue, in capillary walls, and the building up of new tissue. Extensive tissue regeneration, as in burns or mastectomy, may require as much as 1 gm. daily, about fifteen to twenty times the normal requirement. As calories and protein are increased, the B vitamin, thiamine, riboflavin, and niacin, must also be increased to provide essential coenzyme factors to metabolize the carbohydrate and protein. Other B-complex vitamins, folic acid, B_{12}, pyridoxine, and pantothenic acid, also have important metabolic roles in stress situations and in the formation of hemoglobin. Vitamin K is essential to the blood-clotting mechanism.

■ **Why are oral feedings preferred over intravenous therapy as soon as they can be tolerated?**

In some patients the gastrointestinal tract cannot be used and parenteral feeding is the only way to sustain the patient. In such cases solutions of hydrolized protein (amino acids and polypeptides) may be used. Some fat emulsions are available for intravenous therapy but are more difficult to use. However, the majority of patients can and should progress to oral feeding as soon as possible to provide adequate nutrition. A comparison of the nutritive value of an intravenous solution with oral feedings will make it evident that intravenous feeding cannot supply nutrient needs. It can only compete with starvation. For example 1 liter of a 5% dextrose solution contains 50 gm. of sugar with an energy value of 200 calories. Therefore, 3 liters a day at best can supply only 600 calories, and the basal energy requirement is about 700 calories, to say nothing of the increased metabolic demands of the stress of surgical illness. Therefore, rapid return to regular eating should be encouraged and maintained.

■ **What types of formula may be used for tube feedings?**

Tube feedings are indicated in cases where the patient cannot chew or swallow in the normal way, such as following radical neck or facial surgery, or when the patient is comatose or severely debilitated.

Table 16-6. Sample tube feeding formula (2,500 ml., 3,000 calories)

Ingredients	Amount	Protein	Fat	Carbohydrate
Homogenized milk	1 quart	32	40	48
Eggs	3	21	16	
Apple juice	400 ml.			55
Vegetable oil	30 ml.		30	
Strained baby food (4 oz. jars)				
Beef liver	4 cans	56	12	14
Beets	2 cans	3		20
Peaches	2 cans	1	1	59
Sustagen	1½ cups (225 gm.)	52	7	150
(Water as needed to total 2,500 ml.)				
Totals		165	106	346
Total calories			2,998	

Usually a nasogastric tube is used. However, in cases of esophagus obstruction, the tube is inserted into an opening made in the abdominal wall—a gastrostomy. The formula will be prescribed according to the need and tolerance of the individual patient and small amounts will be given initially with a gradual increase. Usually 2 liters of formula are sufficient for a 24-hour period, and the feeding should not exceed 8 to 12 ounces in each 3 to 4 hour interval. Two general types of formula are used:

Table 16-7. Types of tube feedings

Ingredients	Calories	Protein gm.	Fat gm.	Carbohydrate gm.
Regular tube feeding				
6 eggs	452	36.6	33.0	—
1 qt. homogenized milk	666	34.2	38.1	47.8
1 C. nonfat milk solids	434	42.7	1.2	121.3
½ C. Karo syrup				
1 tablet brewers yeast				
75 mg. ascorbic acid				
¼ tsp. salt				
1,500 ml.				
	2,021	113.5	72.3	231.5
Sustagen				
3 C. Sustagen	1,755	105.0	15.0	300.0
4 C. water				
1,200 ml.				
600 gm. Sustagen				
(4 C.)	2,300	140.0	20.0	400.0
1,200 ml. water				
1,400 ml.				
Add for banana Sustagen:				
2 tsp. banana flakes				
or	88	1.2	—	23.0
1 mashed banana				
Low calcium tube feeding				
6 cn. strained meat	540	80.4	25.2	0
1 qt. fruit juice	432	0	2.0	108.0
Karo syrup ¼ c.	234			61.0
ascorbic acid				
brewers yeast				
1,800 cc.				
	1,206	80.4	27.2	169.0
Low sodium tube feeding				
1 qt. low sodium milk	666	34.2	38.1	47.8
Casec 90 gm.—3 oz.	306	75.0		
18 Tbsp.				
Karo syrup ¼ c.	234			61.0
1,000 cc.				
	1,206	109.2	38.1	108.8

1. *Prepared formula.* A variety of commercial preparations are available for simple dilution with water or milk. These include nutrient materials in powdered form, such as Sustagen, a protein hydrolysate, or Lonolac, a low-sodium product. These are simple to use when mixed with water in the desired proportions. However, in the higher calorie formula requirements, the amount of the nutrient material needed to fill the calorie requirement renders too concentrated an amount of carbohydrate and diarrhea may result. In such cases a planned formula of balanced ingredients would achieve a more desirable ratio of nutrients.

2. *A calculated and blended food mixture.* In cases where a more desirable ratio is needed, an individual formula may be calculated and mixed in a blender. For example, a planned formula such as that given in Table 16-6 would give a 3,000 calorie tube feeding with a balanced ratio of nutrient ingredients. In comparison, a 3,000 calorie formula using Sustagen alone would require about 5 cups to 2,500 ml. of water and render a nutrient ratio of 180 gm. of protein, 500 gm. of carbohydrate, and 30 gm. of fat. Other mixtures of food may be liquefied in a blender and sometimes are preferred by patients because they feel they are getting regular foods. Any foods that will liquefy can be used, or strained baby food may be used to simplify the mixing. The usual ingredients include a milk base with additions of egg, strained meat, vegetable, fruit, fruit juices, nonfat dry milk, cream, brewers yeast, and ascorbic acid. These formulas may be compared with other sample mixtures given in Table 16-7.

■ **How is the initial feeding program for the immediate period following a gastrectomy managed?**

A number of nutritional problems may develop following gastric surgery, depending on the type of surgical procedure and the patient's individual response. There must be care in planning the diet following a total gastrectomy, otherwise serious nutritional deficits will ensue. When a vagotomy is performed also, there may be increased gastric fullness and distention. The stomach becomes atonic and empties poorly so that food fermentation follows, producing flatus and diarrhea. Following gastric surgery about 50% of the patients fail to regain weight to optimum levels. Generally, however following surgery there is a very *gradual* resumption of oral feedings according to the individual patient's tolerances. A typical pattern of dietary progression (see box below) will cover about a 2-week period.

The basic principles of diet therapy for this postgastrectomy period are (1) size of meals—small, frequent, and (2) type of food—simple, easily digested, mild, and low in bulk.

■ **What is the "dumping syndrome"?**

The "dumping syndrome" is a complication sometimes encountered following ini-

---

Postgastrectomy diet pattern

First 24 to 48 hours	Nothing by mouth, intravenous therapy
Days 2 to 4	Ice chips, sips of water (temperature adjusted to patient response, some tolerate warm water better)
Day 5	1 to 2 oz. water every even hour, and 1 to 2 oz. milk each odd hour between
Day 6	Same feedings—increase to 3 oz. each
Day 7	Same feedings—increase to 4 oz. each
Day 8	Same feedings—add a soft-cooked egg at 8:00 a.m. and 6:00 p.m. feedings
Days 9 to 16	Water as desired, progress to a six-feeding ulcer-type diet
Day 16	Full bland diet; small meals with interval snacks

tial recovery from a gastrectomy when the patient begins to eat food in greater volume and variety. He may experience increasing discomfort following meals. About 10 to 15 minutes after he has eaten he has a cramping, full feeling, his pulse is rapid, he feels a wave of weakness, cold sweating, and dizziness. Frequently he becomes nauseated and vomits. Such distressing reaction to food intake increases his anxiety and he eats less and less. He continues to lose weight and becomes increasingly malnourished. This postgastrectomy complex of symptoms may more precisely be termed the *jejunal hyperosmolic syndrome*. It is more likely to occur in patients who have had total gastrectomies.

The symptoms of shock result when a meal containing a high proportion of readily hydrolyzed carbohydrate rapidly enters the jejunum. This entering food mass is a concentrated hyperosmolar solution in relation to the surrounding extracellular fluid. To achieve an osmotic balance, water is drawn from the blood into the intestine, causing a rapid shrinking of the vascular fluid compartment. The blood pressure drops, and signs of cardiac insufficiency appear—rapid pulse, sweating, weakness, and tremors.

A second sequence of events may follow about 2 hours later. The concentrated solution of carbohydrate is rapidly digested and absorbed, causing a postparandial rise in the blood glucose. The glucose load stimulates an overproduction of insulin, which in turn leads to an eventual drop in the blood sugar below normal fasting levels. As a result, symptoms of mild hypoglycemia result.

Dramatic relief of these distressing symptoms and gradual regain of lost weight follows careful control of the diet. Characteristics of this diet are listed in the box at the bottom of the page.

■ **What diet measures are helpful to a colostomy or ileostomy patient?**

The control of an ileostomy is more difficult than that of a colostomy. In an ileostomy the opening in the abdominal wall is higher up in the intestine where the intestinal contents are unformed, more liquid, and irritating or corrosive to the skin. The ileostomy drains freely almost continuously and should never be irrigated. Thus, it is difficult for many patients to develop a reasonable degree of regularity in relation to meals. The colostomy is more manageable. The normal contents of the intestine at this point are solid or semisolid because absorption of water and electrolytes has occurred in the proximal colon. The consistency of the discharge and its less irritating nature create fewer problems. Often the sigmoid colostomy can be adequately controlled by simple dietary measures and periodic irrigation. Dietary measures may include the use of a low-residue diet immediately after surgery. However, as soon as possible the diet

---

Principles of diet for the "dumping syndrome"

1. Five or six small meals a day
2. Liquids between meals only; avoid fluids for at least one hour before and after meals
3. No milk, no sugar, sweets, or desserts, no alcohol, or sweet carbonated beverages
4. Relatively low carbohydrate content to prevent rapid passage of quickly utilized foods
5. Relatively high fat content to retard passage of food and help maintain weight
6. High protein content (meat, egg, cheese) to rebuild tissue and maintain weight
7. Relatively low roughage foods; raw foods as tolerated

should be advanced to a regular pattern of food, to provide optimum nutrition and physical rehabilitation and to provide an additional means of psychologic support. Individual tolerances for specific foods may be accommodated in the diet, and the patient can avoid those few foods that may cause him individual discomfort.

■ **How is nutritional therapy planned for the patient with extensive burns?**

The nutritional care of the burned patient is adjusted to individual needs and follows three distinct periods after the injury:

1. *The immediate shock period (days 1 to 3).* A massive flooding edema occurs at the burn site during the first hours after the second day. Loss of enveloping skin surface and exposure of extracellular fluids leads to immediate loss of interstitial water and electrolytes, mainly sodium, and large protein depletion. In an effort to balance this loss the water shifts from the extracellular spaces in other parts of the body, only to add to the continuous loss at the burn site. As the result, vascular fluid is decreased in volume and pressure, and there is hemoconcentration and diminished urine output. Cellular dehydration follows, as intracellular water is drawn out to balance extracellular fluid losses. Cell potassium is also withdrawn, and circulating serum potassium levels rise.

Immediate intravenous fluid therapy seeks to replace:

1. Colloid (protein) through blood or plasma transfusion or by plasma expanders such as dextran
2. Electrolyte sodium and chlorine by use of a saline solution, lactated Ringer's solution
3. Water (dextrose solution) to cover additional insensible losses

The amount of replacement therapy is calculated by the "rule of nines" and a formula such as that of Evans' (1 ml. colloid plus 1 ml. electrolyte solution for each 1% of surface burned and each kilogram of body weight). The rate of flow should be carefully monitored. Half of the calculated fluid and electrolyte needs to be given during the first 8 hours, one fourth during the second 8 hours, and one fourth during the third 8 hours. During the second 24-hour period the patient will require about half the amount of fluid given during the first 24 hours.

2. *Recovery period (days 3 to 5).* As the initial replacement fluid and electrolytes are gradually reabsorbed into the general circulation, balance is established and the pattern of massive tissue loss is reversed. At this point there is a sudden diuresis that indicates successful therapy. Intravenous therapy should then be discontinued and oral solutions such as Holdrane's may be used: 3 to 4 gm. (½ teaspoon) salt, 1.5 to 2 gm. (1½ teaspoons) sodium bicarbonate (baking soda), 1,000 ml. (1 quart) water, flavor with lemon juice and chill. A careful check of fluid intake and output is essential, and constant checks for signs of dehydration and overhydration should be made.

3. *Secondary feeding period (days 6 to 15).* Despite the patient's depression and anorexia, his life may well depend on rigorous nutritional therapy during the secondary feeding period. He may need to be fed by a tube, but oral feeding should be encouraged and supported as much as possible. He needs a high protein intake, 150 gm. to as high as 400 gm., to counteract tissue destruction by the burn, tissue catabolism following with continued nitrogen losses, and increased metabolic demands of infection or fever. From 3,500 to 5,000 calories with a high percentage of carbohydrate is necessary to meet these demands. Extra vitamin C therapy, 1 to 2 gm., is needed for tissue regeneration. Increased thiamine, riboflavin, and niacin are necessary to supply oxidative enzyme systems to metabolize extra carbohydrate and protein. Optimum tissue health is necessary for the subsequent grafting to be successful. Since these nutritional needs are so vital, a careful record of protein and calorie value and the amount of food consumed is a necessary tool for planning care. After

initial liquid feedings using concentrated protein hydrolysates, a soft-to-regular diet will probably be taken by the second week or so. Much continued support and effort is needed to encourage the patient to eat, supplying items he likes.

4. *Follow-up reconstruction period (weeks 2 to 5 and following).* Grafting and plastic surgery may follow at this point.

Continued optimum nutrition is essential to maintain tissue integrity for successful results of reconstructive efforts.

In the rehabilitation period that follows the patient needs continued physical, nutritional, and personal care to minimize or avoid any possible disfigurement or disability.

Appendixes

Nutritive values of the edible part of foods[1]

Food, approximate measure, and weight (in grams)		Food energy	Protein	Fat (total lipid)	Fatty acids			Carbohydrate	Calcium	Iron	Vitamin A value	Thiamine	Riboflavin	Niacin	Ascorbic acid
					Saturated (total)	Unsaturated									
						Oleic	Linoleic								
	gm.	(Calories)	(gm.)	(gm.)	(gm.)	(gm.)	(gm.)	(gm.)	(mg.)	(mg.)	(I.U.)	(mg.)	(mg.)	(mg.)	(mg.)
Milk, cream, cheese (related products)															
Milk, cow's															
Fluid, whole (3.5% fat) 1 cup	244	160	9	9	5	3	Trace	12	288	0.1	350	0.08	0.42	0.1	2
Fluid, nonfat (skim) 1 cup	246	90	9	Trace	—	—	—	13	298	.1	10	.10	.44	.2	2
Buttermilk, cultured, from skim milk 1 cup	246	90	9	Trace	—	—	—	13	298	.1	10	.09	.44	.2	2
Evaporated, unsweetened, undiluted 1 cup	252	345	18	20	11	7	1	24	635	.3	820	.10	.84	.5	3
Condensed, sweetened, undiluted 1 cup	306	980	25	27	15	9	1	166	802	.3	1,090	.23	1.17	.5	3
Dry, whole 1 cup	103	515	27	28	16	9	1	39	936	.5	1,160	.30	1.50	.7	6
Dry, nonfat, instant 1 cup	70	250	25	Trace	—	—	—	36	905	.4	20	.24	1.25	.6	5
Milk, goat's															
Fluid, whole 1 cup	244	165	8	10	6	2	Trace	11	315	.2	390	.10	.27	.7	2
Cream															
Half-and-half (cream and milk) 1 cup	242	325	8	28	16	9	1	11	261	.1	1,160	.08	.38	.1	2
1 tbsp.	15	20	Trace	2	1	1	Trace	1	16	Trace	70	Trace	.02	Trace	Trace
Light, coffee or table 1 cup	240	505	7	49	27	16	1	10	245	.1	2,030	.07	.36	.1	2
1 tbsp.	15	30	Trace	3	2	1	Trace	1	15	Trace	130	Trace	.02	Trace	Trace
Whipping, unwhipped (volume about double when whipped)															
Light 1 cup	239	715	6	75	41	25	2	9	203	.1	3,070	.06	.30	.1	2
1 tbsp.	15	45	Trace	5	3	2	Trace	1	13	Trace	190	Trace	.02	Trace	Trace
Heavy 1 cup	238	840	5	89	49	29	3	7	178	.1	3,670	.05	.26	.1	2
1 tbsp.	15	55	Trace	6	3	2	Trace	Trace	11	Trace	230	Trace	.02	Trace	Trace

Food	Amount															
Cheese																
Blue or Roquefort type	1 oz.	28	105	6	9	5	3	Trace	1	89	.1	350	.01	.17	.1	0
Cheddar or American																
Ungrated	1 inch cube	17	70	4	5	3	2	Trace	Trace	128	.2	220	Trace	.08	Trace	0
Grated	1 cup	112	445	28	36	20	12	2	2	840	1.1	1,470	.03	.51	.1	0
	1 tbsp.	7	30	2	2	1	1	Trace	Trace	52	.1	90	Trace	.03	Trace	0
Cheddar, process	1 oz.	28	105	7	9	5	3	Trace	1	219	.3	350	Trace	.12	Trace	0
Cheese foods, Cheddar	1 oz.	28	90	6	7	4	2	Trace	2	162	.2	280	.01	.16	Trace	0
Cottage cheese, from skim milk																
Creamed	1 cup	225	240	31	9	5	3	Trace	7	212	0.7	380	0.07	0.56	0.2	0
	1 oz.	28	30	4	1	1	Trace	Trace	1	27	.1	50	.01	.07	Trace	0
Uncreamed	1 cup	225	195	38	1	Trace	Trace	Trace	6	202	.9	20	.07	.63	.2	0
	1 oz.	28	25	5	Trace	—	—	—	1	26	.1	Trace	.01	.08	Trace	0
Cream cheese	1 oz.	28	105	2	11	6	4	Trace	1	18	.1	440	Trace	.07	Trace	0
	1 tbsp.	15	55	1	6	3	2	Trace	Trace	9	Trace	230	Trace	.04	Trace	0
Swiss (domestic)	1 oz.	28	105	8	8	4	3	Trace	1	262	.3	320	Trace	.11	Trace	0
Milk beverages																
Cocoa	1 cup	242	235	9	11	6	4	Trace	26	286	.9	390	.09	.45	.4	2
Chocolate-flavored milk drink (made with skim milk)	1 cup	250	190	8	6	3	2	Trace	27	270	.4	210	.09	.41	.2	2
Malted milk	1 cup	270	280	13	12	—	—	—	32	364	.8	670	.17	.56	.2	2
Milk desserts																
Cornstarch pudding, plain (blanc mange)	1 cup	248	275	9	10	5	3	Trace	39	290	.1	390	.07	.40	.1	2
Custard, baked	1 cup	248	285	13	14	6	5	1	28	278	1.0	870	.10	.47	.2	1
Ice cream, plain, factory packed																
Slice or cut brick, 1/8 of quart brick	1 slice or cut brick	71	145	3	9	5	3	Trace	15	87	.1	370	.03	.13	.1	1
Container	3½ fld. oz.	62	130	2	8	4	3	Trace	13	76	.1	320	.03	.12	.1	1
Container	8 fld. ozs.	142	295	6	18	10	6	1	29	175	.1	740	.06	.27	.1	1
Ice milk	1 cup	187	285	9	10	6	3	Trace	42	292	.2	390	.09	.41	.2	2
Yogurt, from partially skimmed milk	1 cup	246	120	8	4	2	1	Trace	13	295	.1	170	.09	.43	.2	2

[1] Reprinted from Nutritive value of foods, U.S. Department of Agriculture, Home and Garden Bulletin No. 72.
Dashes show that no basis could be found for imputing a value although there was some reason to believe that a measurable amount of the constituent might be present.

Food, approximate measure, and weight (in grams)	gm.	Food energy (Calories)	Protein (gm.)	Fat (total lipid) (gm.)	Fatty acids Saturated (total) (gm.)	Fatty acids Unsaturated Oleic (gm.)	Fatty acids Unsaturated Linoleic (gm.)	Carbohydrate (gm.)	Calcium (mg.)	Iron (mg.)	Vitamin A value (I.U.)	Thiamine (mg.)	Riboflavin (mg.)	Niacin (mg.)	Ascorbic acid (mg.)
Eggs															
Eggs, large, 24 ounces per dozen															
Raw															
Whole, without shell	1 egg	50	80	6	6	2	3	Trace	Trace	27	1.1	590	.05	.15	Trace	0
White of egg	1 white	33	15	4	Trace	—	—	—	Trace	3	Trace	0	Trace	.09	Trace	0
Yolk of egg	1 yolk	17	60	3	5	2	2	Trace	Trace	24	.9	580	.04	.07	Trace	0
Cooked															
Boiled, shell removed	2 eggs	100	160	13	12	4	5	1	1	54	2.3	1,180	.09	.28	.1	0
Scrambled, with milk and fat	1 egg	64	110	7	8	3	3	Trace	1	51	1.1	690	.05	.18	Trace	0
Meat, poultry, fish, shellfish (related products)															
Bacon, broiled or fried, crisp	2 slices	16	100	5	8	3	4	1	1	2	.5	0	.08	.05	.8	—
Beef, trimmed to retail basis[2], cooked															
Cuts braised, simmered, or pot-roasted															
Lean and fat	3 oz.	85	245	23	16	8	7	Trace	0	10	2.9	30	.04	.18	3.5	—
Lean only	2.5 oz.	72	140	22	5	2	2	Trace	0	10	2.7	10	.04	.16	3.3	—
Hamburger (ground beef), broiled															
Lean	3 oz.	85	185	23	10	5	4	Trace	0	10	3.0	20	.08	.20	5.1	—
Regular	3 oz.	85	245	21	17	8	8	Trace	0	9	2.7	30	.07	.18	4.6	—
Roast, oven-cooked, no liquid added															
Relatively fat, such as rib															
Lean and fat	3 oz.	85	375	17	34	16	15	1	0	8	2.2	70	.05	.13	3.1	—
Lean only	1.8 oz.	51	125	14	7	3	3	Trace	0	6	1.8	10	.04	.11	2.6	—
Relatively lean, such as heel of round															
Lean and fat	3 oz.	85	165	25	7	3	3	Trace	0	11	3.2	10	.06	.19	4.5	—
Lean only	2.7 oz.	78	125	24	3	1	1	Trace	0	10	3.0	Trace	.06	.18	4.3	—
Steak, broiled															
Relatively fat, such as sirloin															
Lean and fat	3 oz.	85	330	20	27	13	12	1	0	9	2.5	50	.05	.16	4.0	—
Lean only	2.0 oz.	56	115	18	4	2	2	Trace	0	7	2.2	10	.05	.14	3.6	—
Relatively lean, such as round															
Lean and fat	3 oz.	85	220	24	13	6	6	Trace	0	10	3.0	20	.07	.19	4.8	—
Lean only	2.4 oz.	68	130	21	4	2	2	Trace	0	9	2.5	10	.06	.16	4.1	—

Food	Measure	Weight (g)	Food energy (cal.)	Protein (g)	Fat (g)	Saturated	Oleic	Linoleic	Carbohydrate	Calcium (mg)	Iron (mg)	Vitamin A (I.U.)	Thiamin	Riboflavin	Niacin	Ascorbic acid
Beef, canned																
Corned beef	3 oz.	85	185	22	10	5	4	Trace	0	17	3.7	20	.01	.20	2.9	—
Corned beef hash	3 oz.	85	155	7	10	5	4	Trace	9	11	1.7	—	.01	.08	1.8	—
Beef, dried or chipped	2 oz.	57	115	19	4	2	2	Trace	0	11	2.9	—	.04	.18	2.2	—
Beef and vegetable stew	1 cup	235	210	15	10	5	4	Trace	15	28	2.8	2,310	.13	.17	4.4	15
Beef potpie, baked: individual pie, 4¼-inch diameter, weight before baking about 8 oz.	1 pie	227	560	23	33	9	20	2	43	32	4.1	1,860	.25	.27	4.5	7
Chicken, cooked																
Flesh only, broiled	3 oz.	85	115	20	3	1	1	1	0	8	1.4	80	0.05	0.16	7.4	—
Breast, fried, ½ breast																
With bone	3.3 oz.	94	155	25	5	1	2	1	1	9	1.3	70	.04	.17	11.2	—
Flesh and skin only	2.7 oz.	76	155	25	5	1	2	1	1	9	1.3	70	.04	.17	11.2	—
Drumstick, fried																
With bone	2.1 oz.	59	90	12	4	1	2	1	Trace	6	.9	50	.03	.15	2.7	—
Flesh and skin only	1.3 oz.	38	90	12	4	1	2	1	Trace	6	.9	50	.03	.15	2.7	—
Chicken, canned, boneless	3 oz.	85	170	18	10	3	4	2	0	18	1.3	200	.03	.11	3.7	3
Chicken potpie—See Poultry potpie																
Chile con carne, canned																
With beans	1 cup	250	335	19	15	7	7	Trace	30	80	4.2	150	.08	.18	3.2	—
Without beans	1 cup	255	510	26	38	18	17	1	15	97	3.6	380	.05	.31	5.6	—
Heart, beef, lean, braised	3 oz.	85	160	27	5	—	—	—	1	5	5.0	20	.21	1.04	6.5	1
Lamb, trimmed to retail basis,[2] cooked																
Chop, thick, with bone, broiled	1 chop, 4.8 oz.	137	400	25	33	18	12	1	0	10	1.5	—	.14	.25	5.6	—
Lean and fat	4.0 oz.	112	400	25	33	18	12	1	0	10	1.5	—	.14	.25	5.6	—
Lean only	2.6 oz.	74	140	21	6	3	2	Trace	0	9	1.5	—	.11	.20	4.5	—
Leg, roasted																
Lean and fat	3 oz.	85	235	22	16	9	6	Trace	0	9	1.4	—	.13	.23	4.7	—
Lean only	2.5 oz.	71	130	20	5	3	2	Trace	0	9	1.4	—	.12	.21	4.4	—
Shoulder, roasted																
Lean and fat	3 oz.	85	285	18	23	13	8	1	0	9	1.0	—	.11	.20	4.0	—
Lean only	2.3 oz.	64	130	17	6	3	2	Trace	0	8	1.0	—	.10	.18	3.7	—
Liver, beef, fried	2 oz.	57	130	15	6	—	—	—	3	6	5.0	30,280	.15	2.37	9.4	15

²Outer layer of fat on the cut was removed to within approximately ½ inch of the lean. Deposits of fat within the cut were not removed.

Food, approximate measure, and weight (in grams)		Food energy	Protein	Fat (total lipid)	Fatty acids			Carbohydrate	Calcium	Iron	Vitamin A value	Thiamine	Riboflavin	Niacin	Ascorbic acid
					Saturated (total)	Unsaturated Oleic	Linoleic								
	gm.	(Calories)	(gm.)	(gm.)	(gm.)	(gm.)	(gm.)	(gm.)	(mg.)	(mg.)	(I.U.)	(mg.)	(mg.)	(mg.)	(mg.)
Pork, cured, cooked Ham, light cure, lean and fat, roasted 3 oz.	85	245	18	19	7	8	2	0	8	2.2	0	.40	.16	3.1	—
Luncheon meat															
Boiled ham, sliced 2 oz.	57	135	11	10	4	4	1	0	6	1.6	0	.25	.09	1.5	—
Canned, spiced or unspiced 2 oz.	57	165	8	14	5	6	1	1	5	1.2	0	.18	.12	1.6	—
Pork, fresh, trimmed to retail basis,[2] cooked															
Chop, thick, with bone 1 chop, 3.5 oz.	98	260	16	21	8	9	2	0	8	2.2	0	.63	.18	3.8	—
Lean and fat 2.3 oz.	66	260	16	21	8	9	2	0	8	2.2	0	.63	.18	3.8	—
Lean only 1.7 oz.	48	130	15	7	2	3	1	0	7	1.9	0	.54	.16	3.3	—
Roast, oven-cooked, no liquid added															
Lean and fat 3 oz.	85	310	21	24	9	10	2	0	9	2.7	0	.78	.22	4.7	—
Lean only 2.4 oz.	68	175	20	10	3	4	1	0	9	2.6	0	.73	.21	4.4	—
Cuts, simmered															
Lean and fat 3 oz.	85	320	20	26	9	11	2	0	8	2.5	0	.46	.21	4.1	—
Lean only 2.2 oz.	63	135	18	6	2	3	1	0	8	2.3	0	.42	.19	3.7	—
Poultry potpie (based on chicken potpie). Individual pie, 4¼-inch diameter, weigh before baking 1 pie	227	535	23	31	10	15	3	42	68	3.0	3,020	.25	.26	4.1	5
Sausage															
Bologna, slice, 4.1 by 0.1 inch 8 slices	227	690	27	62	—	—	—	2	16	4.1	—	.36	.49	6.0	—
Frankfurter, cooked 1	51	155	6	14	—	—	—	1	3	.8	—	.08	.10	1.3	—
Pork, links or patty, cooked 4 oz.	113	540	21	50	18	21	5	Trace	8	2.7	0	.89	.39	4.2	—
Tongue, beef, braised 3 oz.	85	210	18	14	—	—	—	Trace	6	1.9	—	.04	.25	3.0	—
Turkey potpie. See Poultry potpie															
Veal, cooked															
Cutlet, without bone, broiled 3 oz.	85	185	23	9	5	4	Trace	—	9	2.7	—	.06	.21	4.6	—
Roast, medium fat, medium done; lean and fat 3 oz.	85	230	23	14	7	6	Trace	0	10	2.9	—	.11	.26	6.6	—

Fish and shellfish

Bluefish, baked or broiled	3 oz.	85	135	22	4	—	—	—	0	25	.6	40	.09	.08	1.6	—
Clams																
Raw, meat only	3 oz.	85	65	11	1	—	—	—	2	59	5.2	90	.08	.15	1.1	8
Canned, solids and liquid	3 oz.	85	45	7	1	—	—	—	2	47	3.5	—	.01	.09	.9	—
Crabmeat, canned	3 oz.	85	85	15	2	—	5	—	1	38	.7	—	.07	.07	1.6	—
Fish sticks, breaded, cooked, frozen; stick 3.8 by 1.0 by 0.5 inch	10 sticks or 8 oz. package	227	400	38	20	10	—	—	15	25	.9	—	.09	.16	3.6	—
Haddock, fried[3]	3 oz.	85	140	17	5	—	1	3	5	34	1.0	—	0.03	0.06	2.7	2
Mackerel																
Broiled, Atlantic	3 oz.	85	200	19	13	—	—	—	0	5	1.0	450	.13	.23	6.5	—
Canned, Pacific, solids and liquid[3]	3 oz.	85	155	18	9	—	—	—	0	221	1.9	20	.02	.28	7.4	—
Ocean perch, breaded (egg and bread-crumbs), fried	3 oz.	85	195	16	11	—	—	—	6	28	1.1	—	.08	.09	1.5	—
Oysters, meat only. Raw, 13-19 medium selects	1 cup	240	160	20	4	—	—	—	8	226	13.2	740	.33	.43	6.0	—
Oyster stew, 1 part oysters to 3 parts milk by volume, 3-4 oysters	1 cup	230	200	11	12	—	—	—	11	269	3.3	640	.13	.41	1.6	—
Salmon, pink, canned	3 oz.	85	120	17	5	Trace	1	—	0	[4]167	.7	60	.03	.16	6.8	—
Sardines, Atlantic, canned in oil, drained solids	3 oz.	85	175	20	9	—	—	—	0	372	2.5	190	.02	.17	4.6	—
Shad, baked	3 oz.	85	170	20	10	—	—	—	0	20	.5	20	.11	.22	7.3	—
Shrimp, canned, meat only	3 oz.	85	100	21	1	—	—	—	1	98	2.6	50	.01	.03	1.5	—
Swordfish, broiled with butter or margarine	3 oz.	85	150	24	5	—	—	—	0	23	1.1	1,780	.03	.04	9.3	—
Tuna, canned in oil, drained solids	3 oz.	85	170	24	7	—	—	—	0	7	1.6	70	.04	.10	10.1	—
Mature dry beans and peas, nuts, peanuts (related products)																
Almonds, shelled	1 cup	142	850	26	77	7	52	15	28	332	6.7	0	.34	1.31	5.0	Trace

[2]Outer layer of fat on the cut was removed to within approximately ½ inch of the lean. Deposits of fat within the cut were not removed.

[3]Vitamin values based on drained solids.

[4]Based on total contents of can. If bones are discarded, value will be greatly reduced.

Food, approximate measure, and weight (in grams)		Food energy (Calories)	Protein (gm.)	Fat (total lipid) (gm.)	Fatty acids			Carbohydrate (gm.)	Calcium (mg.)	Iron (mg.)	Vitamin A value (I.U.)	Thiamine (mg.)	Riboflavin (mg.)	Niacin (mg.)	Ascorbic acid (mg.)
					Saturated (total) (gm.)	Unsaturated Oleic (gm.)	Unsaturated Linoleic (gm.)								
Beans, dry															
Common varieties, such as Great Northern, navy, and others, canned:															
Red	1 cup	230	15	1	—	—	—	42	74	4.6	Trace	.13	.10	1.5	—
White, with tomato sauce															
With pork	1 cup	320	16	7	3	3	1	50	141	4.7	340	.20	.08	1.5	5
Without pork	1 cup	310	16	1	—	—	—	60	177	5.2	160	.18	.09	1.5	5
Lima, cooked	1 cup	260	16	1	—	—	—	48	56	5.6	Trace	.26	.12	1.3	Trace
Brazil nuts	1 cup	915	20	94	19	45	24	15	260	4.8	Trace	1.34	.17	2.2	—
Cashew nuts, roasted	1 cup	760	23	62	10	43	4	40	51	5.1	140	.58	.33	2.4	—
Coconut															
Fresh, shredded	1 cup	335	3	34	29	2	Trace	9	13	1.6	0	.05	.02	.5	3
Dried, shredded, sweetened	1 cup	340	2	24	21	2	Trace	33	10	1.2	0	.02	.02	.2	0
Cowpeas or blackeye peas, dry, cooked	1 cup	190	13	1	—	—	—	34	42	3.2	20	.41	.11	1.1	Trace
Peanuts, roasted, salted															
Halves	1 cup	840	37	72	16	31	21	27	107	3.0	—	.46	.19	24.7	0
Chopped	1 tbsp.	55	2	4	1	2	1	2	7	.2	—	.03	.01	1.5	0
Peanut butter	1 tbsp.	95	4	8	2	4	2	3	9	.3	—	.02	.02	2.4	0
Peas, split, dry, cooked	1 cup	290	20	1	—	—	—	52	28	4.2	100	.37	.22	2.2	—
Pecans															
Halves	1 cup	740	10	77	5	48	15	16	79	2.6	140	.93	.14	1.0	2
Chopped	1 tbsp.	50	1	5	Trace	3	1	1	5	.2	10	.06	.01	.1	Trace
Walnuts, shelled															
Black or native, chopped	1 cup	790	26	75	4	26	36	19	Trace	7.6	380	.28	.14	.9	—
English or Persian															
Halves	1 cup	650	15	64	4	10	40	16	99	3.1	30	.33	.13	.9	3
Chopped	1 tbsp.	50	1	5	Trace	1	3	1	8	.2	Trace	.03	.01	.1	Trace
Vegetables and vegetable products															
Asparagus															
Cooked, cut spears	1 cup	35	4	Trace	—	—	—	6	37	1.0	1,580	.27	.32	2.4	46
Canned spears, medium															
Green	6 spears	20	2	Trace	—	—	—	3	18	1.8	770	.06	.10	.8	14
Bleached	6 spears	20	2	Trace	—	—	—	4	15	1.0	80	.05	.06	.7	14

Food	Measure	Grams	Calories	Protein	Fat	Sat.	Oleic	Linoleic	Carbohydrate	Calcium	Iron	Vitamin A	Thiamine	Riboflavin	Niacin	Ascorbic acid
Beans																
Lima, immature, cooked	1 cup	160	180	12	1	—	—	—	32	75	4.0	450	.29	.16	2.0	28
Snap, green																
Cooked																
In small amount of water, short time	1 cup	125	30	2	Trace	—	—	—	7	62	.8	680	.08	.11	.6	16
In large amount of water, long time	1 cup	125	30	2	Trace	—	—	—	7	62	0.8	680	0.07	0.10	0.4	13
Canned																
Solids and liquid	1 cup	239	45	2	Trace	—	—	—	10	81	2.9	690	.08	.10	.7	9
Strained or chopped (baby food)	1 oz.	28	5	Trace	Trace	—	—	—	1	9	.3	110	.01	.02	.1	Trace
Bean sprouts. See Sprouts																
Beets, cooked, diced	1 cup	165	50	2	Trace	—	—	—	12	23	.8	40	.04	.07	.5	11
Broccoli spears, cooked	1 cup	150	40	5	Trace	—	—	—	7	132	1.2	3,750	.14	.29	1.2	135
Brussels sprouts, cooked	1 cup	130	45	5	1	—	—	—	8	42	1.4	680	.10	.18	1.1	113
Cabbage																
Raw																
Finely shredded	1 cup	100	25	1	Trace	—	—	—	5	49	.4	130	.05	.05	.3	47
Coleslaw	1 cup	120	120	1	9	2	2	5	9	52	.5	180	.06	.06	.3	35
Cooked																
In small amount of water, short time	1 cup	170	35	2	Trace	—	—	—	7	75	.5	220	.07	.07	.5	56
In large amount of water, long time	1 cup	170	30	2	Trace	—	—	—	7	71	.5	200	.04	.04	.2	40
Cabbage, celery or Chinese Raw, leaves and stalk, 1-inch pieces	1 cup	100	15	1	Trace	—	—	—	3	43	.6	150	.05	.04	.6	25
Cabbage, spoon (or pakchoy), cooked	1 cup	150	20	2	Trace	—	—	—	4	222	.9	4,650	.07	.12	1.1	23
Carrots																
Raw																
Whole, 5½ by 1 inch, (25 thin strips)	1	50	20	1	Trace	—	—	—	5	18	.4	5,500	.03	.03	.3	4
Grated	1 cup	110	45	1	Trace	—	—	—	11	41	.8	12,100	.06	.06	.7	9
Cooked, diced	1 cup	145	45	1	Trace	—	—	—	10	48	.9	15,220	.07	.08	.7	9
Canned, strained or chopped (baby food)	1 oz.	28	10	Trace	Trace	—	—	—	2	7	.1	3,690	.01	.01	.1	1
Cauliflower, cooked, flowerbuds	1 cup	120	25	3	Trace	—	—	—	5	25	.8	70	.11	.10	.7	66

Food, approximate measure, and weight (in grams)		gm.	Food energy (Calories)	Protein (gm.)	Fat (total lipid) (gm.)	Fatty acids			Carbo-hydrate (gm.)	Cal-cium (mg.)	Iron (mg.)	Vita-min A value (I.U.)	Thia-mine (mg.)	Ribo-flavin (mg.)	Niacin (mg.)	Ascor-bic acid (mg.)
						Satu-rated (total) (gm.)	Unsaturated Oleic (gm.)	Linoleic (gm.)								
Celery, raw																
Stalk, large outer, 8 by about 1½ inches, at root end	1 stalk	40	5	Trace	Trace	—	—	—	2	16	.1	100	.01	.01	.1	4
Pieces, diced	1 cup	100	15	1	Trace	—	—	—	4	39	.3	240	.03	.03	.3	9
Collards, cooked	1 cup	190	55	5	1	—	—	—	9	289	1.1	10,260	.27	.37	2.4	87
Corn, sweet																
Cooked, ear 5 by 1¾ inches[5]	1 ear	140	70	3	1	—	—	—	16	2	.5	[6]310	.09	.08	1.0	7
Canned, solids and liquid	1 cup	256	170	5	2	—	—	—	40	10	1.0	[6]690	.07	.12	2.3	13
Cowpeas, cooked, immature seeds	1 cup	160	175	13	1	—	—	—	29	38	3.4	560	.49	.18	2.3	28
Cucumbers, 10 oz., 7½ by about 2 inches																
Raw, pared		207	30	1	Trace	—	—	—	7	35	.6	Trace	.07	.09	.4	23
Raw, pared, center slice ⅛-inch thick	6 slices	50	5	Trace	Trace	—	—	—	2	8	.2	Trace	.02	.02	.1	6
Dandelion greens, cooked	1 cup	180	60	4	1	—	—	—	12	252	3.2	21,060	.24	.29	—	32
Endive, curly (including escarole)	2 oz.	57	10	1	Trace	—	—	—	2	46	1.0	1,870	.04	.08	.3	6
Kale, leaves including stems, cooked	1 cup	110	30	4	1	—	—	—	4	147	1.3	8,140	—	—	—	68
Lettuce, raw																
Butterhead, as Boston types; head, 4-inch diameter	1 head	220	30	3	Trace	—	—	—	6	77	4.4	2,130	.14	.13	.6	18
Crisphead, as Iceberg; head, 4¾-inch diameter	1 head	454	60	4	Trace	—	—	—	13	91	2.3	1,500	.29	.27	1.3	29
Looseleaf, or bunching varieties, leaves	2 large	50	10	1	Trace	—	—	—	2	34	.7	950	.03	.04	.2	9
Mushrooms, canned, solids and liquid	1 cup	244	40	5	Trace	—	—	—	6	15	1.2	Trace	.04	.60	4.8	4
Mustard greens, cooked	1 cup	140	35	3	1	—	—	—	6	193	2.5	8,120	.11	.19	.9	68
Okra, cooked, pod 3 by ⅝ inch	8 pods	85	25	3	Trace	—	—	—	5	78	.4	420	.11	.15	.8	17

Food	Measure	Weight (g)	Food energy (Calories)	Protein (g)	Fat (g)	Fatty acids – Saturated (total) (g)	Fatty acids – Unsaturated Oleic (g)	Fatty acids – Unsaturated Linoleic (g)	Carbohydrate (g)	Calcium (mg)	Iron (mg)	Vitamin A (I.U.)	Thiamine (mg)	Riboflavin (mg)	Niacin (mg)	Ascorbic acid (mg)
Onions																
Mature																
Raw, onion 2½-inch diameter	1	110	40	2	Trace	—	—	—	10	30	0.6	40	0.04	0.04	0.2	11
Cooked	1 cup	210	60	3	Trace	—	—	—	14	50	.8	80	.06	.06	.4	14
Young green, small, without tops	6	50	20	1	Trace	—	—	—	5	20	.3	Trace	.02	.02	.2	12
Parsley, raw, chopped	1 tbsp.	3.5	1	Trace	Trace	—	—	—	Trace	7	.2	300	Trace	.01	Trace	6
Parsnips, cooked	1 cup	155	100	2	1	—	—	—	23	70	.9	50	.11	.13	.2	16
Peas, green																
Cooked	1 cup	160	115	9	1	—	—	—	19	37	2.9	860	.44	.17	3.7	33
Canned, solids and liquid	1 cup	249	165	9	1	—	—	—	31	50	4.2	1,120	.23	.13	2.2	22
Canned, strained (baby food)	1 oz.	28	15	1	Trace	—	—	—	3	3	.4	140	.02	.02	.4	3
Peppers, hot, red, without seeds, dried (ground chili powder, added seasonings)	1 tbsp.	15	50	2	2	—	—	—	8	40	2.3	9,750	.03	.17	1.3	2
Peppers, sweet																
Raw, medium, about 6 per pound																
Green pod without stem and seeds	1 pod	62	15	1	Trace	—	—	—	3	6	.4	260	.05	.05	.3	79
Red pod without stem and seeds	1 pod	60	20	1	Trace	—	—	—	4	8	.4	2,670	.05	.05	.3	122
Canned, pimentos, medium	1 pod	38	10	Trace	Trace	—	—	—	2	3	.6	870	.01	.02	.1	36
Potatoes, medium (about 3 per pound raw)																
Baked, peeled after baking	1	99	90	3	Trace	—	—	—	21	9	.7	Trace	.10	.04	1.7	20
Boiled																
Peeled after boiling	1	136	105	3	Trace	—	—	—	23	10	.8	Trace	.13	.05	2.0	22
Peeled before boiling	1	122	80	2	Trace	—	—	—	18	7	.6	Trace	.11	.04	1.4	20
French-fried, piece 2 by ½ by ½ inch																
Cooked in deep fat	10 pieces	57	155	2	7	2	2	4	20	9	.7	Trace	.07	.04	1.8	12
Frozen, heated	10 pieces	57	125	2	5	1	1	2	19	5	1.0	Trace	.08	.01	1.5	12
Mashed																
Milk added	1 cup	195	125	4	1	—	—	—	25	47	.8	50	.16	.10	2.0	19
Milk and butter added	1 cup	195	185	4	8	4	3	Trace	24	47	.8	330	.16	.10	1.9	18

[5] Measure and weight apply to entire vegetable or fruit including parts not usually eaten.
[6] Based on yellow varieties; white varieties contain only a trace of cryptoxanthin and carotenes, the pigments in corn that have biological activity.

Food, approximate measure, and weight (in grams)		gm.	Food energy (Calories)	Protein (gm.)	Fat (total lipid) (gm.)	Fatty acids			Carbo-hydrate (gm.)	Cal-cium (mg.)	Iron (mg.)	Vita-min A value (I.U.)	Thia-mine (mg.)	Ribo-flavin (mg.)	Niacin (mg.)	Ascor-bic acid (mg.)
						Satu-rated (total) (gm.)	Unsaturated Oleic (gm.)	Linoleic (gm.)								
Potato chips, medium, 2-inch diameter	10 chips	20	115	1	8	3	2	4	10	8	.4	Trace	.04	.01	1.0	3
Pumpkin, canned	1 cup	228	75	2	1	—	—	—	18	57	.9	14,590	.07	.12	1.3	12
Radishes, raw, small, without tops	4	40	5	Trace	Trace	—	—	—	1	12	.4	Trace	.01	.01	.1	10
Sauerkraut, canned, solids and liquid	1 cup	235	45	2	Trace	—	—	—	9	85	1.2	120	.07	.09	.4	33
Spinach																
Cooked	1 cup	180	40	5	1	—	—	—	6	167	4.0	14,580	.13	.25	1.0	50
Canned, drained solids	1 cup	180	45	5	1	—	—	—	6	212	4.7	14,400	.03	.21	.6	24
Canned, strained or chopped (baby food)	1 oz.	28	10	1	Trace	—	—	—	2	18	.2	1,420	.01	.04	.1	2
Sprouts, raw																
Mung bean	1 cup	90	30	3	Trace	—	—	—	6	17	1.2	20	.12	.12	.7	17
Soybean	1 cup	107	40	6	2	—	—	—	4	46	.7	90	.17	.16	.8	4
Squash																
Cooked																
Summer, diced	1 cup	210	30	2	Trace	—	—	—	7	52	.8	820	.10	.16	1.6	21
Winter, baked, mashed	1 cup	205	130	4	1	—	—	—	32	57	1.6	8,610	.10	.27	1.4	27
Canned, winter, strained and chopped (baby food)	1 oz.	28	10	Trace	Trace	—	—	—	2	7	.1	510	.01	.01	.1	1
Sweetpotatoes																
Cooked, medium, 5 by 2 inches, weight raw about 6 oz.																
Baked, peeled after baking	1	110	155	2	1	—	—	—	36	44	1.0	8,910	.10	.07	.7	24
Boiled, peeled after boiling	1	147	170	2	1	—	—	—	39	47	1.0	11,610	.13	.09	.9	25
Candied, 3½ by 2¼ inches	1	175	295	2	6	2	3	1	60	65	1.6	11,030	.10	.08	.8	17
Canned, vacuum or solid pack	1 cup	218	235	4	Trace	—	—	—	54	54	1.7	17,000	.10	.10	1.4	30

Food	Approximate measure	Weight (g)	Food energy (cal.)	Protein (g)	Fat (g)	Saturated fatty acids (g)	Unsat. oleic (g)	Unsat. linoleic (g)	Carbohydrate (g)	Calcium (mg)	Iron (mg)	Vitamin A (I.U.)	Thiamine (mg)	Riboflavin (mg)	Niacin (mg)	Ascorbic acid (mg)
Tomatoes																
Raw, medium, 2 by 2½ inches, about 3 per pound	1	150	35	2	Trace	—	—	—	7	20	.8	1,350	.10	.06	1.0	[7] 34
Canned	1 cup	242	50	2	Trace	—	—	—	10	15	1.2	2,180	.13	.07	1.7	40
Tomato juice, canned	1 cup	242	45	2	Trace	—	—	—	10	17	2.2	1,940	.13	.07	1.8	39
Tomato catsup	1 tbsp.	17	15	Trace	Trace	—	—	—	4	4	.1	240	.02	.01	.3	3
Turnips, cooked, diced	1 cup	155	35	1	Trace	—	—	—	8	54	.6	Trace	.06	.08	.5	33
Turnip greens																
Cooked																
In small amount of water, short time	1 cup	145	30	3	Trace	—	—	—	5	267	1.6	9,140	.21	.36	.8	100
In large amount of water, long time	1 cup	145	25	3	Trace	—	—	—	5	252	1.4	8,260	.14	.33	.8	68
Canned, solids and liquid	1 cup	232	40	3	1	—	—	—	7	232	3.7	10,900	.04	.21	1.4	44
Fruits and fruit products																
Apples, raw, medium, 2½-inch diameter, about 3 per pound[5]	1	150	70	Trace	Trace	—	—	—	18	8	.4	50	.04	.02	.1	3
Apple brown betty	1 cup	230	345	4	8	4	3	Trace	68	41	1.4	230	.13	.10	.9	3
Apple juice, bottled or canned	1 cup	249	120	Trace	Trace	—	—	—	30	15	1.5	—	.01	.04	.2	2
Applesauce, canned																
Sweetened	1 cup	254	230	Trace	Trace	—	—	—	60	10	1.3	100	.05	.03	.1	3
Unsweetened or artificially sweetened	1 cup	239	100	Trace	Trace	—	—	—	26	10	1.2	100	.04	.02	.1	2
Applesauce and apricots, canned, strained or junior (baby food)	1 oz.	28	25	Trace	Trace	—	—	—	6	1	.1	170	Trace	Trace	Trace	1
Apricots																
Raw, about 12 per pound[5]	3 apricots	114	55	1	Trace	—	—	—	14	18	.5	2,890	.03	.04	.7	10
Canned in heavy syrup[5]																
Halves and syrup	1 cup	259	220	2	Trace	—	—	—	57	28	.8	4,510	.05	.06	.9	10
Halves (medium) and syrup	4 halves; 2 tbsp. syrup	122	105	1	Trace	—	—	—	27	13	.4	2,120	.02	.03	.4	5

[5] Measure and weight apply to entire vegetable or fruit including parts not usually eaten.

[7] Year-round average. Samples marketed from November through May average around 15 milligrams per 150-gram tomato; from June through October, around 39 milligrams.

Food, approximate measure, and weight (in grams)		gm.	Food energy	Pro-tein	Fat (total lipid)	Fatty acids			Carbo-hydrate	Cal-cium	Iron	Vita-min A value	Thia-mine	Ribo-flavin	Niacin	Ascor-bic acid
						Satu-rated (total)	Unsaturated									
							Oleic	Linoleic								
			(Calo-ries)	(gm.)	(gm.)	(gm.)	(gm.)	(gm.)	(gm.)	(mg.)	(mg.)	(I.U.)	(mg.)	(mg.)	(mg.)	(mg.)
Apricots—cont'd																
Dried																
Uncooked, 40 halves, small	1 cup	150	390	8	1	—	—	—	100	100	8.2	16,350	.02	.23	4.9	19
Cooked, unsweetened, fruit and liquid	1 cup	285	240	5	1	—	—	—	62	63	5.1	8,550	.01	.13	2.8	8
Apricot nectar, canned	1 cup	250	140	1	Trace	—	—	—	36	22	.5	2,380	.02	.02	.5	7
Avocados, raw																
California varieties, mainly Fuerte																
10-ounce avocado, about 3½ by 4¼ inches, peeled, pitted	½	108	185	2	18	4	8	2	6	11	.6	310	.12	.21	1.7	15
½-inch cubes	1 cup	152	260	3	26	5	12	3	9	15	.9	440	.16	.30	2.4	21
Florida varieties																
13 oz. avocado, about 4 by 3 inches, peeled, pitted	½	123	160	2	14	3	6	2	11	12	.7	360	.13	.24	2.0	17
½-inch cubes	1 cup	152	195	2	17	3	8	2	13	15	.9	440	.16	.30	2.4	21
Bananas, raw, 6 by 1½ inches, about 3 per pound[5]	1	150	85	1	Trace	—	—	—	23	8	.7	190	.05	.06	.7	10
Blackberries, raw	1 cup	144	85	2	1	—	—	—	19	46	1.3	290	.05	.06	.5	30
Blueberries, raw	1 cup	140	85	1	1	—	—	—	21	21	1.4	140	.04	.08	.6	20
Cantaloups, raw; medium, 5-inch diameter, about 1⅔ pounds[5]	½	385	60	1	Trace	—	—	—	14	27	.8	[8] 6,540	.08	.06	1.2	63
Cherries																
Raw, sweet, with stems[5]	1 cup	130	80	2	Trace	—	—	—	20	26	.5	130	.06	.07	.5	12
Canned, red, sour, pitted, heavy syrup	1 cup	260	230	2	1	—	—	—	59	36	.8	1,680	.07	.06	.4	13
Cranberry juice cocktail, canned	1 cup	250	160	Trace	Trace	—	—	—	41	12	.8	Trace	.02	.02	.1	(⁹)

Food	Measure															
Cranberry sauce, sweetened, canned, strained	1 cup	277	405	Trace	1	—	—	—	104	17	.6	40	.03	0.3	.1	5
Dates, domestic, natural and dry, pitted, cut	1 cup	178	490	4	1	—	—	—	130	105	5.3	90	.16	.17	3.9	0
Figs																
Raw, small, 1½-inch diameter, about 12 per pound	3 figs	114	90	1	Trace	—	—	—	23	40	.7	90	.07	.06	.5	2
Dried, large, 2 by 1 inch	1 fig	21	60	1	Trace	—	—	—	15	26	.6	20	.02	.02	.1	0
Fruit cocktail, canned in heavy syrup, solids and liquid	1 cup	256	195	1	1	—	—	—	50	23	1.0	360	.04	.03	1.1	5
Grapefruit																
Raw, medium, 4¼-inch diameter, size 64																
White⁵	½	285	55	1	Trace	—	—	—	14	22	.6	10	.05	.02	.2	52
Pink or red⁵	½	285	60	1	Trace	—	—	—	15	23	.6	640	.05	.02	.3	52
Raw sections, white	1 cup	194	75	1	Trace	—	—	—	20	31	.8	20	.07	.03	.3	72
Canned, white																
Syrup pack, solids and liquid	1 cup	249	175	1	Trace	—	—	—	44	32	.7	20	.07	.04	.5	75
Water pack, solids and liquid	1 cup	240	70	1	Trace	—	—	—	18	31	.7	20	.07	.04	.5	72
Grapefruit juice																
Fresh	1 cup	246	95	1	Trace	—	—	—	23	22	.5	(¹⁰)	.09	.04	.4	92
Canned, white																
Unsweetened	1 cup	247	100	1	Trace	—	—	—	24	20	1.0	20	.07	.04	.4	84
Sweetened	1 cup	250	130	1	Trace	—	—	—	32	20	1.0	20	.07	.04	.4	78
Frozen, concentrate, unsweetened																
Undiluted, can, 6 fluid oz.	1 can	207	300	4	1	—	—	—	72	70	.8	60	.29	.12	1.4	286
Diluted with 3 parts water, by volume	1 cup	247	100	1	Trace	—	—	—	24	25	.2	20	.10	.04	.5	96
Frozen, concentrate, sweetened																
Undiluted, can, 6 fluid oz.	1 can	211	350	3	1	—	—	—	85	59	.6	50	.24	.11	1.2	245
Diluted with 3 parts water, by volume	1 cup	249	115	1	Trace	—	—	—	28	20	.2	20	.08	.03	.4	82

⁵Measure and weight apply to entire vegetable or fruit including parts not usually eaten.
⁸Value based on varieties with organ-colored flesh, for green-fleshed varieties value is about 540 I.U. per ½ melon.
⁹About 5 milligrams per 8 fluid ounces is from cranberries. Ascorbic acid is usually added to approximately 100 milligrams per 8 fluid ounces.
¹⁰For white-fleshed varieties value is about 20 I.U. per cup; for red-fleshed varieties, 1,080 I.U. per cup.

Food, approximate measure, and weight (in grams)	gm.	Food energy (Calories)	Protein (gm.)	Fat (total lipid) (gm.)	Fatty acids Saturated (total) (gm.)	Fatty acids Unsaturated Oleic (gm.)	Fatty acids Unsaturated Linoleic (gm.)	Carbohydrate (gm.)	Calcium (mg.)	Iron (mg.)	Vitamin A value (I.U.)	Thiamine (mg.)	Riboflavin (mg.)	Niacin (mg.)	Ascorbic acid (mg.)
Grapefruit juice—cont'd															
Dehydrated															
Crystals, can, net weight 4 oz. 1 can	114	430	5	1	—	—	—	103	99	1.1	90	.41	.18	2.0	399
Prepared with water (1 pound yields about 1 gal.) 1 cup	247	100	1	Trace	—	—	—	24	22	.2	20	.10	.05	.5	92
Grapes, raw															
American type (slip skin), such as Concord, Delaware, Niagara, Catawba, and Scuppernong[5] 1 cup	153	65	1	1	—	—	—	15	15	.4	100	.05	.03	.2	3
European type (adherent skin), such as Malaga, Muscat, Thompson Seedless, Emperor, and Flame Tokay[5] 1 cup	160	95	1	Trace	—	—	—	25	17	.6	140	.07	.04	.4	6
Grape juice, bottled or canned 1 cup	254	165	1	Trace	—	—	—	42	28	.8	—	.10	.05	.6	Trace
Lemons, raw, medium, 2½-inch diameter, size 150[5] 1 lemon	106	20	1	Trace	—	—	—	6	18	.4	10	.03	.01	.1	38
Lemon juice															
Fresh 1 cup	246	60	1	Trace	—	—	—	20	17	.5	40	.08	.03	.2	113
1 tbsp.	15	5	Trace	Trace	—	—	—	1	1	Trace	Trace	Trace	Trace	Trace	7
Canned, unsweetened 1 cup	245	55	1	Trace	—	—	—	19	17	.5	40	.07	.03	.2	102
Lemonade concentrate, frozen, sweetened															
Undiluted, can, 6 fluid oz. 1 can	220	430	Trace	Trace	—	—	—	112	9	.4	40	.05	.06	.7	66
Diluted with 4½ parts water, by volume 1 cup	248	110	Trace	Trace	—	—	—	28	2	.1	10	.01	.01	.2	17
Lime juice															
Fresh 1 cup	246	65	1	Trace	—	—	—	22	22	.5	30	.05	.03	.03	80
Canned 1 cup	246	65	1	Trace	—	—	—	22	22	.5	30	.05	.03	.3	52

Food	Measure	Weight (g)	Food energy	Protein (g)	Fat (g)				Carbohydrate (g)	Calcium (mg)	Iron (mg)	Vitamin A (I.U.)	Thiamine (mg)	Riboflavin (mg)	Niacin (mg)	Ascorbic acid (mg)
Limeade concentrate, frozen, sweetened																
Undiluted, can, 6 fluid oz.	1 can	218	410	Trace	Trace	—	—	—	108	11	.2	Trace	.02	.02	.3	26
Diluted with 4⅓ parts water, by volume	1 cup	248	105	Trace	Trace	—	—	—	27	2	Trace	Trace	Trace	Trace	Trace	6
Oranges, raw																
California, Navel (winter), 2⁴/₅-inch diameter, size 88[5]	1 orange	180	60	2	Trace	—	—	—	16	49	.5	240	.12	.05	.5	75
Florida, all varieties, 3-inch diameter[5]	1	210	75	1	Trace	—	—	—	19	67	.3	310	.16	.06	.6	70
Orange juice																
Fresh																
California, Valencia (summer)	1 cup	249	115	2	1	—	—	—	26	27	.7	500	.22	.06	.9	122
Florida varieties																
Early and mid-season	1 cup	247	100	1	Trace	—	—	—	23	25	.5	490	.22	.06	.9	127
Late season, Valencia	1 cup	248	110	1	Trace	—	—	—	26	25	.5	500	.22	.06	.9	92
Canned, unsweetened	1 cup	249	120	2	Trace	—	—	—	28	25	1.0	500	.17	.05	.6	100
Frozen concentrate																
Undiluted, can, 6 fluid oz.	1 can	210	330	5	Trace	—	—	—	80	69	.8	1,490	.63	.10	2.4	332
Diluted with 3 parts water, by volume	1 cup	248	110	2	Trace	—	—	—	27	22	.2	500	.21	.03	.8	112
Dehydrated																
Crystals, can, net weight 4 oz.	1 can	113	430	6	2	—	—	—	100	95	1.9	1,900	.76	.24	3.3	406
Prepared with water, 1 lb. yields about 1 gal.	1 cup	248	115	1	Trace	—	—	—	27	25	.5	500	.20	.06	.9	108
Orange and grapefruit juice																
Frozen concentrate																
Undiluted, can, 6 fluid oz.	1 can	209	325	4	1	—	—	—	78	61	.8	790	.47	.06	2.3	301
Diluted with 3 parts water, by volume	1 cup	248	110	1	Trace	—	—	—	26	20	.3	270	.16	.02	.8	102
Papayas, raw, ½-inch cubes	1 cup	182	70	1	Trace	—	—	—	18	36	.5	3,190	.07	.08	.5	102

[5]Measure and weight apply to entire vegetable or fruit including parts not usually eaten.

Food, approximate measure, and weight (in grams)	gm.	Food energy (Calories)	Protein (gm.)	Fat (total lipid) (gm.)	Fatty acids Saturated (total) (gm.)	Unsaturated Oleic (gm.)	Linoleic (gm.)	Carbohydrate (gm.)	Calcium (mg.)	Iron (mg.)	Vitamin A value (I.U.)	Thiamine (mg.)	Riboflavin (mg.)	Niacin (mg.)	Ascorbic acid (mg.)
Peaches															
Raw															
Whole, medium, 2-inch diameter, about 4 per pound[5]	114	35	1	Trace	—	—	—	10	9	.5	[11]1,320	.02	.05	1.0	7
Sliced	1 cup 168	65	1	Trace	—	—	—	16	15	.8	[11]2,230	.03	.08	1.6	12
Canned, yellow-fleshed, solids and liquid															
Syrup pack, heavy															
Halves or slices	1 cup 257	200	1	Trace	—	—	—	52	10	.8	1,100	.02	.06	1.4	7
Halves (medium) and 2 tbsp. syrup	117	90	Trace	Trace	—	—	—	24	5	.4	500	.01	.03	.7	3
Water pack	1 cup 245	75	1	Trace	—	—	—	20	10	.7	1,100	.02	.06	1.4	7
Strained or chopped (baby food)	1 oz. 28	25	Trace	Trace	—	—	—	6	2	.1	140	Trace	.01	.2	1
Dried															
Uncooked	1 cup 160	420	5	1	—	—	—	109	77	9.6	6,240	.02	.31	8.5	28
Cooked, unsweetened, 10-12 halves and 6 tbsp. liquid	1 cup 270	220	3	1	—	—	—	58	41	5.1	3,290	.01	.15	4.2	6
Frozen															
Carton, 12 oz., not thawed	1 carton 340	300	1	Trace	—	—	—	77	14	1.7	2,210	.03	.14	2.4	[12]135
Can, 16 oz., not thawed	1 can 454	400	2	Trace	—	—	—	103	18	2.3	2,950	.05	.18	3.2	[12]181
Peach nectar, canned	1 cup 250	120	Trace	Trace	—	—	—	31	10	.5	1,080	.02	.05	1.0	1
Pears															
Raw, 3 by 2½-inch diameter[5]	182	100	1	1	—	—	—	25	13	.5	30	.04	.07	.2	7
Canned, solids and liquid															
Syrup pack, heavy															
Halves or slices	1 cup 255	195	1	1	—	—	—	50	13	.5	Trace	.03	.05	.3	4
Halves (medium) and 2 tbsp. syrup	117	90	Trace	Trace	—	—	—	23	6	.2	Trace	.01	.02	.2	2

Food	Measure	Weight (g)	Food energy	Protein	Fat			Carbohydrate	Calcium	Iron	Vitamin A	Thiamine	Riboflavin	Niacin	Ascorbic acid
Water pack	1 cup	243	80	Trace	Trace	—	—	—	20	12	.5	Trace	.02	.05	.3	4
Strained or chopped (baby food)	1 oz.	28	20	Trace	Trace	—	—	—	5	2	.1	10	Trace	.01	.1	1
Pear nectar, canned	1 cup	250	130	1	Trace	—	—	—	33	8	.2	Trace	.01	.05	Trace	1
Persimmons, Japanese or kaki, raw, seedless, 2½-inch diameter[5]	1	125	75	1	Trace	—	—	—	20	6	.4	2,740	.01	.02	.1	11
Pineapple																
Raw, diced	1 cup	140	75	1	Trace	—	—	—	19	24	.7	100	.12	.04	.3	24
Canned, heavy syrup pack, solids and liquid																
Crushed	1 cup	260	195	1	Trace	—	—	—	50	29	.8	120	.20	.06	.5	17
Sliced, slices and juice	2 small or 1 large and 2 tbsp. juice	122	90	Trace	Trace	—	—	—	24	13	.4	50	.09	.03	.2	8
Pineapple juice, canned	1 cup	249	135	1	Trace	—	—	—	34	37	.7	120	.12	.04	.5	22
Plums, all except prunes																
Raw, 2-inch diameter, about 2 ounces[5]	1	60	25	Trace	Trace	—	—	—	7	7	.3	140	.02	.02	.3	3
Canned, syrup pack (Italian prunes)																
Plums (with pits) and juice[5]	1 cup	256	205	1	Trace	—	—	—	53	22	2.2	2,970	.05	.05	.9	4
Plums (without pits) and juice	3 plums and 2 tbsp. juice	122	100	Trace	Trace	—	—	—	26	11	1.1	1,470	.03	.02	.5	2
Prunes, dried, "softenized," medium																
Uncooked[5]	4	32	70	1	Trace	—	—	—	18	14	1.1	440	.02	.04	.4	1
Cooked, unsweetened, 17-18 prunes and ⅓ cup liquid[5]	1 cup	270	295	2	1	—	—	—	78	60	4.5	1,860	.08	.18	1.7	2
Prunes with tapioca, canned, strained or junior (baby food)[5]	1 oz.	28	25	Trace	Trace	—	—	—	6	2	.3	110	.01	.02	.1	1
Prune juice, canned	1 cup	256	200	1	Trace	—	—	—	49	36	10.5	—	.02	.03	1.1	4
Raisin, dried	1 cup	160	460	4	Trace	—	—	—	124	99	5.6	30	.18	.13	.9	2

[5]Measure and weight apply to entire vegetable or fruit including parts not usually eaten.

[11]Based on yellow-fleshed varieties; for white-fleshed varieties value is about 50 I.U. per 114-gram peach and 80 I.U. per cup of sliced peaches.

[12]Average weighted in accordance with commercial freezing practices. For products without added ascorbic acid, value is about 37 milligrams per 12-ounce carton and 50 milligrams per 16-ounce can; for those with added ascorbic acid, 139 milligrams per 12 ounces and 186 milligrams per 16 ounces.

Food, approximate measure, and weight (in grams)		gm.	Food energy	Protein	Fat (total lipid)	Fatty acids Saturated (total)	Unsaturated Oleic	Unsaturated Linoleic	Carbohydrate	Calcium	Iron	Vitamin A value	Thiamine	Riboflavin	Niacin	Ascorbic acid
		gm.	(Calories)	(gm.)	(gm.)	(gm.)	(gm.)	(gm.)	(gm.)	(mg.)	(mg.)	(I.U.)	(mg.)	(mg.)	(mg.)	(mg.)
Raspberries, red																
Raw	1 cup	123	70	1	1	—	—	—	17	27	1.1	160	.04	.11	1.1	31
Frozen, 10 oz. carton, not thawed	1 carton	284	275	2	1	—	—	—	70	37	1.7	200	.06	.17	1.7	59
Rhubarb, cooked, sugar added	1 cup	272	385	1	Trace	—	—	—	98	212	1.6	220	.06	.15	.7	17
Strawberries																
Raw, capped	1 cup	149	55	1	1	—	—	—	13	31	1.5	90	.04	.10	1.0	88
Frozen, 10-oz. carton, not thawed	1 carton	284	310	1	1	—	—	—	79	40	2.0	90	.06	.17	1.5	150
Frozen, 16-ounce can, not thawed	1 can	454	495	2	1	—	—	—	126	64	3.2	150	.09	.27	2.4	240
Tangerines, raw, medium, 2½-inch diameter, about 4 per pound[5]		114	40	1	Trace	—	—	—	10	34	.3	350	.05	.02	.1	26
Tangerine juice																
Tangerine juice																
Canned, unsweetened	1 cup	248	105	1	Trace	—	—	—	25	45	.5	1,040	.14	.04	.3	56
Frozen concentrate Undiluted, can, 6 fluid oz.	1 can	210	340	4	1	—	—	—	80	130	1.5	3,070	.43	.12	.9	202
Diluted with 3 parts water, by volume	1 cup	248	115	1	Trace	—	—	—	27	45	.5	1,020	.14	.04	.3	67
Watermelon, raw, wedge, 4 by 8 inches (1/16 of 10 by 16-inch melon, about 2 pounds with rind)[5]	1 wedge	925	115	2	1	—	—	—	27	30	2.1	2,510	.13	.13	.7	30
Barley, pearled, light, uncooked	1 cup	203	710	17	2	Trace	1	1	160	32	4.1	0	.25	.17	6.3	0
Biscuits, baking powder with enriched flour, 2½-inch diameter	1	38	140	3	6	2	3	1	17	46	.6	Trace	.08	.08	.7	Trace
Bran flakes (40 percent bran) added thiamine	1 oz.	28	85	3	1	—	—	—	23	20	1.2	0	.11	.05	1.7	0

Food	Measure															
Bread																
Boston brown bread, slice, 3 by ¾ inch	1 slice	48	100	3	1	—	—	—	22	43	.9	0	.05	.03	.6	0
Cracked-wheat bread																
Loaf, 1-pound, 20 slices	1 loaf	454	1,190	39	10	2	5	2	236	399	5.0	Trace	.53	.42	5.8	Trace
Slice	1	23	60	2	1	—	—	—	12	20	.3	Trace	.03	.02	.3	Trace
French or Vienna bread																
Enriched, 1-pound loaf	1 loaf	454	1,315	41	14	3	8	2	251	195	10.0	Trace	1.26	.98	11.3	Trace
Unenriched, 1-pound loaf	1 loaf	454	1,315	41	14	3	8	2	251	195	3.2	Trace	.39	.39	3.6	Trace
Italian bread																
Enriched, 1-pound loaf	1 loaf	454	1,250	41	4	Trace	1	2	256	77	10.0	0	1.31	.93	11.7	0
Unenriched, 1-pound loaf	1 loaf	454	1,250	41	4	Trace	1	2	256	77	3.2	0	.39	.27	3.6	0
Raisin bread																
Loaf, 1-pound, 20 slices	1 loaf	454	1,190	30	13	3	8	2	243	322	5.9	Trace	.24	.42	3.0	Trace
Slice	1	23	60	2	1	—	—	—	12	16	.3	Trace	.01	.02	.2	Trace
Rye bread																
American, light (⅓ rye, ⅔ wheat)																
Loaf, 1-pound, 20 slices	1 loaf	454	1,100	41	5	—	—	—	236	340	7.3	0	.81	.33	6.4	0
Slice	1	23	55	2	Trace	—	—	—	12	17	.4	0	.04	.02	.3	0
Pumpernickel, loaf, 1 pound	1 loaf	454	1,115	41	5	—	—	—	241	381	10.9	0	1.05	.63	5.4	0
White bread, enriched																
1 to 2 percent nonfat dry milk																
Loaf, 1-pound, 20 slices	1 loaf	454	1,225	39	15	3	8	2	229	318	10.9	Trace	1.13	.77	10.4	Trace
Slice	1	23	60	2	1	Trace	Trace	Trace	12	16	.6	Trace	.06	.04	.5	Trace
3 to 4 percent nonfat dry milk[13]																
Loaf, 1-pound	1	454	1,225	39	15	3	8	2	229	381	11.3	Trace	1.13	.95	10.8	Trace
Slice, 20 per loaf	1	23	60	2	1	Trace	Trace	Trace	12	19	.6	Trace	.06	.05	.6	Trace
Slice, toasted	1	20	60	2	1	Trace	Trace	Trace	12	19	.6	Trace	.05	.05	.6	Trace
Slice, 26 per loaf	1	17	45	1	1	Trace	Trace	Trace	9	14	.4	Trace	.04	.04	.4	Trace

[5] Measure and weight apply to entire vegetable or fruit including parts not usually eaten.
[13] When the amount of nonfat dry milk in commercial white bread is unknown, values for bread with 3 to 4% nonfat dry milk are suggested.

Food, approximate measure, and weight (in grams)		gm.	Food energy (Calories)	Pro-tein (gm.)	Fat (total lipid) (gm.)	Fatty acids			Carbo-hydrate (gm.)	Cal-cium (mg.)	Iron (mg.)	Vita-min A value (I.U.)	Thia-mine (mg.)	Ribo-flavin (mg.)	Niacin (mg.)	Ascor-bic acid (mg.)
						Satu-rated (total) (gm.)	Unsaturated Oleic (gm.)	Unsaturated Linoleic (gm.)								
Bread—cont'd																
White bread, enriched—cont'd																
5 to 6 percent nonfat dry milk																
Loaf, 1-pound, 20 slices	1 loaf	454	1,245	41	17	4	10	2	228	435	11.3	Trace	1.22	.91	11.0	Trace
Slice	1	23	65	2	1	Trace	Trace	Trace	12	22	.6	Trace	.06	.05	.6	Trace
White bread, unenriched																
1 to 2 percent nonfat dry milk																
Loaf, 1-pound, 20 slices	1 loaf	454	1,225	39	15	3	8	2	229	318	3.2	Trace	.40	.36	5.6	Trace
Slice	1	23	60	2	1	Trace	Trace	Trace	12	16	.2	Trace	.02	.02	.3	Trace
3 to 4 percent nonfat dry milk[13]																
Loaf, 1-pound	1 loaf	454	1,225	39	15	3	8	—	229	381	3.2	Trace	.31	.39	5.0	Trace
Slice, 20 per loaf	1 slice	23	60	2	1	Trace	Trace	Trace	12	19	.2	Trace	.02	.02	.3	Trace
Slice, toasted	1	20	60	2	1	Trace	Trace	Trace	12	19	.2	Trace	.01	.02	.3	Trace
Slice, 26 per loaf	1 slice	17	45	1	1	Trace	Trace	Trace	9	14	.1	Trace	.01	.01	.2	Trace
5 to 6 percent nonfat dry milk																
Loaf, 1-pound, 20 slices	1 loaf	454	1,245	41	17	4	10	2	228	435	3.2	Trace	.32	.39	4.1	Trace
Slice	1	23	65	2	1	Trace	Trace	Trace	12	22	.2	Trace	.02	.03	.2	Trace
Whole-wheat bread, made with 2 percent nonfat dry milk																
Loaf, 1-pound, 20 slices	1 loaf	454	1,105	48	14	3	6	3	216	449	10.4	Trace	1.17	.56	12.9	Trace
Slice	1	23	55	2	1	Trace	Trace	Trace	11	23	.5	Trace	.06	.03	.7	Trace
Slice, toasted	1	19	55	2	1	Trace	Trace	Trace	11	22	.5	Trace	.05	.03	.6	Trace
Breadcrumbs, dry, grated	1 cup	88	345	11	4	1	2	1	65	107	3.2	Trace	.19	.26	3.1	Trace
Cakes[14]																
Angelfood cake; sector, 2-inch (1/12 of 8-inch-diameter cake)	1 sector	40	110	3	Trace	—	—	—	24	4	.1	0	Trace	.06	.1	0
Chocolate cake, chocolate icing; sector, 2-inch (1/16 of 10-inch-diameter layer cake)	1 sector	120	445	5	20	8	10	1	67	84	1.2	[15]190	.03	.12	.3	Trace

Food	Measure															
Fruitcake, dark (made with enriched flour); piece, 2 by 2 by ½ inch	1 piece	30	115	1	5	1	3	1	18	22	.8	[15]40	.04	.04	.2	Trace
Gingerbread (made with enriched flour); piece, 2 by 2 by 2 inches	1 piece	55	175	2	6	1	4	Trace	29	37	1.3	50	.06	.06	.5	0
Plain cake and cupcakes, without icing																
Piece, 3 by 2 by 1½ inches	1	55	200	2	8	2	5	1	31	35	.2	[15]90	.01	.05	.1	Trace
Cupcake, 2¾-inch diameter	1	40	145	2	6	1	3	Trace	22	26	.2	[15]70	.01	.03	.1	Trace
Plain cake and cupcakes, with chocolate icing																
Sector, 2-inch (1/16 of 10-inch-layer cake)	1	100	370	4	14	5	7	1	59	63	.6	[15]180	.02	.09	.2	Trace
Cupcake, 2¾-inch diameter	1	50	185	2	7	2	4	Trace	30	32	.3	[15]90	.01	.04	.1	Trace
Poundcake, old-fashioned (equal weights flour, sugar, fat, eggs); slice, 2¾ by 3 by ⅝ inch	1 slice	30	140	2	9	2	5	1	14	6	.2	[15]80	.01	.03	.1	0
Sponge cake; sector, 2-inch (1/12 of 8-inch-diameter cake)	1	40	120	3	2	1	1	Trace	22	12	.5	180	.02	.06	.1	Trace
Cookies																
Plain and assorted, 3-inch diameter	1 cooky	25	120	1	5	—	—	—	18	9	.2	20	.01	.01	.1	Trace
Fig bars, small	1	16	55	1	1	—	—	—	12	12	.2	20	.01	.01	.1	Trace
Corn, rice and wheat flakes, mixed, added nutrients	1 oz.	28	110	2	Trace	—	—	—	24	11	.5	0	.11	—	.9	0
Corn flakes, added nutrients																
Plain	1 oz.	28	110	2	Trace	—	—	—	24	5	.4	0	.12	.02	.6	0
Sugar-covered	1 oz.	28	110	1	Trace	—	—	—	26	3	.3	0	.12	.01	.5	0

[13]When the amount of nonfat dry milk in commercial white bread is unknown, values for bread with 3 to 4% nonfat dry milk are suggested.

[14]Unenriched cake flour and vegetable cooking fat used unless otherwise specified.

[15]If the fat used in the recipe is butter or fortified margarine, the vitamin A value for chocolate icing will be 490 I.U. per 2-inch sector; 100 I.U. for fruitcake; for chocolate cake with chocolate icing, 440 I.U. per 2-inch sector; 220 I.U. per cupcake; for plain cake without icing, 300 I.U. per piece; 220 I.U. per cupcake; for plain cake with icing, 440 I.U. per 2-inch sector; 220 I.U. per cupcake; and 300 I.U. for poundcake.

Food, approximate measure, and weight (in grams)		Food energy	Pro-tein	Fat (total lipid)	Fatty acids			Carbo-hydrate	Cal-cium	Iron	Vita-min A value	Thia-mine	Ribo-flavin	Niacin	Ascor-bic acid
					Satu-rated (total)	Unsaturated Oleic	Linoleic								
	gm.	(Calo-ries)	(gm.)	(gm.)	(gm.)	(gm.)	(gm.)	(gm.)	(mg.)	(mg.)	(I.U.)	(mg.)	(mg.)	(mg.)	(mg.)
Corn grits, degermed, cooked															
Enriched 1 cup	242	120	3	Trace	—	—	—	27	2	[16].7	[17]150	[16].10	[16].07	[16]1.0	0
Unenriched 1 cup	242	120	3	Trace	—	—	—	27	2	.2	[17]150	.05	.02	.5	0
Cornmeal, white or yellow, dry															
Whole ground, unbolted 1 cup	118	420	11	5	1	2	2	87	24	2.8	[17]600	.45	.13	2.4	0
Degermed, enriched 1 cup	145	525	11	2	Trace	1	1	114	9	[16]4.2	[17]640	[16].64	[16].38	[16]5.1	0
Corn muffins, made with enriched degermed cornmeal and enriched flour; muffin, 2¾-inch diameter 1 muffin	48	150	3	5	2	2	Trace	23	50	.8	[18]80	.09	.11	.8	Trace
Corn, puffed, pre-sweetened, added nutrients 1 oz.	28	110	1	Trace	—	—	—	26	3	.5	0	.12	.05	.6	0
Corn, shredded, added nutrients 1 oz.	28	110	2	Trace	—	—	—	25	1	.7	0	.12	.05	.6	0
Crackers															
Graham, plain 4 small or 2 medium	14	55	1	1	—	—	—	10	6	.2	0	.01	.03	.2	0
Saltines, 2 inches squares 2 crackers	8	35	1	1	—	—	—	6	2	.1	0	Trace	Trace	.1	0
Soda															
Cracker, 2½ inches square 2 crackers	11	50	1	1	Trace	1	Trace	8	2	.2	0	Trace	Trace	.1	0
Oyster crackers 10 crackers	10	45	1	1	Trace	1	Trace	7	2	.2	0	Trace	Trace	.1	0
Cracker meal 1 tbsp.	10	45	1	1	Trace	1	Trace	7	2	.1	0	.01	Trace	.1	0
Doughnuts, cake type 1 doughnut	32	125	1	6	1	4	Trace	16	13	[19].4	30	[19].05	[19].05	[19].4	Trace
Farina, regular, enriched, cooked 1 cup	238	100	3	Trace	—	—	—	21	10	[16].7	0	[16].11	[16].07	[16]1.0	0
Macaroni, cooked															
Enriched															
Cooked, firm stage (8 to 10 minutes; undergoes additional cooking in a food mixture) 1 cup	130	190	6	1	—	—	—	39	14	[16]1.4	0	[16].23	[16].14	[16]1.9	0

Food	Measure															
Cooked until tender	1 cup	140	155	5	1	—	—	—	32	11	[16]1.3	0	[16].19	[16].11	[16]1.5	0
Unenriched Cooked, firm stage (8 to 10 minutes; undergoes additional cooking in a food mixture)	1 cup	130	190	6	1	—	—	—	39	14	.6	0	.02	.02	.5	0
Cooked until tender	1 cup	140	155	5	1	—	—	—	32	11	.6	0	.02	.02	.4	0
Macaroni (enriched) and cheese, baked	1 cup	220	470	18	24	11	10	1	44	398	2.0	950	.22	.44	2.0	Trace
Muffins, with enriched white flour; muffin, 2¾-inch diameter	1	48	140	4	5	1	3	Trace	20	50	.8	50	.08	.11	.7	Trace
Noodles (egg noodles), cooked																
Enriched	1 cup	160	200	7	2	1	1	Trace	37	16	[16]1.4	110	[16].23	[16].14	[16]1.8	0
Unenriched	1 cup	160	200	7	2	1	1	Trace	37	16	1.0	110	.04	.03	.7	0
Oats (with or without corn) puffed, added nutrients	1 oz.	28	115	3	2	Trace	1	1	21	50	1.3	0	.28	.05	.5	0
Oatmeal or rolled oats, regular or quick-cooking, cooked	1 cup	236	130	5	2	Trace	1	1	23	21	1.4	0	.19	.05	.3	0
Pancakes (griddlecakes), 4-inch diameter																
Wheat, enriched flour (home recipe)	1 cake	27	60	2	2	Trace	1	Trace	9	27	.4	30	.05	.06	.3	Trace
Buckwheat (buckwheat pancake mix, made with egg and milk)	1 cake	27	55	2	2	1	1	Trace	6	59	.4	60	.03	.04	.2	Trace
Piecrust, plain, baked Enriched flour																
Lower crust, 9-inch shell	1	135	675	8	45	10	29	3	59	19	2.3	0	.27	.19	2.4	0
Double crust, 9-inch pie	1	270	1,350	16	90	21	58	7	118	38	4.6	0	.55	.39	4.9	0

[16]Iron, thiamine, riboflavin, and niacin are based on the minimum levels of enrichment specified in standards of identity promulgated under the Federal Food, Drug, and Cosmetic Act.

[17]Vitamin A value based on yellow product. White product contains only a trace.

[18]Based on recipe using white cornmeal; if yellow cornmeal is used, the vitamin A value is 140 I.U. per muffin.

[19]Based on product made with enriched flour. With unenriched flour, approximate values per doughnut are: Iron, 0.2 milligram; thiamine, 0.01 milligram; riboflavin, 0.03 milligram; niacin, 0.2 milligram.

Food, approximate measure, and weight (in grams)		gm.	Food energy (Calories)	Protein (gm.)	Fat (total lipid) (gm.)	Fatty acids			Carbohydrate (gm.)	Calcium (mg.)	Iron (mg.)	Vitamin A value (I.U.)	Thiamine (mg.)	Riboflavin (mg.)	Niacin (mg.)	Ascorbic acid (mg.)
						Saturated (total) (gm.)	Unsaturated Oleic (gm.)	Linoleic (gm.)								
Piecrust, plain, baked—cont'd																
Unenriched flour																
Lower crust, 9-inch shell	1	135	675	8	45	10	29	3	59	19	.7	0	.04	.04	.6	0
Double crust, 9-inch pie	1	270	1,350	16	90	21	58	7	118	38	1.4	0	.08	.07	1.3	0
Pies (piecrust made with unenriched flour); sector, 4-inch, 1/7 of 9-inch-diameter pie																
Apple	1 sector	135	345	3	15	4	9	1	51	11	.4	40	.03	.02	.5	1
Cherry	1 sector	135	355	4	15	4	10	1	52	19	.4	590	.03	.03	.6	1
Custard	1 sector	130	280	8	14	5	8	1	30	125	.8	300	.07	.21	.4	0
Lemon meringue	1 sector	120	305	4	12	4	7	1	45	17	.6	200	.04	.10	.2	4
Mince	1 sector	135	365	3	16	4	10	1	56	38	1.4	Trace	.09	.05	.5	1
Pumpkin	1 sector	130	275	5	15	5	7	1	32	66	.6	3,210	.04	.13	.6	Trace
Pizza (cheese); 5½-inch sector; ⅛ of 14-inch-diameter pie	1 sector	75	185	7	6	2	3	Trace	27	107	.7	290	.04	.12	.7	4
Popcorn, popped, with added oil and salt	1 cup	14	65	1	3	2	Trace	Trace	8	1	.3	—	—	.01	.2	0
Pretzels, small stick	5 sticks	5	20	Trace	Trace	—	—	—	4	1	0	0	Trace	Trace	Trace	0
Rice, white (fully milled or polished), enriched, cooked																
Common commercial varieties, all types	1 cup	168	185	3	Trace	—	—	—	41	17	[20] 1.5	0	[20] .19	[20] .01	[20] 1.6	0
Long grain, parboiled	1 cup	176	185	4	Trace	—	—	—	41	33	[20] 1.4	0	[20] .19	[20] .02	[20] 2.0	0
Rice, puffed, added nutrients (without salt)	1 cup	14	55	1	Trace	—	—	—	13	3	.3	0	.06	.01	.6	0
Rice flakes, added nutrients	1 cup	30	115	2	Trace	—	—	—	26	9	.5	0	.10	.02	1.6	0
Rolls																
Plain, pan; 12 per 16 ounces																
Enriched	1 roll	38	115	3	2	Trace	1	Trace	20	28	.7	Trace	.11	.07	.8	Trace
Unenriched	1 roll	38	115	3	2	Trace	1	Trace	20	28	.3	Trace	.02	.03	.3	Trace
Hard, round; 12 per 22 oz.	1 roll	52	160	5	2	Trace	1	Trace	31	24	.4	Trace	.03	.05	.4	Trace
Sweet; pan; 12 per 18	1 roll	43	135	4	4	1	2	Trace	21	37	.3	30	.03	.06	.4	Trace

Food	Measure															
Rye wafers, whole-grain, 1⅛ by 3½ inches	2 wafers	13	45	2	Trace	—	—	—	10	7	.5	0	.04	.03	.2	0
Spaghetti																
Cooked, tender stage (14 to 20 minutes)																
Enriched	1 cup	140	155	5	1	—	—	—	32	11	[16]1.3	0	[16].19	[16].11	[16]1.5	0
Unenriched	1 cup	140	155	5	1	—	—	—	32	11	.6	0	.02	.02	.4	0
Spaghetti with meat balls in tomato sauce (home recipe)	1 cup	250	335	19	12	4	6	1	39	125	3.8	1,600	.26	.30	4.0	22
Spaghetti in tomato sauce with cheese (home recipe)	1 cup	250	260	9	9	2	5	1	37	80	2.2	1,080	.24	.18	2.4	14
Waffles, with enriched flour, ½ by 4½ by 5½ inches	1	75	210	7	7	2	4	1	28	85	1.3	250	.13	.19	1.0	Trace
Wheat, puffed																
With added nutrients (without salt)	1 oz.	28	105	4	Trace	—	—	—	22	8	1.2	0	.15	.07	2.2	0
With added nutrients, with sugar and honey	1 oz.	28	105	2	1	—	—	—	25	7	.9	0	.14	.05	1.8	0
Wheat, rolled; cooked	1 cup	236	175	5	1	—	—	—	40	19	1.7	0	.17	.06	2.1	0
Wheat, shredded, plain (long, round, or bite-size)	1 oz.	28	100	3	1	—	—	—	23	12	1.0	0	.06	.03	1.2	0
Wheat and malted barley flakes, with added nutrients	1 oz.	28	110	2	Trace	—	—	—	24	14	.7	0	.13	.03	1.1	0
Wheat flakes, with added nutrients	1 oz.	28	100	3	Trace	—	—	—	23	12	1.2	0	.18	.04	1.4	0
Wheat flours																
Whole-wheat, from hard wheats, stirred	1 cup	120	400	16	2	Trace	1	1	85	49	4.0	0	.66	.14	5.2	0
All-purpose or family flour																
Enriched, sifted	1 cup	110	400	12	1	Trace	Trace	Trace	84	18	[16]3.2	0	[16].48	[16].29	[16]3.8	0
Unenriched, sifted	1 cup	110	400	12	1	Trace	Trace	Trace	84	18	.9	0	.07	.05	1.0	0
Self-rising, enriched	1 cup	110	385	10	1	Trace	Trace	Trace	82	292	[16]3.2	0	[16].49	[16].29	[16]3.9	0
Cake or pastry flour, sifted	1 cup	100	365	8	1	Trace	Trace	Trace	79	17	.5	0	.03	.03	.7	0
Wheat germ, crude, commercially milled	1 cup	68	245	18	7	2	2	4	32	49	6.4	0	1.36	.46	2.9	0

[16]Iron, thiamine, riboflavin, and niacin are based on the minimum levels of enrichment specified in standards of identity promulgated under the Federal Food, Drug, and Cosmetic Act.

[20]Iron, thiamine, and niacin are based on unenriched rice. When the minimum level of enrichment for riboflavin specified in the standards of identity becomes effective the value will be 0.12 milligram per cup of parboiled rice and of white rice.

Food, approximate measure, and weight (in grams)		Food energy	Protein	Fat (total lipid)	Fatty acids			Carbohydrate	Calcium	Iron	Vitamin A value	Thiamine	Riboflavin	Niacin	Ascorbic acid
					Saturated (total)	Unsaturated									
						Oleic	Linoleic								
	gm.	(Calories)	(gm.)	(gm.)	(gm.)	(gm.)	(gm.)	(gm.)	(mg.)	(mg.)	(I.U.)	(mg.)	(mg.)	(mg.)	(mg.)
Fats, oils															
Butter, 4 sticks per pound															
Sticks, 2	1 cup	1,625	1	184	101	61	6	1	45	0	[21] 7,500	—	—	—	0
Stick, 1/8	1 tbsp.	100	Trace	11	6	4	Trace	Trace	3	0	[21] 460	—	—	—	0
Pat or square (64 per pound)	1	50	Trace	6	3	2	Trace	Trace	1	0	[21] 230	—	—	—	0
Fats, cooking															
Lard	1 cup	1,985	0	220	84	101	22	0	0	0	0	0	0	0	0
Lard	1 tbsp.	125	0	14	5	6	1	0	0	0	0	0	0	0	0
Vegetable fats	1 cup	1,770	0	200	46	130	14	0	0	0	—	0	0	0	0
Vegetable fats	1 tbsp.	110	0	12	3	8	1	0	0	0	—	0	0	0	0
Margarine, 4 sticks per pound															
Sticks, 2	1 cup	1,635	1	184	37	105	33	1	45	0	[22] 7,500	—	—	—	0
Stick, 1/8	1 tbsp.	100	Trace	11	2	6	2	Trace	3	0	[22] 460	—	—	—	0
Pat or square (64 per pound)	1 pat	50	Trace	6	1	3	1	Trace	1	0	[22] 230	—	—	—	0
Oils, salad or cooking															
Corn	1 tbsp.	125	0	14	1	4	7	0	0	0	—	0	0	0	0
Cottonseed	1 tbsp.	125	0	14	4	3	7	0	0	0	—	0	0	0	0
Olive	1 tbsp.	125	0	14	2	11	1	0	0	0	—	0	0	0	0
Soybean	1 tbsp.	125	0	14	2	3	7	0	0	0	—	0	0	0	0
Salad dressings															
Blue cheese	1 tbsp.	80	1	8	2	2	4	1	13	Trace	30	Trace	.02	Trace	Trace
Commercial, mayonnaise type	1 tbsp.	65	Trace	6	1	1	3	2	2	Trace	30	Trace	Trace	Trace	—
French	1 tbsp.	60	Trace	6	1	1	3	3	2	.1	—	—	—	—	—
Home cooked, boiled	1 tbsp.	30	1	2	1	1	Trace	3	15	.1	80	.01	.03	—	Trace
Mayonnaise	1 tbsp.	110	Trace	12	2	3	6	Trace	3	.1	40	Trace	.01	Trace	—
Thousand island	1 tbsp.	75	Trace	8	1	2	4	2	2	.1	50	Trace	Trace	Trace	Trace
Sugars, sweets															
Candy															
Caramels	1 oz.	115	1	3	2	1	Trace	22	42	.4	Trace	.01	.05	Trace	Trace
Chocolate, milk, plain	1 oz.	150	2	9	5	3	Trace	16	65	.3	80	.02	.09	.1	Trace
Fudge, plain	1 oz.	115	1	3	2	1	Trace	21	22	.3	Trace	.01	.03	.1	Trace

Food	Measure	Weight (g)	Food energy (cal.)	Protein (g)	Fat (g)	Saturated fatty acids (g)	Unsaturated, Oleic (g)	Unsaturated, Linoleic (g)	Carbohydrate (g)	Calcium (mg)	Iron (mg)	Vitamin A (I.U.)	Thiamine (mg)	Riboflavin (mg)	Niacin (mg)	Ascorbic acid (mg)
Hard candy	1 oz.	28	110	0	Trace	—	—	—	28	6	.5	0	0	0	0	0
Marshmallows	1 oz.	28	90	1	Trace	—	—	—	23	5	.5	0	0	Trace	Trace	0
Chocolate sirup, thin type	1 tbsp.	20	50	Trace	Trace	Trace	Trace	Trace	13	3	.3	—	Trace	.01	.1	0
Honey, strained or extracted	1 tbsp.	21	65	Trace	0	—	—	—	17	1	.1	0	Trace	.01	.1	Trace
Jams and preserves	1 tbsp.	20	55	Trace	Trace	—	—	—	14	4	.2	Trace	Trace	.01	Trace	Trace
Jellies	1 tbsp.	20	55	Trace	Trace	—	—	—	14	4	.3	Trace	Trace	.01	Trace	1
Molasses, cane																
Light (first extraction)	1 tbsp.	20	50	—	—	—	—	—	13	33	.9	—	.01	.01	Trace	—
Blackstrap (third extraction)	1 tbsp.	20	45	—	—	—	—	—	11	137	3.2	—	.02	.04	.4	—
Sirup, table blends (chiefly corn, light and dark)	1 tbsp.	20	60	0	0	—	—	—	15	9	.8	0	0	0	0	0
Sugars (cane or beet)																
Granulated	1 cup	200	770	0	0	—	—	—	199	0	.2	0	0	0	0	0
	1 tbsp.	12	45	0	0	—	—	—	12	0	Trace	0	0	0	0	0
Lump, 1 1/8 by 3/4 by 3/8	1 lump	6	25	0	0	—	—	—	6	0	Trace	0	0	0	0	0
Powdered, stirred before measuring	1 cup	128	495	0	0	—	—	—	127	0	.1	0	0	0	0	0
	1 tbsp.	8	30	0	0	—	—	—	8	0	Trace	0	0	0	0	0
Brown, firm-packed	1 cup	220	820	0	0	—	—	—	212	187	7.5	0	.02	.07	.4	0
	1 tbsp.	14	50	0	0	—	—	—	13	12	.5	0	Trace	Trace	Trace	0
Miscellaneous items																
Beer (average 3.6 percent alcohol by weight)	1 cup	240	100	1	0	—	—	—	9	12	Trace	—	.01	.07	1.6	—
Beverages, carbonated																
Cola type	1 cup	240	95	0	0	—	—	—	24	—	—	0	0	0	0	0
Ginger ale	1 cup	230	70	0	0	—	—	—	18	—	—	0	0	0	0	0
Bouillon cube, 5/8 inch	1 cube	4	5	1	Trace	Trace	Trace	Trace	Trace	—	—	—	—	—	—	—
Chili powder. See Vegetables, peppers																
Chili sauce (mainly tomatoes)	1 tbsp.	17	20	Trace	Trace	—	—	—	4	3	.1	240	.02	.01	.3	3
Chocolate																
Bitter or baking	1 oz.	28	145	3	15	8	6	Trace	8	22	1.9	20	.01	.07	.4	0
Sweet	1 oz.	28	150	1	10	6	4	Trace	16	27	.4	Trace	.01	.04	.1	Trace
Cider. See Fruits, apple juice																

[21] Year-round average.
[22] Based on the average vitamin A content of fortified margarine. Federal specifications for fortified margarine require a minimum of 15,000 I.U. of vitamin A per pound.

Food, approximate measure, and weight (in grams)		gm.	Food energy	Pro-tein	Fat (total lipid)	Fatty acids			Carbo-hydrate	Cal-cium	Iron	Vita-min A value	Thia-mine	Ribo-flavin	Niacin	Ascor-bic acid
						Satu-rated (total)	Unsaturated									
							Oleic	Linoleic								
			(Calories)	(gm.)	(gm.)	(gm.)	(gm.)	(gm.)	(gm.)	(mg.)	(mg.)	(I.U.)	(mg.)	(mg.)	(mg.)	(mg.)
Gelatin, dry																
Plain	1 tbsp.	10	35	9	Trace	—	—	—	—	—	—	—	—	—	—	—
Dessert powder, 3-oz. package	½ cup	85	315	8	0	—	—	—	75	—	—	—	—	—	—	—
Gelatin dessert, ready-to-eat																
Plain	1 cup	239	140	4	0	—	—	—	34	—	—	—	—	—	—	—
With fruit	1 cup	241	160	3	Trace	—	—	—	40	—	—	—	—	—	—	—
Olives, pickled																
Green	4 medium or 3 extra large or 2 giant	16	15	Trace	2	Trace	2	Trace	Trace	8	.2	40	—	—	—	—
Ripe: Mission	3 small or 2 large	10	15	Trace	2	Trace	2	Trace	Trace	9	.1	10	Trace	Trace	—	—
Pickles, cucumber																
Dill, large, 4 by 1¾ inches	1	135	15	1	Trace	—	—	—	3	35	1.4	140	Trace	.03	Trace	8
Sweet, 2¾ by ¾ inches	1	20	30	Trace	Trace	—	—	—	7	2	.2	20	Trace	Trace	Trace	1
Popcorn. See Grain products																
Sherbet, orange	1 cup	193	260	2	2	—	—	—	59	31	Trace	110	.02	.06	Trace	4
Soups, canned; ready-to-serve (prepared with equal volume of water)																
Bean with pork	1 cup	250	170	8	6	1	2	2	22	62	2.2	650	.14	.07	1.0	2
Beef noodle	1 cup	250	70	4	3	1	1	1	7	8	1.0	50	.05	.06	1.1	Trace
Beef bouillon, broth, consomme	1 cup	240	30	5	0	0	0	0	3	Trace	.5	Trace	Trace	.02	1.2	—
Chicken noodle	1 cup	250	65	4	2	Trace	1	1	8	10	.5	50	.02	.02	.8	Trace
Clam chowder	1 cup	255	85	2	3	—	—	5	13	36	1.0	920	.03	.03	1.0	—
Cream soup (mushroom)	1 cup	240	135	2	10	1	3	5	10	41	.5	70	.02	.12	.7	Trace
Minestrone	1 cup	245	105	5	3	—	—	—	14	37	1.0	2,350	.07	.05	1.0	—
Pea, green	1 cup	245	130	6	2	1	1	Trace	23	44	1.0	340	.05	.05	1.0	7
Tomato	1 cup	245	90	2	2	Trace	1	1	16	15	.7	1,000	.06	.05	1.1	12
Vegetable with beef broth	1 cup	250	80	3	2	—	—	—	14	20	.8	3,250	.05	.02	1.2	—

Food	Measure																
Starch (cornstarch)	1 cup	128	465	Trace	Trace	—	—	—	112	0	0	0	0	0	0	0	0
	1 tbsp.	8	30	Trace	Trace	—	—	—	7	0	0	0	0	0	0	0	0
Tapioca, quick-cooking	1 cup	152	535	1	Trace	—	—	—	131	15	.6	0	0	0	0	0	0
granulated, dry, stirred	1 tbsp.	10	35	Trace	Trace	—	—	—	9	1	Trace	0	0	0	0	0	0
before measuring																	
Vinegar	1 tbsp.	15	2	0	—	—	—	—	1	0	.1	—	—	—	—	—	—
White sauce, medium	1 cup	265	430	10	33	18	11	1	23	305	.5	1,220	.12	.44	.6	Trace	Trace
Yeast																		
Baker's																		
Compressed	1 oz.	28	25	3	Trace	—	—	—	3	4	1.4	Trace	.20	.47	3.2	Trace	Trace
Dry active	1 oz.	28	80	10	Trace	—	—	—	11	12	4.6	Trace	.66	1.53	10.4	Trace	Trace
Brewer's, dry, debittered	1 tbsp.	8	25	3	Trace	—	—	—	3	17	1.4	Trace	1.25	.34	3.0	Trace	Trace
Yogurt. See Milk, cream, cheese; related products																		

Cholesterol content of foods

Foods of plant origin, such as fruits, vegetables, cereal grains, legumes, and nuts, do not have cholesterol. The following list indicates the *approximate* amount in some foods of animal origin.

Food	Amount in common serving	Cholesterol (milligrams)
Milk, nonfat		—
Nuts		—
Vegetable oils		—
Cottage cheese, creamed	½ cup	15
Bacon fat	1 tablespoon	25
Butter	2 teaspoons	
Cheese, cheddar	1 ounce	
Cream (half and half)	3 tablespoons	30
Cream cheese	2 tablespoons	
Ice cream	½ cup	
Milk, whole	1 cup	
Beef		
Fish	3 ounces cooked	
Lamb	including	70
Pork	lean and fat	
Poultry		
Caviar or fish roe	1 ounce	80
Shrimp	2 ounces ⎫ about	80
Crab meat	2 ounces ⎬ ⅓	80
Lobster	2 ounces ⎭ cup	120
Oysters	2 ounces	120 or more
Liver	2 ounces, cooked	250
Kidney	2 ounces, cooked	250
Egg yolk	1	300
Brains	2 ounces, cooked	1,350 or more

C Calorie values of some common snack foods

Food	Weight gm.	Approximate measure	Calories
Beverages			
Carbonated, cola type	180	1 bottle, 6 ounces	70
Malted milk	405	1 regular (1½ cups)	420
Chocolate milk (made with skim milk)	250	1 cup	190
Cocoa	200	1 cup	235
Soda, vanilla ice cream	242	1 regular	260
Cake			
Angel food	40	2-inch sector	110
Cupcake, chocolate, iced	50	1 cake, 2¾ inches in diameter	185
Fruit cake	30	1 piece, 2 by 2 by ½ inch	115
Candy and popcorn			
Butterscotch	15	3 pieces	60
Candy bar, plain	57	1 bar	295
Caramels	30	3 medium	120
Chocolate coated creams	30	2 average	130
Fudge	28	1 piece	115
Peanut brittle	30	1 ounce	125
Popcorn with oil added	14	1 cup	65
Cheese			
Camembert	28	1 ounce	85
Cheddar	28	1 ounce	105
Cream	28	1 ounce	105
Swiss (domestic)	28	1 ounce	105
Cookies			
Brownies	30	1 piece, 2 by 2 by ¾ inch	140
Cookies, plain and assorted	25	1 cooky, 3 in. in diameter	120
Crackers			
Cheese	18	5 crackers	85
Graham	14	2 medium	55
Saltines	16	4 crackers	70
Rye	13	2 crackers	45
Dessert type cream puff and doughnuts			
Cream puff—custard filling	105	1 average	245
Doughnut, cake type, plain	32	1 average	125
Doughnut, jelly	65	1 average	225
Doughnut, raised	30	1 average	120

Food	Weight gm.	Approximate measure	Calories
Miscellaneous			
Hamburger and bun	96	1 average	330
Ice cream, vanilla	62	3½ ounce container	130
Sherbet	96	½ cup	120
Jams, jellies, marmalades, preserves	20	1 tablespoon	55
Syrup, blended	80	¼ cup	240
Waffles	75	1 waffle, 4½ by 5½ by ½ inch	210
Nuts			
Mixed, shelled	15	8-12	95
Peanut butter	16	1 tablespoon	95
Peanuts, shelled, roasted	144	1 cup	840
Pie			
Apple	135	4-inch sector	345
Cherry	135	4-inch sector	355
Custard	130	4-inch sector	280
Lemon meringue	120	4-inch sector	305
Mince	135	4-inch sector	365
Pumpkin	130	4-inch sector	275
Potato chips			
Potato chips	20	10 chips, 2 inches in diameter	115
Sandwiches			
Bacon, lettuce, tomato	150	1 sandwich	280
Egg salad	140	1 sandwich	280
Ham	80	1 sandwich	280
Liverwurst	90	1 sandwich	250
Peanut butter	85	1 sandwich	330
Soups, commercial canned			
Bean with pork	250	1 cup	170
Beef noodle	250	1 cup	70
Chicken noodle	250	1 cup	65
Cream (mushroom)	240	1 cup	135
Tomato	245	1 cup	90
Vegetable with beef broth	250	1 cup	80

D Composition of beverages—alcoholic and carbonated nonalcoholic per 100 grams[1]

	Food energy	Protein	Carbo- hydrate	Calcium	Phos- phorus	Iron	Thiamine	Ribo- flavin	Niacin
Beverages, alcoholic and carbonated non-alcoholic									
Alcoholic									
Beer, alcohol 4.5% by volume (3.6% by weight)	42	.3	3.8	5	30	Trace	Trace	.03	.6
Gin, rum, vodka, whisky:									
80-proof (33.4% alcohol by weight)	231	—	Trace	—	—	—	—	—	—
86-proof (36.0% alcohol by weight)	249	—	Trace	—	—	—	—	—	—
90-proof (37.9% alcohol by weight)	263	—	Trace	—	—	—	—	—	—
94-proof (39.7% alcohol by weight)	275	—	Trace	—	—	—	—	—	—
100-proof (42.5% alcohol by weight)	295	—	Trace	—	—	—	—	—	—
Wines									
Dessert, alcohol 18.8% by volume (15.3% by weight)	137	.1	7.7	8	—	—	.01	.02	.2
Table, alcohol 12.2% by volume (9.9% by weight)	85	.1	4.2	9	10	.4	Trace	.01	.1
Carbonated, non-alcoholics									
Carbonated waters:									
sweetened (quinine sodas)	31	—	8	—	—	—	—	—	—
unsweetened (club sodas)	—	—	—	—	—	—	—	—	—
Cola type	39	—	10	—	—	—	—	—	—
Cream sodas	43	—	11	—	—	—	—	—	—
Fruit-flavored sodas (citrus, cherry, grape, strawberry, Tom Collins mixer, other) (10%-13% sugar)	46	—	12	—	—	—	—	—	—
Ginger ale, pale dry and golden	31	—	8	—	—	—	—	—	—
Root beer	41	—	10.5	—	—	—	—	—	—
Special dietary drinks with artificial sweetener (less than 1 calorie per ounce)	—	—	—	—	—	—	—	—	—

[1]From Watt, B. K., and Merrill, A. L.: Composition of foods—raw, processed, prepared, U.S. Department of Agriculture, Agriculture Handbook, No. 8, December, 1963.

Food and Nutrition Board, National Academy of Sciences —National Research Council recommended daily dietary allowances[1] (revised 1968)

DESIGNED FOR THE MAINTENANCE OF GOOD NUTRITION OF PRACTICALLY ALL HEALTHY PEOPLE IN THE U.S.A.

Age[2] (years)	Weight (kg)	Weight (lbs)	Height (cm)	Height (in.)	kcal	Protein (gm)	Fat-soluble vitamins Vitamin A activity (IU)	Vitamin D (IU)	Vitamin E activity (mg)	Water-soluble vitamins Ascorbic acid (mg)	Folacin[3] (mg)	Niacin (mg equiv)[4]	Riboflavin (mg)	Thiamine (mg)	Vitamin B_6 (mg)	Vitamin B_{12} (μg)	Minerals Calcium (g)	Phosphorus (g)	Iodine (μg)	Iron (mg)	Magnesium (mg)
Infants																					
0–1/6	4	9	55	22	kg × 120	kg × 2.2[5]	1,500	400	5	35	0.05	5	0.4	0.2	0.2	1.0	0.4	0.2	25	6	40
1/6–1/2	7	15	63	25	kg × 110	kg × 2.0[5]	1,500	400	5	35	0.05	7	0.5	0.4	0.3	1.5	0.5	0.4	40	10	60
1/2–1	9	20	72	28	kg × 100	kg × 1.8[5]	1,500	400	5	35	0.1	8	0.6	0.5	0.4	2.0	0.6	0.5	45	15	70
Children																					
1–2	12	26	81	32	1,100	25	2,000	400	10	40	0.1	8	0.6	0.6	0.5	2.0	0.7	0.7	55	15	100
2–3	14	31	91	36	1,250	25	2,000	400	10	40	0.2	8	0.7	0.6	0.6	2.5	0.8	0.8	60	15	150
3–4	16	35	100	39	1,400	30	2,500	400	10	40	0.2	9	0.8	0.7	0.7	3	0.8	0.8	70	10	200
4–6	19	42	110	43	1,600	30	2,500	400	10	40	0.2	11	0.9	0.8	0.9	4	0.8	0.8	80	10	200
6–8	23	51	121	48	2,000	35	3,500	400	15	40	0.2	13	1.1	1.0	1.0	4	0.9	0.9	100	10	250
8–10	28	62	131	52	2,200	40	3,500	400	15	40	0.3	15	1.2	1.1	1.2	5	1.0	1.0	110	10	250

Males

Age (years)																				
10–12	35	77	140	55	2,500	45	4,500	400	20	40	0.4	17	1.3	1.3	1.4	5	1.2	1.2	125	10	300
12–14	43	95	151	59	2,700	50	5,000	400	20	45	0.4	18	1.4	1.4	1.6	5	1.4	1.4	135	18	350
14–18	59	130	170	67	3,000	60	5,000	400	25	55	0.4	20	1.5	1.5	1.8	5	1.4	1.4	150	18	400
18–22	67	147	175	69	2,800	60	5,000	400	30	60	0.4	18	1.6	1.4	2.0	5	0.8	0.8	140	10	400
22–35	70	154	175	69	2,800	65	5,000	—	30	60	0.4	18	1.7	1.4	2.0	5	0.8	0.8	140	10	350
35–55	70	154	173	68	2,600	65	5,000	—	30	60	0.4	17	1.7	1.3	2.0	5	0.8	0.8	125	10	350
55–75+	70	154	171	67	2,400	65	5,000	—	30	60	0.4	14	1.7	1.2	2.0	6	0.8	0.8	110	10	350

Females

Age (years)																				
10–12	35	77	142	56	2,250	50	4,500	400	20	40	0.4	15	1.3	1.1	1.4	5	1.2	1.2	110	18	300
12–14	44	97	154	61	2,300	50	5,000	400	20	45	0.4	15	1.4	1.2	1.6	5	1.3	1.3	115	18	350
14–16	52	114	157	62	2,400	55	5,000	400	25	50	0.4	16	1.4	1.2	1.8	5	1.3	1.3	120	18	350
16–18	54	119	160	63	2,300	55	5,000	400	25	50	0.4	15	1.5	1.2	2.0	5	1.3	1.3	115	18	350
18–22	58	128	163	64	2,000	55	5,000	400	25	55	0.4	13	1.5	1.0	2.0	5	0.8	0.8	100	18	350
22–35	58	128	163	64	2,000	55	5,000	—	25	55	0.4	13	1.5	1.0	2.0	5	0.8	0.8	100	18	300
35–55	58	128	160	63	1,850	55	5,000	—	25	55	0.4	13	1.5	1.0	2.0	5	0.8	0.8	90	18	300
55–75+	58	128	157	62	1,700	55	5,000	—	25	55	0.4	13	1.5	1.0	2.0	6	0.8	0.8	80	10	300

Pregnancy				+200	65	6,000	400	30	60	0.8	15	1.8	+0.1	2.5	8	+0.4	+0.4	125	18	450
Lactation				+1,000	75	8,000	400	30	60	0.5	20	2.0	+0.5	2.5	6	+0.5	+0.5	150	18	450

[1] The allowance levels are intended to cover individual variations among most normal persons as they live in the United States under usual environmental stresses. The recommended allowances can be attained with a variety of common foods, providing other nutrients for which human requirements have been less well defined. See text for more detailed discussion of allowances and of nutrients not tabulated.

[2] Entries on lines for age range 22–35 years represent the reference man and woman at age 22. All other entries represent allowances for the midpoint of the specified age range.

[3] The folacin allowances refer to dietary sources as determined by Lactobacillus casei assay. Pure forms of folacin may be effective in doses less than ¼ of the RDA.

[4] Niacin equivalents include sources of the vitamin itself plus 1 mg equivalent for each 60 mg of dietary tryptophan.

[5] Assumes protein equivalent to human milk. For proteins not 100 percent utilized factors should be increased proportionately.

References

The health practitioner will find a number of references useful in his daily encounter with nutritional needs. From these he will want to select several for his personal library and read excerpts from others as he has opportunity and need. This listing of journals, magazines, and basic texts will provide a recommended cross section of helpful resources.

Journals
American Journal of Clinical Nutrition
American Journal of Public Health
Journal of the American Dietetic Association
Journal of Nutrition Education
Nutrition Today

Education journals (useful references in nutrition education)
Adult Leadership
Change
Educational Technology
Today's Education

Magazines (useful references for lay readership and perspective)
Family Health
Today's Health

Journals of related disciplines
American Journal of Nursing
Journal of the American Medical Association
New England Journal of Medicine
Nursing Outlook
Preventive Medicine

Basic texts
Bogert, L. J., Briggs, G., and Calloway, D.: Nutrition and physical fitness, ed. 9, Philadelphia, 1972, W. B. Saunders Co.
Best, C. H., and Taylor, N. B.: The physiological basis of medical practice, Baltimore, 1966, The Williams and Wilkins Co.
Fomon, S. J.: Infant nutrition, Philadelphia, 1967, W. B. Saunders Co.
Guthrie, H. A.: Introductory nutrition, St. Louis, 1971, The C. V. Mosby Co.

Ganong, W. F.: Review of medical physiology, Los Altos, 1971, Lange Medical Publications.
Goodman, L. S., and Gilman, A.: The pharmacological basis of therapeutics, New York, 1965, The Macmillan Co.
Guyton, A. C.: Textbook of medical physiology, Philadelphia, 1971, W. B. Saunders Co.
Harper, H. A.: Review of physiological chemistry, Los Altos, 1971, Lange Medical Publications.
Lowenberg, M. E., and others: Food and man, New York, 1968, John Wiley & Sons, Inc.
Nizel, A. E.: The science of nutrition and its application in clinical dentistry, Philadelphia, 1966, W. B. Saunders Co.
Williams, S. R.: Nutrition and diet therapy, ed. 2, St. Louis, 1973, The C. V. Mosby Co.
Williams, S. R.: Nutrition and diet therapy: a learning guide for students, St. Louis, 1973, The C. V. Mosby Co.
Wohl, M., and Goodhart, R., editors: Modern nutrition in health and disease, Philadelphia, 1968, Lea and Febiger.

References for basic calculations
Composition of foods, Agriculture Handbook No. 8, Agricultural Research Service, U. S. Department of Agriculture, Washington, D. C., 1963, Government Printing Office.
Church, C. F., and Church, H. N.: Food values of portions commonly used, ed. 11, Philadelphia, 1970, J. B. Lippincott Co.
Recommended dietary allowances, ed. 7, 1968, Food and Nutrition Board, National Research Council, National Academy of Sciences, Washington, D. C.

General books for lay readers
Deutsch, R. M.: The family guide to better food and better health, Des Moines, Iowa, 1971, Meredith Corp.
Deutsch, R. M.: Nuts among the berries, New York, 1962, Ballantine Books, Inc.
Jacobson, M. F.: Eater's digest: the consumer's factbook of food additives, Garden City, N. Y., 1972, Doubleday and Co.
Lappé, F. M.: Diet for a small planet, New York, 1971, Ballantine Books, Inc.

Turner, J. S.: The chemical feast, New York, 1970, Grossman Publishers.

United States Department of Agriculture Yearbooks: 1959, Food; 1966, Protecting Our Food; 1969, Food For Us All, Washington, D. C., Government Printing Office.

General references for nutrition education

Brown, J. W., Lewis, R. B., and Harcleroad, F. F.: AV instruction: materials and methods, New York, 1964, McGraw-Hill Book Co.

Coles, R., and Clayton, A.: Still hungry in America, New York, 1969, New American Library, World Publishing Co.

Dale, E.: AV methods in teaching, ed. 3, New York, 1969, Holt, Reinhart and Winston, Inc.

DeKeiffer, R. E.: Audiovisual instruction, New York, 1965, Center for Applied Research in Education.

Duff, R. S., and Hollingshead, A. B.: Sickness and society, New York, 1968, Harper and Row, Publishers.

Erikson, E.: Childhood and society, ed. 2, New York, 1963, W. W. Norton and Co.

Erikson, E.: Identity: youth and crisis, New York, 1968, W. W. Norton and Co., Inc.

Gagné, R. M.: The conditions of learning, New York, 1965, Holt, Reinhart and Winston, Inc.

Garrett, A.: Interviewing: its principles and methods, New York, 1942, Family Service Association of America.

Ginther, J. R.: Educational diagnosis of patients, J. American Dietetic Association 59(6):560, 1971.

Granick, S., and Patterson, R., editors: Human aging II: an eleven year follow-up biomedical and behavioral study, Pub. No. (HSM) 71-9037, Washington, D. C., 1972, Government Printing Office.

Kotz, N.: Let them eat promises: the politics of hunger in America, Englewood Cliffs, N. J., 1969, Prentice-Hall, Inc.

Mager, R. F.: Developing attitudes toward learning, Palo Alto, 1968, Fearon Publishers.

Mager, R. F.: Developing vocational instruction, Palo Alto, 1967, Fearon Publishers.

Mager, R. F.: Preparing instructional objectives, Palo Alto, 1962, Fearon Publishers.

Maslow, A. H.: The farther reaches of human nature, New York, 1971, The Viking Press, Inc.

Mead, M.: Culture and commitment, New York, 1970, Natural History Press.

Neugarten, B. L.: Middle age and aging: a reader in social psychology, Chicago, 1968, University of Chicago Press.

Parker, J. C., and Rubin, L. J.: Process as content, Chicago, 1966, Rand McNally & Co.

Rogers, C.: Freedom to learn, Columbus, Ohio, 1969, Charles E. Merrill Publishing Co.

Somers, A. R.: Health care in transition: directions for the future, Chicago, 1971, Hospital Research and Educational Trust.

Townsend, C.: Old age: the last segregation, New York, 1970, Grossman Publishers.

Index